OXFORD MEDICAL PUBLICATIONS

Oxford Handbook of
Cardiology

Oxford Handbook of
Cardiology

Punit Ramrakha

Consultant Cardiologist, Stoke Mandeville Hospital,
Aylesbury and Hammersmith Hospital, London, UK

and

Jonathan Hill

Clinical Senior Lecturer and Consultant Cardiologist,
King's College Hospital, King's College London, UK

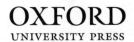

OXFORD
UNIVERSITY PRESS

OXFORD
UNIVERSITY PRESS

Great Clarendon Street, Oxford OX2 6DP

Oxford University Press is a department of the University of Oxford.
It furthers the University's objective of excellence in research, scholarship,
and education by publishing worldwide in

Oxford New York

Auckland Cape Town Dar es Salaam Hong Kong Karachi
Kuala Lumpur Madrid Melbourne Mexico City Nairobi
New Delhi Shanghai Taipei Toronto

With offices in

Argentina Austria Brazil Chile Czech Republic France Greece
Guatemala Hungary Italy Japan Poland Portugal Singapore
South Korea Switzerland Thailand Turkey Ukraine Vietnam

Oxford is a registered trade mark of Oxford University Press
in the UK and in certain other countries

Published in the United States
by Oxford University Press, Inc., New York

British Library Cataloguing in Publication Data
Data available

Library of Congress Cataloging in Publication Data

Data available

Typeset by Newgen Imaging Systems (P) Ltd., Chennai, India
Printed in Italy
on acid-free paper by
LegoPrint s.r.l.

ISBN 0–19–852597–4   978–0–19–852597–4

10 9 8 7 6 5 4 3 2 1

"Perfect as the wing of a bird may be, it will never enable the bird to fly if unsupported by the air. Facts are the air of science. Without them a man of science can never rise"

Ivan Pavlov

Dedication

PR "For Sabine"
JH "For my family"

Preface

The pace of cardiological progress in the 21st century continues to accelerate. Yet the health-care resources of both the developed world and developing world seem to be consumed at an even greater rate by the global pandemic of cardiovascular disease. At the turn of the century the World Health Organisation estimates suggest that 1 person in every 3 died of a cardiovascular cause. Nearly 4 in every 5 of these deaths were in low or middle income countries. By 2010 cardiovascular disease will be the leading cause of death in developing countries. As countries undergo economic transition diseases predominantly found in the developing world such as rheumatic heart disease are merely traded for those of a developed country such as coronary artery disease. Far from being the disease of developed world all those involved in care of the cardiovascular patient must realise that heart disease has no geographic, gender or socio-economic boundaries.

In this book we have tried to span the range of cardiovascular disease with an emphasis on all aspects of practical cardiac care ranging from the latest in electrophysiological techniques to the management of rheumatic fever. We have attempted to give as complete coverage as is possible in a book of this size and hope that there is sufficient detail not only for practical day to day advice at the bedside for patients with cardiac problems. This book will appeal to anyone involved in the specialist care of the cardiology patient, whether on the coronary care unit, cardiac catheterisation suite, outpatient clinic or in the accident and emergency rooms in every hospital.

First editions are never perfect and the rapid pace of progress can often overtake the speed of publication. However we have endeavoured to give as contemporary a view as possible of modern cardiological practice, without forgetting the basic facts that we all rely on. As with all books in the Oxford Handbook series we invite you the reader to give your personal feedback and recommendations for future editions.

Foreword

"It gives me great pleasure to support the publication of the Oxford Handbook of Cardiology. It's an important book on a very important subject. The death toll from cardiovascular disease across the world is enormous and growing as we successfully tackle other major global killers.

The fact that the majority of such deaths are already preventable underlines the responsibility of governments and health services in every country to work harder to improve care and reduce cardiovascular risk factors. In the United Kingdom, the Government and the National Health Service has taken very seriously - and with real success – this responsibility in recent years but we also recognise there is a great deal more to do.

As a politician, I am, of course, very aware of the importance of good cardiac care. But it was as a patient myself that I recently witnessed first hand the skills and dedication of NHS cardiologists and their colleagues. What I saw reinforced my respect for the expertise and commitment within our health service and my determination to continue helping the NHS to improve care."

With millions of people now dying prematurely and unnecessarily from heart disease across the world, it's obviously important that knowledge and expertise are spread as widely as possible. That's the purpose of this book by Punit Ramrakha and Jonathan Hill. Their hope is that it can play its part in informing and inspiring doctors, nurses and other health professionals to continue improving the quality and standards of care for patients with heart disease worldwide."

Tony Blair

Acknowledgements

We would like to record our most sincere thanks to all who have contributed to the production of this book. It has been a long process and has required the help and expertise from many people. All the chapter contributors deserve special thanks and are listed on the previous page.

JH would like to thank the consultants and teachers from the London Chest and St Bartholomew's hospitals who offered guidance and support throughout his specialist registrar training, especially (but in no particular order) Dr PG Mills, Dr J Hogan, Dr T Crake, Dr S Banim, Dr J Sayer, Dr AW Nathan, Dr C Knight, Prof AD Timmis, Dr A Mathur, Prof MT Rothman, Dr DS Dymond, Dr JR Dawson, Dr T Koh, Dr A Deaner, Dr R Aggarwal. He would also like to extend a huge thank you to his wife and family, Jayne, Thomas, Mathhew, JJ, Caitlin and Joseph.

PR would like to thank his wife for infinite patience and perseverance over long weekends where she was left to her own devices while he toiled over the manuscript.

Finally we would both like to extend a huge thank you to all the staff at OUP for their phenomenal patience and dedication for seeing this first edition through to completion.

Contents

Contributors

David Begley
Specialist Registrar in Cardiology,
Northern Deanery, UK

Shay Cullen
Consultant Cardiologist,
Specialist in Adult Congenital
Heart Disease, The Heart
Hospital, University College
London Hospitals, London, UK

Ceri Davies
Specialist Registrar in Cardiology,
Barts and the London NHS Trust,
London, UK

Mehul Dhinoja
Specialist Registrar in Cardiology,
Heart Hospital, London, UK

Mark Earley
Consultant Cardiologist,
Manchester Heart Centre, UK

John Graham
Specialist Registrar in Cardiology,
London Deanery; currently
Cardiology Fellow, Sunnybrook &
Women's College Health Sciences
Centre, Toronto, Canada

Julian Halcox
Al Maktoum British Heart
Foundation, Senior Lecturer
in Cardiology, University College
London; Honorary Consultant
Cardiologist, University College
London Hospitals, London, UK

Stuart Harris
Consultant Cardiologist,
St Bartholomew's Hospital,
London, UK

Ajay Jain
Specialist Registrar in Cardiology,
Barts and the London
NHS Trust, London, UK

Tat Koh
Consultant Cardiologist,
Cardiology Department,
London Chest Hospital,
London, UK

Bongani Mayosi
The Cardiac Clinic,
Department of Medicine,
Groote Schuur Hospital &
University of Cape Town,
Cape Town,
South Africa

Catherine Nelson-Piercy
Consultant Obsteric Physician,
Guys & St Thomas' Hospital,
London, UK

Jonathan Plehn
Professor of Medicine, George
Washington University Medical
Centre, USA

Mrin Saha
Specialist Registrar in Cardiology,
St Bartholomew's Hospital,
London, UK

Abbreviations

AA	aortic annulus
AAD	antirrhythmic drugs
AAI	demand atrial pacing
ACAB	atraumatic coronaiy artery bypass
ACC	American College of Cardiologists
ACE	angiotensin-converting enzyme
ACS	acute coronary syndrome
ADA	adenosine deaminase
ADH	anti-diuretic hormone
AEG	atrial electrical activity
AFB	acid-fast bacilli
AFT	alpha-feto protein
AHA	American Heart Association
AOO	asynchronous atrial pacing
APC	antigen presenting cells
APTT	activated partial thromboplastin time
AR	aortic regurgitation
ARB	angiotensin II receptor antagonist
ARDS	acute respiratory distress syndrome
ARVC	arrhythmogenic right ventricular cardiomyopathy
AS	aortic stenosis
ASB	assisted spontaneous breathing
ASD	atrial septal defect
ATP	adenosine triphosphate
AVN	atrioventricular node
AVNERP	atrio-ventricular nodal effective refractory period
AVNRT	atrio-ventricular nodal reentrant tachycardia
AVR	aortic valve replacement
AVRT	atrio-ventricular reentrant tachycardia
AWCL	anterograde Wenckebach cycle length
BAR	binary angiographic restenosis
BARI	balloon angioplasty revascularization
BCT	broad complex tachycardia
BIMA	bilateral internal mammary artery

BiPAP	biphasic positive pressure ventilation
BiVAD	biventricular assist device
BP	blood pressure
Ca	calcium
CABG	coronary arteiy bypass graft
CAD	coronary artery disease
CAVH	continuous arteriovenous haemofiltration
CCF	congestive cardiac failure
CC-TGA	congenitally corrected transposition of the great arteries
CEA	carcinoembryonic antigen
CHB	complete heart block
CHF	chronic heart failure
CLR	culprit lesion revascularization
cm	centimetre
CMV	controlled mechanical ventilation
COAD	chronic obstructive airways disease
COPD	chronic obstructive pulmonary disease
CPAP	continuous positive airway pressure
CPB	cardiopulmonary bypass
CPR	cardiorespiratory resuscitation
CRT	cardiac resynchronization therapy
CS	coronary stenosis
CTO	chronic total occlusion
CVD	cardiovascular disease
CWH	continuous venovenous haemofiltration
CXR	chest X-ray
DALY	disability-adjusted life years
DCM	dilated cardiomyopathy
DFT	defibrillation threshold
DSWI	deep sternal wound infection
DVI	dual chamber
DVT	deep vein thrombosis
EDV	end-diastolic volume
ELISPOT	enzyme-linked immunospot
EP	electrophysiology
ERP	effective refractory period
FAt	focal atrial tachycardia
FBC	full blood count
Fe	iron

FFP	fresh frozen plasma
FFR	fractional flow reserve
FO	fossa ovalis
g	gram
GFR	glomerular filtration rate
GI	gastrointestinal
HCM	hypertrophic cardiomyopathy
HF	heart failure
HOCM	hypertrophic obstructive cardiomyopathy
hr	hour
IABP	intra-aortic balloon pump
IAP	incremental atrial pacing
ICD	implantable cardiac defibrillator
im	intramuscular
IMA	internal mammary artery
INPV	intermittent negative pressure ventilation
Int	intermediate
ITU	intensive care unit
iv	intravenous
IVC	inferior vena cava
IVP	incremental ventricular pacing
IVUS	intravascular ultrasound
K	potassium
kg	kilogram
L	litre
LA	left atrium
LAD	left anterior descending coronary artery
LAM	left anterior mediastinoscopy
LAO	left anterior oblique
LAP	left atrial pressure
LCA	left coronary artery
LCB	left coronary bypass
LFT	liver function test
LFV	left femoral vein
LIMA	left internal mammary artery
LMS	left main stem
LPA	left pulmonary artery
LQTS	long QT syndrome
LSV	long saphenous vein

LV	left ventricular/ventricle
LV	left ventricle
LVAD	left ventricular assist device
LVB	lateral ventricular branches
LVEDP	left ventricular end-diastolic pressure
LVEDV	left ventricular end-diastolic volume
LVH	left ventricular hypertrophy
MAP	mean arterial pressure
mcg	microgram
mg	milligram
MI	myocardial infarction
min	minutes
ml	millilitre
MLD	minimum luminal diameter
mmol	millimole
MRA	magnetic resonance angiography
MRI	magnetic resonance imaging
MV	mitral valve
MVR	mitral valve replacement
Na	sodium
NCD	non-communicable disease
NCT	narrow complex tachycardia
NIPPV	non-invasive intermittent positive pressure ventilation
NO	nitric oxide
NSAID	non-steroidal anti-inflammatory drug
NYHA	New York Heart Association
OPCAB	off-pump coronary artery bypass
PA	pulmonary artery
PAP	pulmonary artery pressure
PAPVD	partial anomalous pulmonary venous drainage
PAWP	pulmonary artery wedge pressure
PCWP	pulmonary capillary wedge pressure
PDA	posterior descending artery
PDA	patient ductus arteriosus
PDEI	phosphodiesterase inhibitors
PE	pulmonary embolism
PEEP	positive end-expiratory pressure
PET	positron emission topography
Plts	platelets

PMV	percutaneous mitral valvuloplasty
po	per os (by mouth)
POBA	plain old balloon angioplasty
PPM	permanent pacemaker
prn	pro re nata (as required)
PS	pressure support
PSV	pressure support ventilation
PVARP	post-ventricular atrial refractory period
PVR	peripheral vascular resistance
QCA	quantitative coronary analysis
qds	quater die sumendus (to be taken 4 times a day)
QIVUS	quantitative intravascular ultrasound
RA	right atrium
RAM	right anterior mediastinoscopy
RAP	right atrial pressure
RBB	right bundle branch
RBC	red blood cell
RCA	right coronary artery
RFA	radiofrequency ablation
RFV	right femoral vein
RHD	rheumatic heart disease
RIMA	right internal mammary artery
RPA	right pulmonary artery
RSPV	right superior pulmonary vein
RSV	respiratory syncitial virus
RV	right ventricle
RVAD	right ventricular assist device
RVD	reference vessel diameter
RVEDP	right ventricular end-diastolic pressure
RVEDV	right ventricular end-diastolic volume
RVOT	right ventricular outflow tract
RWCL	retrograde Wenckebach cycle length
S	seconds
SA	sinoatrial
SAM	systolic anterior motion
SAN	sinoatrial node
SC	subcutaneous
SCD	sudden cardiac death
SIADH	syndrome of inappropriate anti-diuretic hormone secretion

SIMV	synchronized intermittent mandatory ventilation
SSV	short saphenous vein
SV	single ventricle
SVC	superior vena cava
SWI	superficial wound infection
TA	truncus arteriosu
TAPVD	total anomalous pulmonary venous drainage
TDI	tissue Doppler imaging
TOP	Torsades des pointes
tds	ter die sumendus (to be taken 3 times a day)
TEC	transluminal extraction catheter
TGA	transposition of the great arteries
TIA	transient ischaemic attack
TIF	tracheoinnominate fistula
TIVA	total intravenous anaethesia
TLR	target lesion revascularization
TOE	transoesophageal echocardiography
TOF	tetralogy of Fallot
TOS	tracheoesophagal fistula
TTE	transthoracic echocardiography
TV	tricuspid valve
TVR	target vessel revascularization
U&E	urea and electrolytes
U/S	ultrasound
URTI	upper respiratory tract infection
VAD	ventricular assist device
VF	ventricular fibrillation
VOO	asynchronous ventricular pacing
VPC	ventricular premature complexes
VSD	ventricular septal defect
VT	ventricular tachycardia

Cardiac investigations

Exercise ECG

A commonly used test involving a treadmill, BP measurement, and continuous ECG monitoring. Overall sensitivity for coronary heart disease is around 68% and specificity is 77%. This increases when considering prognostically significant disease which has a sensitivity of 86%. The test improves to have a predictive accuracy of >90% in intermediate to high risk patients (older men with ischaemic symptoms). The test is of least value in populations who are least likely to be suffering from ischaemic heart disease e.g. asymptomatic middle-aged women have a positive predictive value of <50%.

Indications

- Diagnosis of IHD: Intermediate or high probability IHD, vasospastic angina.
- Post-MI: Pre-discharge (sub maximal test in days 4–7 to assess prognosis, decide upon exercise programme and evaluate treatment), late post-discharge (symptom-limited 3–6 weeks).
- Pre and post-revascularization.
- Evaluation of arrhythmias: Optimizing rate-responsive pacemaker function, evaluation of known or suspected exercise-induced arrhythmias, and evaluation of treatment of above.

Contraindications

- Fever/acute viral illness.
- Myo/pericarditis.
- Severe aortic stenosis.
- Aortic dissection.
- Uncontrolled hypertension.
- Overt cardiac failure.
- Unstable angina or acute phase of MI.
- Significant resting arrhythmia (e.g. uncontrolled atrial fibrillation or complete heart block).
- Known severe left main stem (LMS) or LMS equivalent disease.
- Physical disability.
- ECG abnormality rendering interpretation of ST segment difficult (e.g. LBBB, LVH with strain or digoxin ECG changes).

When to stop

- Target heart rate achieved. (Tests have better sensitivity and specificity if the target heart rate is reached (>85% of 220 minus age in years for men or 210 minus age in years for women).)
- Worsening angina or excessive breathlessness.
- Dizziness.
- Fatigue/patient requests to stop.
- Atrial arrhythmia other than ectopic beats.
- Frequent ventricular ectopic beats or VT.
- Worsening ST segment shift (elevation or depression) at least 2 mm. depression but up to 5 mm depression.
- BP fall or failure to rise.
- Exaggerated hypertensive response to exercise (SBP >220 mmHg).
- New high-grade AV block or bundle branch block.

Criteria for a positive test

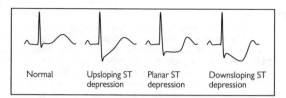

Normal   Upsloping ST   Planar ST   Downsloping ST
depression   depression   depression

- **Planar or downsloping ST depression** of at least 1 mm 80 ms after the J point (junction between the QRS and ST segment).
- ST elevation*.
- Increase in QRS voltage (ischaemic LV dilatation).
- Failure of BP to rise during exercise (ischaemic LV dysfunction)*.
- Ventricular arrhythmias*.
- Typical ischaemic symptoms during exercise.
- Inability to increase heart rate.

Features which are indications for urgent angiography
- Also ST depression at low workload (<<6 minutes Bruce) in multiple lead groups, persisting into recovery, >2 mm, down-sloping pattern.

Causes of false positive tests

- Cardiomyopathies
- Hypertension
- LVOT obstruction
- Mitral valve prolapse syndrome
- Hyperventilation
- Resting ECG abnormality (LBBB, pre-excitation, digoxin)
- Electrolyte abnormalities (hypokalaemia)
- Tricyclic antidepressants
- Syndrome X
- Coronary artery spasm
- Sympathetic overactivity.

Transthoracic echocardiography

Introduction

Despite dramatic advances in new cardiac imaging technologies, echocardiography remains the most important diagnostic imaging tool in clinical practice. Since its development by Edler and Herz almost five decades ago, and routine clinical implementation a decade later, echocardiography has developed into an intuitive, comprehensible and practical method to rapidly and repeatedly evaluate cardiac morphology and function. Competent interpretation of the echocardiographic examination first requires an understanding of the physical principles underlying the various technique modalities.

Ultrasound Physics

All forms of ultrasonic imaging are based on generation of high frequency (>1 mHz) acoustic pressure waves from a transducer comprised of one or more piezoelectric crystals. Current is passed across the latter leading to material deformation and wave transmission. The piezoelectric element also serves as a receiver and waves returning from insonified objects (e.g. walls, valves) deform the crystal(s) which, in turn, generate a current which can be sampled over time. Because the velocity of sound is constant, object location (spatial resolution) can be determined based on timing of the returning signal. The amplitude of the returning signal is based on the angle of incidence (surfaces perpendicular to the ultrasound beam are stronger reflectors) and the interface of acoustic impedances (greater differences such as occurs in the left ventricle at the tissue blood interface lead to greater reflectivity). Returning ultrasound information is processed for maximum image integrity and then mapped to pixels for display and storage. While many institutions continue to store images on videotape, image degradation necessarily incurred by this medium, as well as ease-of-use issues, have led to increased implementation of digital storage primarily on dedicated file servers.

M-mode

This was the first available form of echocardiography and, while still available on modern machines, has largely disappeared from routine use in modern laboratories. M- or 'motion'- mode images depict a single line of ultrasound over time. The information is graphic in nature and requires considerable experience for accurate interpretation. Its advantage lies in its high sampling rate (>1 kHz) and resultant ability to depict rapidly moving structures that may be of interest from a didactic or physiologic perspective.

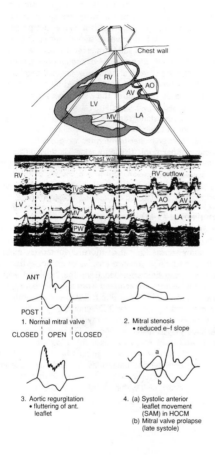

Fig. 1.1 Normal M-mode echocardiogram (RV = right ventricle; LV = left ventricle; AO = aortic valve; LA = left atrium; MV = mitral valve; PW = posterior wall of LV; IVS = interventricular septum). After R Hall *Med International* **17**: 774. Reprinted with permission from Longmore M, Wilkinson I, Rajagopalan S (2004). *Oxford Handbook of Clinical Medicine*. 6th ed. Oxford: Oxford University Press.

Two-dimensional (2-D) or sector scanning

When an ultrasound beam is swept across a chosen cardiac window, rapid sequential sampling can be performed leading to display of multiple 'scan lines' of information and a sector image created nearly instantaneously. Since a finite number of scan lines is possible, interpolation of data between lines is performed and an image slice or sector (hence the term 'sector scanning') is stored in digital form. Through reiterative acquisition over a cardiac cycle, a movie composed of sequentially acquired sectors is created demonstrating structural motion, which can then be displayed on a monitor. Beam sweeping can be performed by mechanical rotation of one or more crystals or through the use of programmed firing of a bank of crystals (phased array). Sampling rates were previously dictated and limited by videotape standards (e.g. PAL or NTSC) but, with digital capabilities appearing in some form on virtually all machines and replacing outdated tape technology, higher frame rates are possible.

The availability of harmonic tissue imaging has substantially improved image resolution by eliminating artifactual 'noise'. Low level signals emanating from tissue and comprising the first harmonic of the transmitted ultrasound are selectively sampled. In this way extraneous reflections such as reverberations are filtered out leaving a cleaner image.

Three-dimensional (3-D) imaging

While 2-D echo presents user-selected sector or tomographic information, 3-D echo has the potential to provide a comprehensive evaluation of cardiac anatomy similar to that of more quantitatively mature technologies such as magnetic resonance imaging or computerized tomography. Three-D echo can be performed using the 'freehand' approach in which multiple 2-D sectors are acquired from a probe that is positionally mapped using a 'spark gap' or magnetic tracking system. Both image and postion data is stored for post-hoc 3-D rendering. The development of rotational and, more recently, matrix array probes, coupled to powerful computer technology, has made post-hoc, 3-D chamber reconstruction a reality with accurate volumetric assessment. Most recently, real-time rendering of spatially limited cardiac segments has been made available. Though there are considerable limitations currently available in limited form from various manufacturers, it is almost certain that this technology will become the standard well within the next decade.

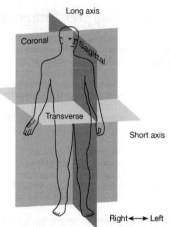

Fig. 1.2 The so-called 'anatomical position'. The subject is upright and facing the observer. Any structure within the body can be described within the references of the three orthogonal planes—two in the long axis and the third in the short axis. Reprinted with permission from Anderson RH, Ho SY, Brecker SJ (2001). Anatomic basis of cross-sectional echocardiography. *Heart* **85**: 716–720.

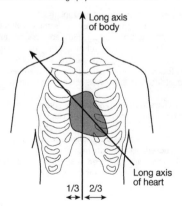

Fig. 1.3 The heart lies in the mediastinum with its own long axis tilted relative to the long axis of the body. Appreciation of this discrepancy is important in the setting of cross-sectional echocardiography. Reprinted with permission from Anderson RH, Ho SY, Brecker SJ (2001). Anatomic basis of cross-sectional echocardiography. *Heart* **85**: 716–720.

Transthoracic Doppler imaging

Quantification of object motion within the heart is performed using Doppler-based technologies. In brief, the same equipment described earlier propagates ultrasound which is aimed at moving red blood cells or tissue.

- Frequencies of returning ultrasound are shifted upwards and downwards by cells travelling towards and away from the transducer, respectively.
- The frequency shift is proportional to an object's velocity.
- The signal intensity is dependent on the number of cells moving at a particular velocity.
- Velocity information is depicted graphically as a spectral pattern over time (similar to the M-mode display) or mapped to pixels as colour overlaying the 2-D or 3-D, image.
- The echo beam must be as parallel as possible to the target with off-axis angulation by >30° leading to significant underestimation of velocities.

Doppler is restricted in its ability to sample high velocities by the *Nyquist limit* which is dependent on the sampling rate (the lower the frequency the higher the evaluable velocity) and object depth (the deeper the object, the lower the sampling rate). When the frequency shift of moving objects (i.e. velocity) exceeds the Nyquist limit, *aliasing* occurs precluding velocity assessment.

Pulsed Doppler permits accurate sampling of blood velocities averaged within a limited region of interest or 'sample volume'. Transducer elements serve both as transmitters and receivers permitting selective sampling of reflected ultrasound and accurate range or spatial information. Pulsed Doppler spectral displays portray velocity vectors over time:

Laminar flow is found within normal vessels and chambers and characterized by a gradual increase in flow velocities from the vessel wall to the vessel centre.

Laminar flow is characterized by a narrow spectral trace representing a relatively discrete population of blood velocities.

Turbulent flow occurs across stenotic or regurgitant orifices (valves, shunts, etc.) where high pressure gradients lead to high red cell kinetic energy and disordered, high velocity motion.

Turbulent flow is graphically portrayed as spectral broadening.

Aliasing often occurs with high velocity jets leading to 'wraparound' or the 'paint brush sign'.

Flow quantitation from pulsed doppler

Quantitation: pulsed Doppler spectral traces can provide important information regarding flow quantitation or timing. E.g. assuming that sampling occurs at an orifice with a relatively fixed area over the cardiac cycled (e.g. the left ventricular outflow tract) by integrating the time velocity spectral curve ('time-velocity integral' or TVI), the area under the curve can be multiplied by the area of the orifice (determined from 2-D echo) and stroke volume determined.

Continuous wave (CW) Doppler involves continuous transmission of ultrasound with one transducer element while a second element serves as a receiver. Higher sampling rates are achieved and, consequently, higher velocities as found in stenotic and regurgitant lesions can be measured. CW Doppler does not permit ranging information to be acquired and all velocities along a scan line are included in the spectral trace. CW Doppler can be performed with **stand-alone (Pedoff) probes** where the operator determines sample location based on familiar spectral patterns.

Imaging CW Doppler permits beam steering. Transducer elements are shared for purposes of CW and intermittent 2-D imaging. A virtual cursor positioned over the 2-D image can be moved to guide and minimize off-axis sampling angulation. CW Doppler velocities are depicted as a filled-in spectral tracing since these represent sampling of all of the velocities in structures along the sampling cursor (or ultrasound beam). Blood cells travelling at the fastest velocities are represented at the outer edge of the spectral trace (peak) or darkest line of the trace (modal) velocities.

Colour Doppler flow imaging employs multigate pulsed Doppler to portray blood flow overlying the 2-D image. Information is used to detect regurgitant or stenotic lesions or shunts and qualitative assessment of velocities is possible using colour maps.
- Pixels are assigned a colour based on user-configurable mapping parameters. Pixel colour is based on average velocity in the pixel region of interest.
- By convention, the BART colour map system is used in all machines with **b**lue colours representing flow **a**way from the transducer and **r**ed colour depicting flow **t**owards the transducer.
- The lighter the colour the higher the velocity.
- Abnormal velocity distributions characteristic of turbulence can be mapped usually by including a green hue ('variance mapping').
- Aliasing is depicted as a mix of colours or a 'mosaic' pattern.

Tissue Doppler imaging (TDI) is used to assess low velocity displacement of structures. A high pass filter excludes higher frequency shifts caused by red cell flow, leaving only low velocity shifts attributable to wall motion.

- Mitral or tricuspid annular motion can be tracked and correlates with systolic and relaxation performance of the associated ventricles.
- Regional wall motion can be assessed for displacement which may be affected by overall cardiac motion or local tethering.

Strain rate imaging can measure regional thickening and thinning independent of external influences described above, which influence tissue Doppler measurements. With strain rate imaging, two sampling sites are simultaneously acquired and inter-sample displacement (strain) over time (strain rate) can be determined.

Calculations from Doppler measurements

Valve gradients. The velocity of blood cells traveling across a narrow orifice is directly proportional to the pressure gradient at that point in time. This relationship is approximated by the simplified Bernoulli formula:-

Gradient (mmHg) = 4 V^2 (where V = peak Doppler velocity in m/sec)

In situations where there are high flow velocities (e.g. aortic stenosis with high LVOT velocities) the flow before the stenosis must be accounted for.

Gradient (mmHg) = $4(V_2^2 - V_1^1)$ (where V_2 = velocity across the lesion and V_1 = pre-lesional velocity)

Both peak and mean gradients can be determined, the latter by integrating the velocity spectra over a cardiac cycle.

Valve area (continuity equation). This is based upon the principle that flow in the pre-valve area (e.g. LV outflow tract, LVOT) = flow across the valve. Generally used for aortic stenosis quantitation though applicable to other stenotic orifices as well.

LVOT flow = LVOT area × LVOT time velocity integral (TVI) by pulsed Doppler

LVOT area = π (maximum LVOT diameter in PLA view)^2

Aortic valve flow = Aortic valve area × Aortic valve TVI by CW Doppler

As aortic valve flow = LVOT flow,

Aortic valve area = LVOT TVI/Aortic valve TVI × LVOT area

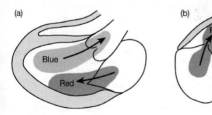

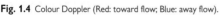

Fig. 1.4 Colour Doppler (Red: toward flow; Blue: away flow).

The standard transthoracic echo

Most laboratories employ imaging protocols incorporating acquisition of images from standard windows, resulting in standard views presented in a fairly standard sequence. Image quality is maximized by avoiding pulmonary artefacts and rib reflections. Pulsed and colour flow Doppler are performed following 2-D imaging in each view. Standard echo windows and views include:

Left parasternal window
- Long axis (PLA): left atrium, ventricle, proximal ascending aorta, mitral and aortic valves and right ventricle.
- Short axis (PSA): 4 levels—aortic valve /left atrial level: includes tricuspid and pulmonic valves and pulmonary artery; mitral valve, papillary muscle, and apex.
- Right ventricular inflow tract (RVIT).
- Right ventricular outflow tract (RVOT).

Apical window
- 4 chamber (A4Ch): atria, ventricles and AV valves, media septal and anterolateral LV walls.
- 5 chamber (A5Ch): A4Ch angled anteriorly to LV outflow tract.
- 2 chamber (A2 Ch): anterior and inferior LV walls.
- 3 chamber/apical long axis (A3Ch): apical version of PLA view with anteroseptal, posterior walls and LV outflow tract.
- Suprasternal window (SS): aortic arch.
- Subcostal window (SC): 4 chamber, Short axis, inferior vena cava.
- Suprasternal window (optional): aortic arch and proximal descending thoracic aorta.
- Right parasternal window (optional): ascending aorta and CW Doppler of aortic valve.

Chamber evaluation
- Chambers are routinely measured from M-mode tracings or, preferably, using digital calipers to perform point-to-point (PTP) assessment from 2-D images.
- Area tracings provide enhanced accuracy but are time-consuming.
- Volumes are derived from 2-D and PTP analysis using geometric modelling. The most common volumetric approaches include the modified Simpson's biplane method of stacked discs, bullet and area–length formulae.
- 3-D volume assessment has been validated but the technology is immature and inappropriate for routine clinical assessment.
- Most clinical labs perform PTP measurements online. End-diastole is usually defined as the beginning of the QRS complex and end-systolic measurements are performed at maximum LV contraction.

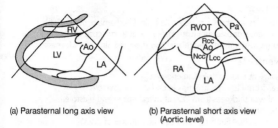

(a) Parasternal long axis view

(b) Parasternal short axis view
(Aortic level)

Fig. 1.5 (a) Parasternal long axis view; (b) Parasternal short axis view (aortic level).

Left atrium

- Measure at ventricular end-systole (min. LV chamber dimension).
- Linear (anteroposterior) from PLA view at aortic cusp level (A4Ch).
- Area (A4Ch) and volume (preferably modified Simpson's formula).

Left ventricle

- Measure at end-diastole and end-systole.
- Linear from PLA at mitral tips in end-diastole/systole.
- Septal wall thickness from PLA at mitral tips in end-diastole.
- Posterior wall thickness.
- Volumes: (modified Simpson's biplane method of discs).
- Derived variables:
  - Fractional shortening: LVIDd-LVIDs/LVIDs where LVID=LV internal diameter in diastole (d) & systole (s).
  - Ejection fraction (from 2-D or 3-D-generated volumes or derived from M-mode [e.g. Teicholz formula])
  - Mass: can be derived from M-mode measures (ASE-modified Penn formula), 2-D volumetric models or 3-D reconstruction. M-mode mass calculations tend to over-quantify LV mass.

Aortic root and ascending aorta

Linear measurements from 2-D PLA view or M-mode. The root is measured at cuspal level, aorta measured at sino-tubular junction and 2 cm above this.

Right atrium

- Area from 2-D A4Ch view.
- Inferior/superior and lateral/medial point to point measurements.

Right ventricle

- PTP measurements are exclusively used.
- Irregularity of chamber configuration makes standardized quantitation difficult.

Pulmonary artery

PTP medial-lateral measurement in PSA at aortic valve level.

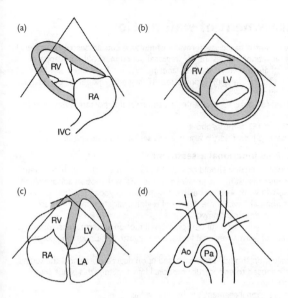

Fig. 1.6 (a) Parasternal long axis view (RV inflow); (b) Parasternal short axis (mitral valve level); (c) Apical 4 chamber view; (d) Suprasternal long axis.

Assessment of wall motion

Assessment is based upon review of multiple cuts as described earlier. In general, abnormalities of LV regional function should be apparent in more than one view. Various labelling systems have been used but the AHA Cardiac Imaging Committee 17 segment model is the standard convention:

- **Basal (6):** anteroseptal, anterior, anterolateral, posterolateral, inferior, inferoseptal.
- **Mid LV (6):** same as above.
- **Apical (5):** anterior, lateral inferior, septal, and true apical.

Regional functional assessment

- Systolic function should be classified as 'normal', 'globally hypokinetic', or demonstrating the presence of 'regional wall motion abnormalities'.
- Global hypokinesis is consistent with cardiomyopathy, either ischemic or non-ischemic. Some degree of regional variation may be present in non-ischemic cardiomyopathy.
- The presence of distinct regional wall motion abnormalities with large areas of normal regional function is suggestive of underlying coronary artery disease.
- Evaluation should ideally be based upon degree of regional thickening as opposed to endocardial motion. Unfortunately, this is not always possible.
- Each regional segment can be qualified as
    1) Hyperkinetic,
    2) normal,
    3) hypokinetic,
    4) akinetic,
    5) dyskinetic.
- Wall motion quantification, based on similar characteristics, may be prognostically useful, but are not useful in routine evaluation.
- Identification of hyper-echogenic, thinned areas suggests the presence of scarring and should be mentioned in the evaluation.
- Scarred segments may demonstrate endocardial motion, without wall thickening, due to tethering by peripheral segments.

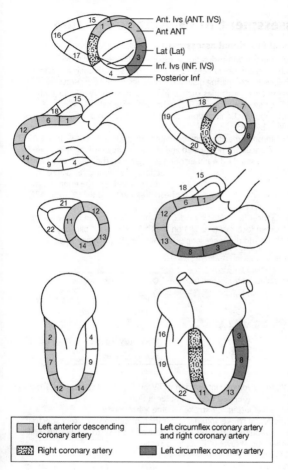

Ant. Ivs (ANT. IVS)
Ant ANT
Lat (Lat)
Inf. Ivs (INF. IVS)
Posterior Inf

| | Left anterior descending coronary artery | | Left circumflex coronary artery and right coronary artery |
| | Right coronary artery | | Left circumflex coronary artery |

Fig. 1.7

Assessment of LV systolic function

Global functional assessment

- Ejection fraction estimation is usually performed qualitatively. Echocardiographers need to routinely 'recalibrate' their assessment abilities by comparing qualitative readings to more accurate quantitative modalities such as MRI, radionuclide ventriculography, 3-D or even quantitative 2-D echo (see table below).
- 2-D echo ejection fractions can be quantitated most efficiently on or offline by the:
  - *Simpson's modified biplane method of stacked discs:* A4Ch and A2Ch LV traces are performed and the apex–annulus length is divided into a standard number of equal segments, the length of which serves as disc height. Cross-sectional disc area is calculated from the elliptical formula (π $r_1 r_2$) where r_1 and r_2 = the endocardial medial-lateral dimension of each segment in the A4Ch and A2Ch views, respectively.
  - *Cylinder hemielipsoid model:* volume is determined by measuring the LV endocardial area (A) on the PSA view at the papillary muscle level and the longest apex-annulus length (L) in any apical view. Volume = 5/6 AL.

LV ejection fraction	Qualitative assessment
>75%	Hyperdynamic
55–75%	Normal
40–54%	Mildy reduced
30–39%	Moderately reduced
<30%	Severly reduced

- *LV stroke volume:* integration of LV outflow tract spectra × LV outflow tract area (derived from diameter in PLA view).
- *Systemic output:* LV stroke volume × heart rate.
- *Pulmonary stroke volume:* integration of pulmonary artery spectral trace × pulmonary artery area (derived from systolic medial-lateral dimension at level of Doppler sampling).
- *RV output:* Pulmonary stroke voume × heart rate.
- *Pulmonic/systemic shunt ratio (Qp/Qs):* pulmonary output/systemic output.
- *Tissue Doppler of mitral and tricuspid annular motion.*

Essential aspects of ECHO assessment in patients with impaired LV systolic function

Anatomy

- LV dimensions (systolic and end diastolic).
- LF ejection fraction.
- Regional wall motion abnormalities.

Doppler characteristics

- E:A ratio (grade according to Fig. 1.8 p22).
- E deceleration time.
- Estimate PA systolic (from TR jet).
- Estimate PA diastolic (from PR jet).
- Estimate pulmonary capacitance (= stroke volume / (Pas–PAd pressures).

Implications for therapy

- Mitral regurgitation at end diastole if AV delay too long.
- Dysynchrony (TDI septum/lateral annulus >60 msec).

Assessment of LV diastolic function

Evaluation of LV diastolic function includes measurement of the various phases of diastole including isovolumic relaxation, early filling, diastasis (atrio-ventricular pressure equilibration without LV filling), and atrial systole. These measures are generally age and heart-rate dependent and effected by LV loading conditions to variable degrees (see Fig. 1.8 pp22–3).

Pulsed Doppler mitral inflow: E wave (peak early diastolic velocity), A wave (peak atrial systolic velocity), E/A ratio and trans-mitral deceleration time. The following should be taken into account when assessing these parameters:

- E/A ratio is particularly dependent on sample volume placement (annulus, mitral tips, etc.) and loading conditions.
- E/A ratio decreases with age and assessment must be age-normalized. An E/A ratio <1.0 is common among the elderly and often represents normal aging.
- Increasing LV filling pressures (e.g. in heart failure) lead to 'pseudonormalization' of the ratio which often reverts to an abnormal pattern following manoeuvres to reduce LV preload (e.g. diuresis) or Valsalva manoeuvre.
- The deceleration time correlates somewhat with invasive measures of LV stiffness whereas other measures largely reflect LV relaxation.

Pulsed Doppler of pulmonary veins: flow into the left atrium can be sampled. S, D, and A waves represent systolic and diastolic atrial filling. The A wave is generated by reverse flow into the pulmonary veins during atrial contraction.

- The S/D ratio increases with age as LV diastolic relaxation declines. A pulmonary vein A wave duration more than 30 msec greater than transmitral A wave durations suggests elevated LV filling pressure.

CW Doppler of LV outflow/mitral inflow: isovolumic relaxation time.

Tissue Doppler of medial and lateral mitral annuli (E', A')

- This is considered the least load-dependent filling variable. There is generally poor correlation between medial and lateral velocities with the lateral annulus measurement being more reproducible.
- The E/ E' ratio correlates roughly with LV end-diastolic pressure and a ratio > 15 is strongly suggestive of elevated filling pressure with a ratio <8 strongly suggestive of normal filling pressure.

Colour Doppler flow propagation (CFP) slope: rate of blood acceleration into the LV from annulus to apex.

Various diastolic profiles combining some of the above parameters have been suggested as indicators of degree or stage of 'diastolic dysfunction'. (see Fig.1.8 pp22–3). In general:

- Markers of impaired relaxation (e.g. decreased E and E' are accompanied by compensatory enhancement of A and A'), reduced pulmonary venous D and reduced CFP slope.
- Increases in LV filling pressure lead to pseudonormalization of the transmitral Doppler E/A ratio with less effect on Doppler with Valsalva manoeuvre and tissue Doppler velocity ratios.
- As compliance decreases or a patient's position on the LV pressure/volume curve advances (operating stiffness), the transmitral DT drops below 130 msec, early Doppler filling velocity is increased and, due to elevated late diastolic LV pressures, atrial contraction and associated velocities are reduced.
- If E/E' ratio <8 and LA is of normal size, symptoms are unlikely to be due to diastolic heart failure.
- Do not miss constriction (see p355). Look for:
  - Septal 'bounce' and dyschrony.
  - IVC dilatation.
  - Hepatic vein expiratory reversal.

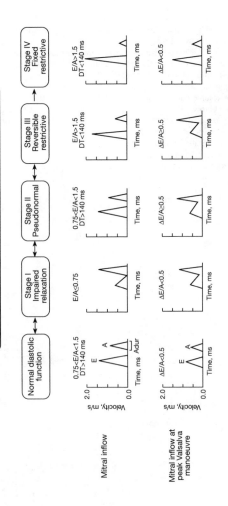

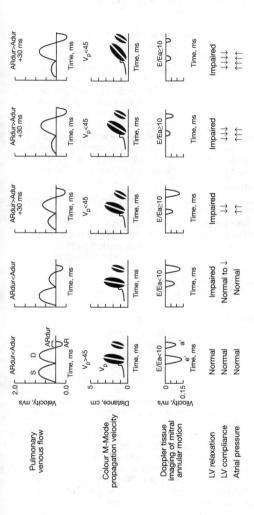

Fig. 1.8 Echocardiographic classification of diastolic dysfunction.

ECHO in aortic stenosis (AS)

Etiology

- AS can be congenital or, more commonly, degenerative. In late stages, severe fibrocalcification precludes etiologic identification even on direct intraoperative visualization. Chronic severe AS is usually accompanied by concentric LV hypertrophy, a product of pressure overload.
- **Bicuspid aortic valve** is diagnosed best on short axis view and can display various configurations. Often a 'raphe' is observed representing the undeveloped commisure where persistent cuspal fusion is present. Systolic cuspal 'doming' is consistent with congenital AS.
- **Degenerative AS** is, typically initiated in the annulus fibrosis (most commonly in the non-coronary cusp area) and gradually proceeds to invade the cuspal bases, body and, in later stages, the tips. Valve thickening without hemodynamic stenosis is often termed 'sclerosis'.

Hemodynamics

- Stenosis is defined as a haemodynamically significant reduction in valve area as indicated by a rise in transvalvular pressure gradient.
- Pressure gradient is dependent upon flow and, in the setting of low cardiac output, may be minimally elevated despite significant stenosis.
- Valve area is generally not indexed to body size in most clinical labs and categorization of severity may vary. One convention is as follows
  - Mild: area >1.5 cm^2 and <2.0 cm^2
  - Moderate: >1.0 and <1.5 cm^2
  - Severe: <1.0 cm^2
  - Critical: <0.7 cm^2

Echo diagnosis

- Assess cuspal separation or presence of doming. A trileaflet valve with one cusp opening fully (approaching edge of the root) is probably not stenotic.
- CW Doppler-derived gradients are reported as instantaneous peak and/or mean. The mean gradient is more reliable in determining stenosis severity.
- Cath lab gradients are 'peak to peak' with pressure measurements that are usually not acquired simultaneously and often do not correlate with Doppler gradients.
- Peak transvalvular velocity >2.5 m/sec (instantaneous gradient of 25 mmHg) suggests some degree of stenosis.
- Elevated cardiac output or significant aortic regurgitation will increase transvalvular flow and gradient but not valve area.
- **The dimensionless obstructive index (DOI)** is the ratio of LV outflow tract velocity (pulsed Doppler)/transvalvular velocity (CW Doppler) and takes into account elevated flow. General guidelines:
  - DOI <50%: significant stenosis.
  - DOI 30–50%: moderate stenosis.
  - DOI <30%: severe stenosis.

Aortic valve area is quantitated by the Continuity Equation. The most common errors in this assessment include:
a) under-measurement of the LVOT and
b) failure to assess LVOT Doppler at angle within 30° of flow vector.

Transoesophageal echocardiography (TOE)

Clinical indications

Transoesophageal echo (TOE) is a semi-invasive test that has advantages over transthoracic echo (TTE). The TOE transducer is closer to the heart and has a higher frequency (5 MHz), thus giving better resolution than TTE (2.5 MHz). The oesophageal approach means that an unobstructed echo window is possible in those patients with poor transthoracic windows, and it also allows the use of TOE in the intraoperative setting without interfering with the operative field. Virtually all TOE probes have multi-plane scanning capability.

Patient preparation

The procedure is performed using local anaesthesia and, if required IV sedation.

Prior to procedure:

- The patient is fasted for 4 hours prior.
- Any dentures are removed and the back of the throat is sprayed with lidocaine (Xylocaine®), taking care not to exceed the maximum dose because absorption of the local anaesthetic can cause systemic effects (nausea, drowsiness and ataxia).
- IV midazolam (dose 2–6 mg) can be given for sedation but in the majority of patients, local anaesthesia will suffice.
- Flumazenil may be required to reverse the effect of midazolam.

Procedure

- Oxygen and wall suction should be available. A nurse should be available to assist in monitoring during and after the procedure. A bite guard is used.
- The patient is placed in the left lateral position with the neck flexed. Oxygen saturation and the ECG are monitored.
- The sheathed TOE probe is lubricated with gel and introduced gently to the pharynx. Once the patient swallows, the probe is advanced into the oesophagus. The patient should be told that the initial gag feeling will ease with the passage of the probe from the pharynx into the oesophagus. Undue force must be avoided.

Post Procedure

- The patient should be 'nil by mouth' for 1 hour post-procedure for the effect of the local anaesthetic to wear off. Some patients such as paediatric or adolescent patients with complex congenital heart disease will require general anaesthesia

Pitfalls

- Serious complications are rare (0.2%) and mortality rate is less than 0.01%. Serious complications include oesophageal rupture, laryngospasm, ventricular arrhythmia, and severe hypoxia.
- The proximal aortic arch and the upper portion of the ascending aorta is a 'blind spot' because of the interposition of the trachea and right bronchus between the heart and oesophagus and dissection could be missed. Due to the resolution of TOE, certain normal structures e.g. Chiari network, aortic valve strands, prosthetic valve sutures might be inadvertently mistaken as pathology.

Indications for transoesophageal echocardiography

- Valve disease
  - Mitral valve prolapse, assess mitral stenosis for mitral valvuloplasty
  - Aortic regurgitation, adjunct to assess aortic stenosis
  - Prosthetic valve dysfunction
- Bacterial endocarditis
- Cardiac source of embolism, including PFO
- Aortic pathology
  - Acute aortic dissection, aortic rupture and aortic aneurysm, atheroma
- Prior to DC cardioversion
- Cardiac masses
- Pericardial disease and masses
- Congenital heart defects
- Intraoperative monitoring of valve procedures, LV and RV function
- ITU setting to determine cause of haemodynamic collapse
- Guiding interventional procedure—ASD closure, mitral valvuloplasty
- Poor transthoracic window.

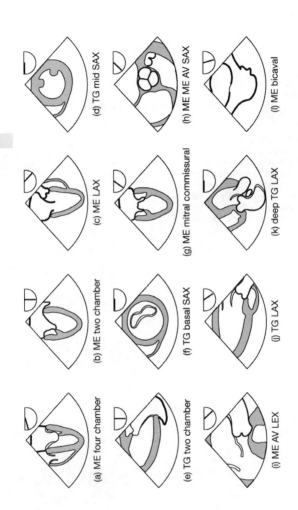

(a) ME four chamber

(b) ME two chamber

(c) ME LAX

(d) TG mid SAX

(e) TG two chamber

(f) TG basal SAX

(g) ME mitral commissural

(h) ME ME AV SAX

(i) ME AV LEX

(j) TG LAX

(k) deep TG LAX

(l) ME bicaval

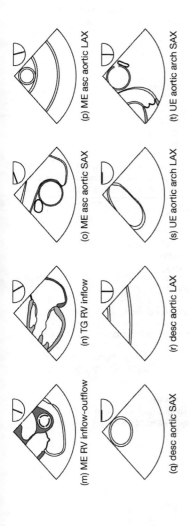

Fig. 1.9 Standard TOE views: ME, mid oesophageal; LAX, long axis; TG, trans-gastric; SAX, short axis; AV, aortic valve; RV, right ventricular. Reprinted with permission from Shanewise JS, Cheung AT, Arouson S et al. (1999). ASE/SCA guidelines for performing a comprehensive intraoperative multiplane transoesophageal echocardiography examination. *J Am Soc Echocardiogr* **12**: 884–900.

TOE for a cardiac source of embolism

Patients who have suffered a cerebral embolic event, especially at a young age (<50 years), may have a cardiac source of emboli that is not evident on transthoracic echo (TTE). Once a TTE has excluded major causes such as mitral valve disease, a TOE should be performed to examine the following areas:

Key views:

- Left atrial clot or spontaneous contrast (0° ME four chamber, 90° ME bicaval).
- Left atrial appendage for clot (90° ME two chamber).
- Patent foramen ovale (90° ME bicaval).
- Atrial septal aneurysm (90° ME bicaval).
- Atrial myxoma (0° ME four chamber, 90° ME two chamber, 90° ME bicaval).
- LV cavity for left ventricular thrombus, including apex (120° TG LAX).
- Aortic atheroma (>4 to 5 mm, mobile and ulcerated aortic plaques have the highest risk of embolization) in ascending, arch and descending aorta.
- Aortic and mitral valves for vegetations.

Diagnosis of patent foramen ovale

- 10 ml of saline is agitated by injecting between 2 syringes connected by a 3-way tap. Some operators report better opacification with colloid (e.g. Haemaccel) rather than saline.
- Position the TOE probe at either 0 or 180 degrees at mid oesophagus level to visualize the right atrium.
- Inject agitated saline.
- Repeat with Valsalva manoeuvre induced by asking the patient to cough or try to blow out the plunger from a 2 ml syringe.
- The presence of bubbles in the left heart chambers 3 cardiac cycles after opacification of the right atrium is required for a diagnosis of PFO.
- Sensitivity of detection of R–L shunt can be improved by injecting into the femoral vein rather than an antecubital vein, but this is not routinely done.

Diagnosis of atrial septal aneurysm

- The base of the aneurysm should measure at least 1.5 cm.
- The excursion of the membrane should be at least 1.5 cm in the direction of either atria.

TOE in aortic dissection

TOE can demonstrate the presence of an intimal flap in the aorta with great accuracy (sensitivity of 99%, specificity 98%). TOE should examine the following:

Key views
- Presence of intimal flap in:
  - ascending aorta (120° ME AV LAX, 0° ME asc aortic SAX).
  - descending aorta (0° desc aortic SAX, 90° desc aortic LAX).
  - aortic arch (0° UE aortic arch LAX, 90° UE aortic arch SAX).
- Coronary artery involvement (0° ME AV SAX).
- Aortic valve for regurgitation, annular diameter, cusp (120° ME AV LAX).
- Site of intimal rupture, colour flow mapping to determine true and false lumen.
- Aortic rupture with collection around aorta and
- Pericardial effusion
- Thrombus or spontaneous contrast in false lumen.

Blood pressure control should be initiated prior to TOE and sedation should generally be given to avoid undue hypertension

Pitfalls
- Blind spots in proximal arch.
- Aortic artefacts especially common in dilated aorta—artefacts are characterized by its position parallel to the aortic wall, blood flow velocities similar on either side of the artefact, and superimposition of the colour flow map over the artefact.
- An equivocal TOE examination should prompt the use of another imaging modality such as CT or MRI.

Aortic intramural haematoma (AIH)

This appears as an area of wall thickness >7 mm with or without the presence of an echolucent space in the aortic wall. It may be difficult to distinguish this entity from an atherosclerotic plaque or penetrating aortic ulcer and other imaging modalities may be required.

Diagnosis of AIH
- ≥7 mm crescent or circular thickening of aortic wall.
- Extending 1–20 cm longitudinal.
- No intimal flap or Doppler flow in thickened aortic wall.

TOE in endocarditis

> TOE is more sensitive **(sensitivity >90%)** than TTE for the detection of vegetations (sensitivity <60%) in infective endocarditis (IE), especially if the vegetations are <5 mm in size.

TOE is the investigation of choice in:
- Patients with poor TTE window.
- Prosthetic valve endocarditis.
- High or intermediate suspicion of IE with negative TTE.
- Detect IE related complications.

Some authorities feel that all patients with IE should have TOE for early detection of complications such as aortic abscess formation, and for *Staphyloccocus aureus* IE, where the risk of complications is high. Note that negative TTE and TOE has a negative predictive value of 95%. If clinical suspicion remains high, *TOE should be repeated in 7–10 days.*

Echocardiographic criteria for diagnosis of IE according to Duke classification
- Vegetations.
- Abscess formation: most commonly occurs in the aortic root followed by ventricular septum, mitral valve, and papillary muscle. TOE has a sensitivity of 80% compared to TTE 30%.
- Prosthetic valve dehiscence.

OR
- New valvular regurgitation.

Others complications include: leaflet perforation, fistula, and chordal rupture.

Key views
- Aortic root abscess seen (60° ME AV SAX)
- Mitral valve views (see p37)
- Tricuspid valve (0° ME four chamber, 120° TG LAX)
- Pulmonary valve (90° ME RV inflow-outflow)

TOE is useful prior to surgery to exclude infection on other valves and to look for abscess formation that will require additional procedures.

Pitfall
Valve strands (Lambl's excrescences), chordal structures from myxomatous degeneration, non-specific valvular thickening may be mistaken as vegetations leading to false positive TOE result.

Echocardiographic features requiring surgical referral

- Acute aortic or mitral regurgitation causing left ventricular failure. There may be associated valve destruction such as perforation or chordal rupture.
- Prosthetic valve dehiscence causing haemodynamic compromise.
- Large abscess formation or extension of abscess despite antibiotics.
- Vegetations—recurrent embolization.
- High risk of embolic events for mitral valve vegetation >10 mm.
- Increase in vegetation size after 4 weeks of antibiotics.

TOE for mitral regurgitation (MR)

- Morphological assessment of mitral valve to determine mechanism of regurgitation:
- Elongation or rupture of chordae.
- Retraction of chord.
- Prolapse or restriction of leaflets.
- Subvalvular apparatus.
- Annular diameter, degree of calcification.
- LV size and regional wall abnormalities.

Key views (see Fig.1.10)
- Leaflet prolapse or restriction (0° ME four chamber, 45° ME mitral commissural, 90° ME two chamber, 120° ME LAX).
- Annular diameter (120° ME LAX).
- Leaflet prolapse (0° TG basal SAX).
- Subvalvular apparatus (90° TG two chamber).

How to assess severity of MR using TOE

- Length of regurgitant jet.
- Timing of mitral regurgitation: early systolic vs. holosystolic by colour M-mode.
- Direction of jet: eccentric wall hugging or central.
- Pulmonary venous flow (see table below).
- Other features of severe mitral regurgitation:
  - Regurgitant jet width at its origin, >/=0.5 cm in 120° view so called 'vena contracta'.
  - Active volume loaded LV.
  - Peak e wave velocity >1.5 m/s

Assessment of severity of MR using pulmonary venous flow

Grade	Length (MR jet/LA size)	Timing	Direction	Pulmonary venous flow
1	1/3	Early	Central	Normal
2	2/3	<Pansystolic	Central	Normal
3	2/3	Pansystolic	Eccentric	Normal or reversed
4	3/3	Pansystolic	Eccentric or central	Reversed

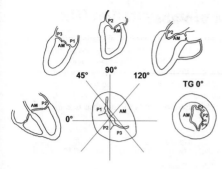

Fig.1.10 Assessment of the mitral valve by TOE. Reprinted with permission from Shanewise JS, Cheung AT, Arouson S et al. (1999). ASE/SCA guidelines for performing a comprehensive intraoperative multiplane transoesophageal echocardiography examinantion. *J Am Soc Echocardiogr* **12**: 884–900.

Mitral valve prolapse

The mitral valve annulus is a non-planar saddle-shaped structure. Mitral valve prolapse (MVP) due to myxomatous change should only be diagnosed if the mitral valve moves beyond the 'high points' of the mitral annular plane—imaged in 120 degree long axis view of mitral valve. The transverse plane 0 degree view images the 'low points' of the annulus (the distance between low and high points averages 1.4 cm) Thus, to avoid overdiagnosis of MVP prolapse the criteria for diagnosis is as follows:

Diagnosis
- *Classical MVP*
  - At least 2 mm displacement of mitral leaflet beyond the mitral annular plane in any view.
  - Mitral valve thickness >5 mm.
- *Non-classical MVP*
  - The prolapsing leaflets are not thickened (<5 mm) and are unaffected by myxomatous degeneration.
  - Such patients are not at increased risk of complications such as severe MR, infective endocarditis, and sudden death as compared to the classical form of MVP.

MVP causes eccentric mitral regurgitation, hence prolapse of the posterior leaflet produces anteriorly directed jet and vice versa. Note that when the MR jet hugs the wall of the left atrium, the reported severity should be upgraded. The left and right pulmonary veins should be sampled with pulse wave to check for systolic flow reversal.

Perioperative assessment of MVP
- Optimise loading conditions
  - Ensure that patient is fully off bypass and loading conditions are optimal with a systolic blood pressure of >120 mmHg before assessing the results of mitral valve repair.
  - Volume replacement or vasoconstrictors may be required.
- Assess coaptation
  - Multiplane interrogation of the zone of coaptation using colour flow mapping.
  - If there are persistent abnormalities of coaptation or apposition with significant MR, revision surgery may be required.
- Assess left ventricular outflow tract
  - LVOT obstruction may occur after mitral valve repair especially after the use of a rigid annuloplasty ring, but is uncommon (1–2%).
  - This phenomenon is exacerbated by hypovolaemia, and the LVOT gradient can be monitored from the transgastric long axis view, while any hypovolaemia is corrected.
  - If LVOT obstruction persists, the annuloplasty ring may have to be removed.

TOE for mitral valve repair

- Mapping of the prolapsing mitral valve segments can be performed to aid surgical planning.
- Two thirds of cases of MVP involve the middle scallop of the posterior leaflet and 70% of these cases can be successfully repaired.
- Ruptured chordae and flail mitral valve leaflets should be noted.
- The mitral annulus diameter is also measured (upper limit normal is 35 mm) and presence of annular calcification noted.

Indications for revision surgery after MV repair

- Grade 2+ MR.
- Persistent LVOT obstruction.
- Mitral stenosis (mean gradient ≥ 6 mmhg, MVA <1.5 cm^2.
- Leaflet perforation.

TOE in chronic ischaemic MR

- Typically the mitral valve is structurally normal and therefore MR is termed 'functional'.
- Remodelling of the LV displaces the papillary muscle towards the apex and traction on the mitral leaflets causes incomplete leaflet closure.
- The zone of coaptation is displaced towards the apex and 'systolic tenting' of the mitral valve is seen.
- LV remodelling and dilatation appears to be necessary for severe MR to develop. Isolated segmental wall motion abnormalities without LV dilatation are not generally associated with severe MR.
- Annular dilatation will exacerbate incomplete leaflet coaptation but does not in isolation cause MR.
- In the presence of an inferior or posterior infarct, the posterobasal wall (site of the posteromedial papillary) of the LV may become aneurysmal. This can exert asymmetrical traction on the chordae resulting in retraction of the posterior leaflet. There is abnormal apposition and an eccentric anteriorly directed jet of MR results.

Key views
- Restriction of leaflet, systolic tenting of MV (0° ME four chamber, 45° ME mitral commissural, 90° ME two chamber, 120° ME LAX).
- Annulus size (120° ME LAX).
- LV assessment especially the posterobasal wall (90° ME two chamber, 0° TG mid SAX).

TOE for mitral stenosis

Assessment for suitability for percutaneous balloon mitral valvuloplasty (PBMV see p68):
- LA and LAA thrombus—relative contraindication
- > grade 2 MR—relative contraindication
- Mitral valve anatomy
  - Mobility.
  - Thickening.
  - Calcification.
  - Subvalvular thickening.

TOE for prosthetic valve dysfunction

TOE is a valuable method for assessing prosthetic valve function and their complications. Prosthetic valve complications detectable on TOE include:
- Paraprosthetic leak.
- Intra-prosthetic leak from degeneration of tissue valve.
- Prosthetic valve obstruction from pannus or thrombus.
- Endocarditis including abscess formation.
- Patient- prosthesis mismatch (when the aortic valve is too small).

TOE assessment of mitral valve prosthesis

TOE is especially sensitive in detecting mitral regurgitation in association with a prosthetic valve because the left atrium is imaged in the foreground and is therefore devoid of the artefacts generated by the metal elements of the prosthetic valve.

Paraprosthetic mitral leak

The sewing ring of the mechanical prosthetic valve appears as a bright ring attached to the mitral annulus. If a significant circumference of the sewing ring has come away (e.g. from endocarditis) a rocking movement of the valve will be evident—this 'rocking prosthetic valve' is characteristic of a partial dehiscence of the valve.

Key views The mitral valve sewing ring should be identified in and interrogated with colour flow and continuous wave Doppler.

• 0° ME four chamber.
• 90° ME two chamber.
• 120° ME LAX views of the mitral valve.

The motion of the prosthetic valve mechanism (e.g. tilting disc) should be assessed to ensure the discs or occluder are moving freely in 120° ME LAX view.

The presence of flow outside the sewing ring (i.e. paraprosthetic) is not normal, although small or mild jets may be seen early after valve implantation. This represents failure of the sutures attaching the valve ring to the annulus either from technical failure or the effect of endocarditis. Paraprosthetic leaks are more likely in the presence of a calcified mitral annulus.

Transprosthetic mitral leak

Mechanical prosthetic valves have regurgitation during closure of the valve which arise within the sewing ring (i.e. intraprosthetic). These 'closing jets' are a normal feature and should not be mistaken as pathological. In general they can be easily distinguished from pathological regurgitation. (see table opposite) Causes for abnormal intraprosthetic leak include pannus or thrombus preventing the occluder from functioning properly.

Tissue mitral prosthesis

Should be assessed in the same way as a mechanical prosthesis. The prosthetic valve leaflet should be assessed for:

• Prolapsing leaflet.
• Flail leaflet.
• Thickened cusps (>3 mm—higher risk of dysfunction).
• The Doppler signal for a flail cusp shows a characteristic striated 'zebra stripe pattern'.

Obstruction of the prosthetic mitral valve

This may be due to thrombus or pannus formation. The diagnosis is made by finding:
- Limited movement of the occluder or disc.
- Haemodynamic confirmation by finding high peak pressure gradient across the mitral valve(>2.5 m/s) or a prolonged pressure half time (>200 ms).

Features of normal closing jets

- Short jets <3 cm length.
- Narrow base <5 mm.
- Early systolic rather than pansystolic leak.

Upper limit of pressure half time (msec) for commonly used valves	
Valve type	**Max t½ (msec)**
Starr–Edwards	170
St Jude	131
CarboMedics	117
Carpentier–Edwards	171
Native valve	60

TOE for aortic valve prosthesis

- The orientation of the aortic valve means that the sewing ring will obstruct the view of the orifice of the valve for mechanical and stented tissue aortic valves. Thus assessment of aortic paraprosthetic leak on 2-D imaging is limited compared to mitral valve assessment.
- Continuous wave interrogation is not possible because the LVOT is orientated perpendicular to the ultrasound beam, when the aortic valve is assessed from the standard mid-oesophageal views.
- A combined TTE and TOE approach is required, because TTE is ideally suited to Doppler interrogation of the aortic valve.

Deep transgastric View

A deep transgastric TOE allows imaging of the aortic valve in the foreground, and allows proper alignment of the Doppler signal from the aortic valve (0° deep TG LAX and 120° TG LAX views). This view is useful to assess:

- Movement of the aortic prosthetic valve mechanism.
- Colour flow Doppler interrogation for aortic regurgitation.
- Continuous wave assessment of aortic regurgitation.
- Continuous wave measurement aortic valve gradient.

The use of the deep transgastric TOE view is especially useful for assessment of aortic prosthetic valve function when mechanical mitral prosthesis is also present. This is because acoustic shadowing from the mitral valve obscures the LVOT in all mid-oesophageal TOE views of the aortic valve. However, this view is not possible in all patients.

Regurgitation is most commonly transprosthetic in aortic tissue valves. The following may be visible on TOE: cusp thickening (>3 mm predicts risk of valve failure), cusp tear, cusp prolapse and flail cusp. Rocking of the aortic prosthesis is due to dehiscence of the valve (40% circumference affected) and best seen in the 0° ME AV SAX and 120° ME AV LAX views.

Key views

The aortic valve prosthesis is assessed in:

- 0° ME AV SAX.
- 120° ME AV LAX.
- 0° deep TG LAX.
- 120° TG LAX.

TOE assessment of normal and dysfunctional aortic prosthetic valves

Normal peak gradient across mechanical aortic valve prosthesis

- St Jude Medical   24 ± 7 mmHg
- Medtronic Hall   21 ± 7 mmHg

Significant stenosis or obstruction likely mechanical aortic valve

- Peak velocity of >4 m/s or mean velocity of 3 m/s are suggestive of obstruction

Tissue aortic valves

- Aortic valve area by continuity equation <1 cm^2.
- Mean gradient >26 mmHg.
- Ratio of LVOT to peak velocity across aortic valve <0.2.

Stentless aortic valves

- (Freestyle or Toronto valve) or aortic homografts do not have the disadvantage of a sewing ring casting an acoustic shadow on the aortic valve orifice and TEE gives excellent views of valve cusps. Some of these valves are indistinguishable from native valves on TOE.

Intraoperative TOE

Indications

AHA Class I indications

- Cardiac valve repair.
- Haemodynamic compromise where LV function is unknown.
- Complex endocarditis surgery where peri-valvular extension is suspected.
- Complex valve replacement such as homograft valve replacement with coronary reimplantation.
- Ascending aortic dissection with aortic valve involvement.
- Posterior or loculated pericardial effusion.
- Congenital heart surgery.
- HOCM surgery.

AHA Class II indications

- Heart valve replacement.
- Cardiac tumour removal.
- Coronary surgery including 'off pump bypass'.
- Cardiac aneurysm repair.
- LV or RV assist device implantation.
- Ascending aortic dissection without aortic valve involvement.
- Cardiac trauma.
- Intracardiac thrombectomy or pulmonary embolectomy.
- Heart and/or lung transplantation to assess anastomotic sites.

Key views (see Fig.1.11)

LV assessment in made on these views:

- 0° ME four chamber.
- 90° ME two chamber.
- 120° ME LAX.
- 0° TG mid SAX.

TOE in the intra-operative and perioperative period (in ITU) to assess haemodynamic instability

- Coronary artery bypass graft failure: examine LV in all 3 coronary distributions. The transgastric view shows all 3 coronary distributions in one view.
- Hypovolaemia: reduced LV cavity size and end systolic cavity obliteration is a sign of hypovolaemia.
- Pericardial collection: any collection can be localized, to say, just the left atrium and need not be a global collection.
- Severe LV dysfunction.
- Right ventricular failure.
- Unsuspected severe mitral regurgitation.
- Unsuspected aortic dissection.

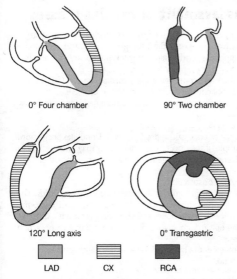

0° Four chamber

90° Two chamber

120° Long axis

0° Transgastric

LAD   CX   RCA

Fig. 1.11 Assessment of LV function by TOE. Reprinted with permission from Shanewise JS, Cheung AT, Arouson S et al. (1999). ASE/SCA guidelines for performing a comprehensive intraoperative multiplane transoesophageal echocardiography examinantion. *J Am Soc Echocardiogr* **12**: 884–900.

TOE for assessment of cardiac masses

- Normal anatomy that should not be mistaken for pathology: Chiari network, eustachian valve near the inferior vena cava, trebeculations in the left atrial appendage, ridge separating left pulmonary vein and left atrial appendage.
- Myxomas are the most common primary cardiac tumour (50% of all tumours) and specific features can be delineated on TOE.
  - Attached by a stalk to the inter-atrial septum near the fossa ovalis in 90% cases.
  - 75% are in the LA.
  - May have a speckled, cystic appearance with frond-like projections.
  - May be multiple. If they occur elsewhere, they may be mistaken for thrombus (tend to be homogeneous in appearance) or other tumours.
  - May cause valve obstruction.
- Fiboelastomas are benign tumours that attach to valve apparatus. They have a frond-like appearance and may mimic vegetations or myxoma.
- Primary malignant cardiac tumours and secondary metastatic disease can infiltrate the epicardium, myocardium, endocardium- or present as intracavity mass.
- Pericardial involvement in malignant disease frequently causes pericardial effusion.

PET scanning

Positron emission tomography (PET) is a nuclear imaging technique that uses short half-life radionuclides incorporated into radiopharmaceuticals allowing quantitative assessment of various aspects of cardiac function in different regions of the heart:

• Global and regional left ventricular function.
• Myocardial blood flow.
• Myocardial metabolism: glucose and fatty acid metabolism; myocardial oxygen consumption.
• Pharmacology: beta adrenergic and muscarinic receptors; sympathetic innervation; myocardial ACE and angiotensin II receptors.
• Myocardial gene expression.

Clinical applications

Identification of myocardial viability

The main clinical application of PET scanning has been determination of *myocardial viability* of patients with impaired left ventricular function secondary to coronary artery disease who may benefit from surgical or percutaneous coronary revascularization. These studies have demonstrated that PET imaging has high sensitivity for predicting recovery of contractile function after revascularization and have also provided major insights into the mechanisms underlying left ventricular dysfunction in patients with coronary artery disease.

Research applications

The large variety of compounds available for study using PET permits interrogation of many facets of cardiac function, providing important in vivo mechanistic information in human disease. These measurements also allow for analysis of the mechanisms underlying the benefit of established and novel therapeutic strategies. Examples include:

• Myocardial blood flow and microvascular function: ischaemic heart disease, hypertrophic cardiomyopathy, dilated cardiomyopathy, aortic stenosis, syndrome X.
• Myocardial metabolism and cardiac energetics: ischaemic cardiomyopathy, dilated cardiomyopathy.
• Cardiac autonomic function: hypertrophic cardiomyopathy, dilated cardiomyopathy, arryhthmogenic right ventricular dysplasia, autonomic neuropathy, long QT syndrome.

Comparison of PET over conventional cardiac nuclear modalities (gamma camera, SPECT)

Advantages

- Short half-life of radionuclides.
- Better spatial resolution.
- Accurate attenuation correction allowing absolute quantification of radiopharmaeutical concentration.
- On site cyclotron.

Disadvantages

- Expensive.
- Limited access.
- Predominantly a research application.

Adapted with permission from de Silva R and Camici PG (1994). Role of positron emission tomography in the investigation of human coronary circulatory function. *Cardiovasc Res* **28**(11): 1595–612.

Cardiac magnetic resonance imaging (CMR)

In the past decade, cardiac magnetic resonance imaging (CMR) has emerged as an important investigative tool in management of all types of cardiovascular disease.

Technique

- Uses signals produced from protons (H^+ ions, abundant in vivo due to large proportion of body being water).
- When magnetic field is applied, the protons align both parallel (majority) and anti-parallel to the field with a net vector between.
- Net vector can be altered by applying differing types of short radiofrequency pulses.
- On cessation of this secondary pulse, the vector returns/relaxes to its original position and releases energy in the form of radiowaves.
- Two forms of net vector relaxation: longitudinal (T1) and transverse (T2).

Types of CMR

- *Spin-echo* used to assess morphology. Higher soft-tissue contrast, flowing blood appears dark.
- *Gradient-echo* used to assess shunts, valvular lesions, great vessels and LV function. Flowing blood (i.e. flowing protons) across magnetic gradient have magnetic vectors with phase shift proportional to flow velocity—hence allowing assessment of these dynamic lesions. Uses lower soft-tissue contrast with blood flow shown by high signal intensity.

Uses of CMR (list of uses rapidly expanding)

- **Congenital heart disease**—useful in assessment (both anatomic and haemodynamic) of complex abnormalities of heart and great vessels.
- **Ventricular function**—particularly useful for assessing RV/LV systolic and diastolic function and ventricular mass. Useful in assessing response to novel therapies (e.g. stem cell therapy).
- **Aortic disease**—at least as good as TOE/CT in diagnosis of acute aortic dissection. Good at delineating anatomy (origin, extent and involvement) of dissection—particularly in patients with previous aortic disease/surgery. Marfan's syndrome—serial scans used to assess progression of aneurysm. Intramural haematoma. Plaque disease.
- **Valvular heart disease**—echocardiography and catheterization remain mainstays of assessment in these patients. CMRI use becoming commoner as specificity/sensitivity improved.
- **Cardiomyopathies**—shows morphological features and assesses haemodynamic function. In HOCM, may see fibrosis and perfusion abnormality. CMRI is examination of choice for ARVC.
- **Cardiac tumours/pericardial disease**—useful in assessing both primary and metastatic intracardiac neoplasia. Gives anatomical localization and indication of extracardiac involvement. Gradient-echo sequence can assess vascularity of tumour. Investigation of choice in diagnosing pericardial disease/effusions.

Cardiac magnetic resonance imaging

Advantages

- Rapid scanning sequences.
- Clinical Information—can give anatomical, haemodynamic and functional information from same scan.
- Non-invasive (for diagnostic imaging)—c.f. angiography, TOE, etc.
- High spatial resolution—c.f. echocardiography, CT.
- No ionizing radiation—c.f. angiography, etc.

Disadvantages

- Claustrophobia—tight enclosed space within scanner.
- Lack of adequate monitoring—due to electrical distortion, makes it difficult to scan haemodynamically unstable patients—who may benefit most from diagnostic accuracy of CMRI. Can be overcome with special extension leads (for monitoring, O_2 therapy, etc) allowing isolation of metallic/electrical equipment.
- Expense/lack of centres—initial high capital expenditure necessary, but becoming more widespread.
- Metallic prosthetic implants—becoming less of a problem (see p54).

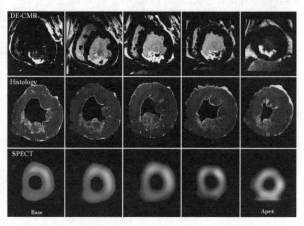

Fig. 1.12 Comparison of in vivo DE-CMR images (upper panel) to histopathology (middle panel) in a canine with subendocardial inferior wall infarction. Corresponding SPECT-sestamibi images are also shown for comparison (bottom panel). Modified from Wagner A, Mahrholdt H, Holly TA, et al. (2003) Lancet **361**: 374–379.

Metallic prostheses and CMR

Ferromagnetism (refers to metallic compounds attracted by a magnetic field) initially referred to ferrous compounds and their properties in a magnetic field i.e. attraction. 4 other metals are also strongly magnetic: cobalt, dysprosium, gadolinium, and nickel. Alloys of these compounds will also exhibit magnetism to some degree. Most human prosthetic implants are not strongly magnetic as they have impurities added to the iron to give them added strength/anti-oxidant properties.

Potential for causing injury with CMR and metallic objects—
there are three main mechanisms for this.

- *Projectile injury* Refers to external adjunctive equipment e.g. O_2 cylinders, forceps, scissors, etc which are in the MR room. Strong magnetic field could launch these across the room with obvious consequences. Ferrous compounds such as these must therefore be barred from the room or special 'MR safe' equipment used.
- *Implanted prostheses* Again injury can result from internal movement of these. Potential for movement will depend on magnetic properties of device and restraining tissue it is surrounded by. Thus hip prosthesis has less potential to cause damage than an intracranial arterial clip.
- *Electrical currents* CMR can induce electrical currents in devices with conductance properties which can cause heating and thermal injury. Examples include pacing wires, guide wires, PA catheters.

Device	Risk*
Coronary stents	Theoretical risk of thermal injury or movement. Clinical studies show CMR safe in this group. Newer cobalt alloy and DES stents still to be evaluated (but probably safe)
Other vascular stents	Similar to coronary stents (manufacturers often advise wait 6/52 post-implant)
Guidewires	May cause thermal injury (newer CMR safe ones developed for CMR intervention)
Prosthetic valves/rings	All valves appear safe (including earlier ball and cage ones)
Pacemakers and ICDs	Potential for movement, thermal injury and electrical inhibition. CMR use is associated with excess mortality. NOT currently recommended although guidelines may change with certain (lower) field strength scanners
Intracardiac catheters	Polyurethane and PVC ones are safe. Those with metallic component (e.g. PA flotation catheters) will cause thermal injury NOT safe
IABP/LVAD	NOT safe due to thermal injury, movement and mechanical malfunction
ECG leads	Standard metallic leads have been associated with burns (may be severe). Newer carbon-based CMR-compatible leads are available
Sternal wires/Epicardial pacing wires	Safe, although may cause artefact

*NB Always check with the MRI dept if concerned.

Valvular heart disease

General considerations

Development

Cardiac valves develop from the mesodermal germ layer between the 4th–7th week of gestation. Any factors affecting embryogenesis during this time can affect development of valves and include infection (German measles/rubella, drugs, etc).

Anatomy

Four cardiac valves: two on the left side of heart (mitral and aortic) and two on the right (tricuspid and pulmonary). Both the mitral and tricuspid valve cusps are tethered to papillary muscles in respective ventricles. All valves have three cusps/leaflets except mitral with two leaflets (anterior and posterior MV leaflets).

Acute rheumatic fever

Epidemiology

- Less than 1 case per 1000 population in developed countries. Around 10 cases per 1000 schoolchildren in developing countries. Although it is becoming rarer in the developed world, it still accounts for almost half of cardiac disease in developing world
- Declining incidence in developed world is most likely multifactorial: improved economic standards and housing conditions, decreased crowding in houses and schools, improved access to medical care, and effective antimicrobials all probably contribute.
- Typically children aged 5–15 years from lower socio-economic class living in crowded conditions. 20% cases in adults. Incidence higher in native Hawaiians and Maoris despite antibiotic prophylaxis.
- No sex difference but chorea and mitral stenosis more common in females.

Pathology

- Typically occurs several weeks after a streptococcal pharyngitis. Usually group A beta haemolytic streptococci: *Streptococcus pyogenes* serotype M. Antigenic mimicry is implicated. Antibodies to carbohydrate in cell wall (anti-M antibodies) of Group A Streptococcus cross react with protein in cardiac valves.
- Delay from acute infection to onset of rheumatic fever (RF) is usually 3–4 weeks. RF is thought to complicate up to 3% of untreated streptococcal sore throats. Previous episodes of RF predispose to further events (up to 50% of streptococcal sore throat complicated by RF if previous episode). Other areas of cross reactivity may explain other signs (e.g. involvement of connective tissue in joints → arthritis, caudate nucleus in brain → Sydenham's chorea).
- Commonly causes a pancarditis. Pericarditis rarely causes haemodynamic instability or constriction. Myocarditis may cause acute heart failure and arrhythmias. Endocarditis affects mitral valve (65–70%), aortic valve (25%), and tricuspid valve (10%, never in isolation) causing acute regurgitation and heart failure but chronic stenosis.
- Pericardium, perivascular regions of myocardium, and endocardium develop perivascular foci of eosinophilic collagen surrounded by lymphocytes, plasma cells and macrophages called Aschoff bodies.

Clinical features

- *Sore throat* 1–5 weeks ago reported in two thirds of cases.
- Fever, abdominal pain and epistaxis.
- Migratory large joint *polyarthritis* starting in the lower limbs in 75% of cases. Duration less than 4 weeks at each site. Severe pain and tenderness in contrast to degree of joint swelling.
- *Pancarditis* in 50% of cases with features of acute heart failure, mitral and aortic regurgitation, an apical, mid-diastolic flow murmur (Carey Coombs murmur) and pericarditis.
- *Chorea* in 10–30%, usually 1–6 months after the index pharyngitis. Patients exhibit difficulties in writing and speaking, generalized weakness, choreiform movements (can be unilateral and stop whilst asleep) and emotional lability. Joints are hyperextended with hypotonia, diminished tendon reflexes, tongue fasciculation, and a relapsing grip (alternate increases and decreases in tension). Full recovery in 2–3 months.
- *Erythema marginatum* is an evanescent rash with serpiginous outlines and central clearings on the trunk and proximal limbs. Seen in 5–13% of cases. Begins as erythematous, non-pruritic papules or macules that spread outwards. Fades and reappears in hours and persists throughout course. See Fig. 2.1.
- *Subcutaneous nodules* seen in 0–8% of cases usually several weeks after the onset of severe pancarditis. Mainly over bony surfaces or prominences and tendons. Commonly elbows, knees, wrists, ankles, Achilles tendons, occiput and vertebral spinous processes. Duration 1–2 weeks.
- There is a danger of overdiagnosing rheumatic fever in children admitted with fever, soft murmurs and arthralgia, all of which are common in childhood. Evidence for an antecedent streptococcal infection is required for the definitive diagnosis—see table opposite.

Treatment

- Oral penicillin V for 10 days (250 mg tds in children and 500 mg tds in adults)
- or intramuscular penicillin G (single dose of 1.2 million units) to treat the acute infection.
- Oral erythromycin, if penicillin allergic, for 10 days (20–40 mg/kg/day qds in children and 250 mg qds in adults). Alternatives include clarithromycin, azithromycin, or cephalexin.
- Oral aspirin 4–8 g daily until ESR and CRP normal.
- Prednisolone 2 mg/kg/day for 2–4 weeks if moderate–severe carditis.
- Oral haloperidol for chorea (0.5–2 mg tds in adults and 0.05–0.15 mg/kg/day in 3–12 year old children).
- Use diuretics, ACE inhibitors, and digoxin for heart failure.

Prognosis
- Determined by level of cardiac involvement and antibiotic prophylaxis (5 years or until 21 years old if no carditis, 10 years or well into adulthood if carditis but no valve disease, 10 years or until 40 years old if valves affected and for all dental and surgical procedures).
- Acute phase duration about 3 months in 80% of cases. Mortality 1–10% in developing countries.
- Recurrence rates are high. Chronic valve disease in one third without and two thirds with recurrent infections.
- Murmurs resolve in 50% of cases up to 5 years after index infection.

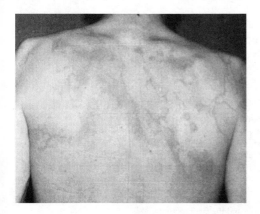

Fig. 2.1 Erythems marginatum.

Diagnostic criteria for rheumatic fever (Jones criteria)

Evidence of group A streptococcal pharyngitis.

Either a positive throat culture or rapid streptococcal antigen test, or an elevated or rising streptococcal antibody titre (samples taken two weeks apart).

Plus two major or one major and two minor Jones criteria.

Major criteria
- Polyarthritis
- Carditis
- Chorea
- Erythema marginatum
- Subcutaneous nodules

Minor criteria
- Fever
- Arthralgia
- Prolonged PR interval
- Elevated ESR and CRP

Mitral stenosis

This is most commonly due to rheumatic fever. Other causes are rare. They include congenital (isolated lesion or in association with an ASD—Lutembacher's syndrome), malignant carcinoid, mucopolysaccharidoses (e.g. Hurler's syndrome) and endocardial fibroelastosis. Stenosis occurs at three levels: chordae (fuse, thicken, and shorten), cusps (thicken and calcify), and commissures (fuse with the valve cusps still mobile).

Pathophysiology

Elevated LA pressure is required to propel the blood through the narrowed mitral valve orifice. This leads to ↑ pulmonary venous pressure and exertional dyspnoea due to ↓ pulmonary compliance. Reactive pulmonary hypertension occurs leading to RV hypertrophy and failure. LV function is unaffected but as filling is impaired, adequate CO cannot always be maintained. The rise in CO during exertion is blunted. Onset of AF is associated with abrupt clinical deterioration, due to both the loss of atrial systole and the fast heart rate.

Clinical features

• Dyspnoea on exertion, orthopnoea, paroxysmal nocturnal dyspnoea.
• Acute pulmonary oedema may be precipitated by uncontrolled AF, exercise, chest infection, anaesthesia, and pregnancy.
• AF increases the risk of thromboembolism. Systemic embolism occurs in 20–30% and usually originates in the dilated LA and LA appendage.
• Fatigue is due to reduced cardiac output reserve and is common in mild–moderate stenosis.
• Haemoptysis can occur for a variety of reasons: alveolar capillary rupture (pink frothy pulmonary oedema); bronchial vein rupture (larger haemorrhage); blood stained sputum of chronic bronchitis; pulmonary infarction (low CO, immobile patients).
• Chest pains similar to angina may occur in patients with pulmonary hypertension and RV hypertrophy, even with normal coronaries.
• The enlarging LA may compress surrounding structures producing hoarse voice (left recurrent laryngeal nerve compression—Ortner's syndrome), dysphagia (oesophageal compression), left lung collapse (left main bronchus compression).

Physical signs

Mitral facies or malar flush. Prominent 'a' waves in JVP. Small volume arterial pulse. Irregularly irregular pulse in AF. 'Tapping' apex beat—palpable S1. Diastolic thrill at apex. Left parasternal heave (due to RVH), palpable pulmonary closure.

Auscultation: S1 loud if in sinus rhythm and valve is pliable. P2 accentuated. Opening snap (OS) of the MV heard best at or medial to the apex in expiration. A2–OS interval varies inversely with severity of stenosis. Low pitched, rumbling, mid-diastolic murmur with pre-systolic accentuation (if in sinus rhythm) heard best at the apex with patient in left lateral position. Early diastolic murmur due to pulmonary regurgitation from pulmonary hypertension (Graham Steell murmur) may be heard.

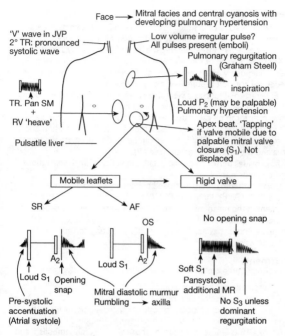

Fig. 2.2 Physical signs in mitral stenosis. Reproduced with permission from Swanton H (2003). *Pocket consultant: cardiology.* 5th ed. Oxford: Blackwell Publishing.

Investigations

- *ECG:* bifid p wave (if in sinus rhythm) due to LA enlargement most prominent in lead II. Tall and peaked p waves in pulmonary hypertension. AF is frequent. Right axis deviation and RV hypertrophy.
- *CXR:* straightening of the left heart border, prominent upper lobe veins, pulmonary artery enlargement, Kerley B lines—interstitial oedema. Large left atrium visible as a double shadow.
- *TTE:* parasternal long axis view shows enlarged left atrium and doming of the valve leaflets due to commissural fusion. In short axis view mitral valve orifice can be calculated by planimetry. Calcification can be visualised. M-mode imaging—restricted valve leaflet separation due to commissural fusion. CW Doppler can be used to estimate the valve area and transvalvular gradient (see p9).
- *TOE* provides better anatomic detail, can visualize small vegetations and thrombi in the LA.
- *Cardiac catheterization:* increased pulmonary capillary wedge pressure (PCWP). Increased PCWP to LV end diastolic pressure gradient. If the mean mitral gradient is low at rest, get the patient to perform exercise on the cath-lab table (e.g. straight-leg raising) to calculate gradient again. Assessment of co-existing coronary and valvular lesions.

Treatment

Medical

- Asymptomatic patients need only infective endocarditis prophylaxis.
- Mild symptoms—salt intake restriction and oral diuretics.
- In AF—digoxin, beta-blocker, or calcium channel blocker for rate control. Restoration of sinus rhythm may be attempted if appropriate.
- Anticoagulants—at least 1 year for those with thromboembolism and life-long if in AF. Patients with low-output states and R heart failure should also be anticoagulated. There is no proven benefit if the patient is in sinus rhythm.

Balloon valvotomy

Moderate to severe symptoms or development of pulmonary hypertension warrants mechanical relief of mitral stenosis. In percutaneous balloon mitral valvotomy, a guide wire is placed in LA after transseptal puncture and a balloon (Inoue balloon) is directed across the valve and inflated at the orifice. This procedure is suitable for patients with pliable valves with minimal MR, no subvalvular distortion and without heavy calcification.

Surgical

- *Closed valvotomy*. Fused cusps separated by a dilator introduced through LV apex.
- *Open valvotomy* with cardiopulmonary bypass is preferred to closed valvotomy. Cusps separated under direct vision. Any fusion of subvalvular apparatus is loosened.
- *Mitral valve replacement* if there is significant MR or the valve is severely diseased or heavily calcified.

Radiographic features of mitral stenosis

PA film

- Straight or convex L heart border
- Double shadow of LA behind RA
- Splaying of carina (> 90°)
- Dilated upper lobe veins
- Prominent pulmonary conus
- Pulmonary haemosiderosis

Lateral film

- LA or RV enlargement
- Valvular calcification
- McCallum's patch (LA calcification)
- Oesophageal indentation on barium swallow

Indications for surgery in mitral stenosis

- Significant symptoms limiting daily activities
- Episode of acute pulmonary oedema with no obvious precipitant
- Recurrent systemic emboli
- Pulmonary oedema in pregnancy (consider emergency valvotomy)
- Deterioration due to AF that does not improve with medical treatment

---

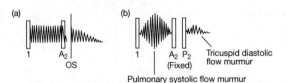

Fig. 2.3 Similarity on auscultation between (a) mixed mitral valve disease and (b) ASD. Reprinted with permission from Swanton H (2003). *Pocket consultant: cardiology.* 5th ed. Oxford: Blackwell Publishing.

Mitral regurgitation

Causes

Acute: infective endocarditis, acute MI, trauma.

Chronic: chronic rheumatic heart disease, mitral valve prolapse, Left ventricular dilatation of any cause. Degeneration of valve cusps, collagen disorders, hypertrophic cardiomyopathy.

Pathophysiology

LV is decompressed into the LA during systole. In acute MR there is little enlargement of LA due to normal compliance. This results in raised LA pressure and can result in pulmonary oedema. In longstanding severe MR there is enlargement of LA, which accommodates the volume overload with minimal rise in LA pressure.

Symptoms

- In acute severe MR—pulmonary oedema is common.
- In chronic MR—Fatigue (due to ↓forward CO), exertional dyspnoea, orthopnoea, systemic embolisation (less common than MS). Palpitation (↑stroke volume/associated AF). Right heart failure in later stages.

Examination

Rapid upstroke in arterial pulse. Prominent 'a' waves in JVP in patients in sinus rhythm. Large 'v' waves if associated TR. Forceful apex displaced laterally. Systolic thrill at apex. Soft first heart sound. Loud mitral valve closure sound helpful in excluding severe MR. Wide splitting of S2 due to premature aortic valve closure. Prominent low pitched S3. A mid-diastolic flow murmur may follow S3 even in the absence of MS. Pansystolic murmur loudest at the apex and radiating into the axilla.

Investigations

- *ECG.* Features of LA enlargement, LVH, RA enlargement in pulmonary hypertension. AF common in chronic MR.
- *CXR.* Cardiomegaly. LA and LV enlargement. Pulmonary venous congestion, calcified mitral annulus may be seen.
- *TTE.* Shows dilated LA, hyper dynamic LV. Colour Doppler to detect and quantify the MR. Assessment of LV function from ejection fraction, end systolic dimension and end diastolic dimension. CW Doppler to assess the velocity of the regurgitant jet.
- *TOE* shows the anatomy in greater detail and allows accurate assessment of the feasibility of valve repair. Should be performed prior to surgery.
- *Cardiac catheterization* confirms the severity of the lesion. Detection and assessment of the associated valve lesions and coronary artery disease.

Prognosis

Outcome is poor in severe symptomatic mitral regurgitation. 33% survival at 8 years without surgical intervention. Death occurs mostly from heart failure but substantial incidents of sudden deaths, which may be arrhythmia related.

Management

Medical management

Infective endocarditis prophylaxis required. Asymptomatic patients with mild MR managed conservatively with serial echocardiograms. Vasodilators in symptomatic patients to increase forward CO and reduce regurgitant volume. In AF—rate control and anticoagulation.

Surgical treatment

This is indicated in patients with severe MR who are symptomatic despite optimum medical management. Asymptomatic patients with severe MR may need surgery if there is worsening of LV function. Timing of the surgery is very important. Reduction of the LV ejection fraction <60% or end systolic dimension of >45 mm indicates LV systolic dysfunction and the need for surgery.

- Mitral valve repair is preferred to valve replacement if technically feasible. Long term anticoagulation and risk of haemorrhage and thromboembolism can be avoided.
- Mitral valve replacement with prosthesis needed if valve leaflets are severely damaged with calcification.

Mitral valve prolapse

(Barlow's syndrome, Floppy mitral valve syndrome)

Causes

Most of the cases are idiopathic. Connective tissue disorders including Marfan's syndrome, Ehlers–Danos syndrome, pseudoe xanthoma elasticum, osteogenesis imperfecta. In 20% of ostium secundum ASD. Can be acquired following rheumatic fever, cardiomyopathies, ischaemic heart disease. ♀>♂

Pathophysiology

Myxomatous degeneration and excess mucopolysaccharides leads to large 'floppy' valve leaflets. Prolapse can be caused by papillary muscle dysfunction, elongated chordae tendinae and enlarged mitral annulus. MV leaflet (usually posterior) prolapses into the LA during ventricular systole. Strain and ischaemia of papillary muscle and MR results.

Symptoms

Mostly asymptomatic. Atypical chest pain, Palpitations resulting from ventricular and supra ventricular arrhythmias. Symptoms of MR if significant.

Examination

Mid or late systolic click due to tensing of the chordae tendinae and the prolapse of the leaflet. Late systolic murmur due to associated MR.

Investigations

ECG is usually normal. Some non-specific changes may be seen. CXR normal if no significant MR TTE. Systolic displacement of 1 or both MV leaflets by >2 mm into the LA beyond the high points of mitral annulus. Assessment of MR.

Treatment

Infective endocarditis prophylaxis if MR or thickening of MV leaflet on TTE. Beta-blocker for chest pain and palpitations. Anticoagulation if in AF. MV repair (rarely replacement) for severe MR.

Aortic stenosis

Incidence

Commonest valve lesion in UK. ♂ > ♀. ↑ with age. 2% of people >65 years have echo features of aortic stenosis (AS). Congenital bicuspid AS presents ~20 years earlier. Becoming commoner (population ageing, improved diagnosis).

Causes

Acquired Degenerative calcific AS (commonest); rheumatic fever, Paget disease of bone, end-stage renal failure, ochronosis.

Congenital Bicuspid aortic valve 1–2% live births. Bicuspid AV results in chronic turbulent flow which results in calcification and fibrosis of leaflets with reduced valve area.

Aetiology

AS can occur at level of valve or above (supravalvular stenosis) or below (subvalvular) the aortic valve. Degenerative calcific AS results from years of normal stress on valve. Similar risk factors as IHD (↑ BP, ↑ lipids, DM). Inflammatory change occurs within valve with calcium deposited along flexion lines causing immobility, reduced excursion and reduced opening area. Rheumatic AS due to adhesion and fusion of commisures with fibrosis and retraction.

Pathophysiology

Progressive narrowing of valve orifice results in worsening LVH (to maintain stroke volume). LVH results in stiff, non-compliant ventricle with elevated end-diastolic pressure (diminished coronary perfusion pressure). Atrial component of LV filling then becomes more significant.

Clinical features

- Angina pectoris (occurs in $^2/_3$—only $^1/_2$ of these have obstructive coronary lesions), dyspnoea, syncope, dizziness, palpitations, heart failure, sudden death.
- Slow rising, small volume pulse (pulsus parvus et tardus)—best felt at carotid. BP—narrow pulse pressure, in advanced AS systolic BP is ↓. Prominent 'a' wave on JVP. Sustained, heaving apical impulse. If CCF develops, apex beat displaced inferolaterally. Systolic thrill felt in aortic area (2nd intercostal space on right) during full expiration.
- Auscultation—S1 normal or soft. S2 in mild AS, normal (i.e. A2 pre-cedes P2). In moderate AS S2 becomes single (closure of AV delayed until it coincides with closure of PV). In severe AS get reversed splitting with A2 after P2. S4 often heard (atria contracting into stiff ventricle) and systolic ejection click (if valve pliable). Ejection systolic murmur heard throughout precordium but best heard in aortic area in full expiration. Radiates to carotids. As AS worsens, murmur extends later through systole and may obscure S2.

Aortic stenosis: management

Investigation

ECG: LVH with strain; BBB (either R or L). *CXR*: calcification in valve or aortic root, post-stenotic dilatation in ascending aorta. *TTE*: will show calcified valve with restricted opening (M-mode). *Colour doppler* to look for concomitant AR, *CW Doppler* to assess velocity (and hence pressure drop) across valve. *Cardiac catheterization*: to assess for concomitant coronary artery disease prior to aortic valve surgery. No need to assess pullback gradient across valve nowadays (significant risk of embolic events with this, CW Doppler accurately assesses gradient and LV function).

Severity

Arbitrary classification of severity according to gradient (assessed by CW Doppler (see p11)) across valve.

Severity	Gradient (mmHg)
Normal/trivial AS	<20
Mild AS	20–40
Moderate AS	40–60
Severe AS	>60

Prognosis

AS is a progressive condition which gradually worsens. Symptoms often not present until severe AS (gradient across valve often >100 mmHg). Once symptoms occur, prognosis worsens (unoperated): of patients who present with symptoms of angina, 50% will die within 5 years; if patients present with syncope, 50% will die in three years; if patients present with dyspnoea, 50% will die within two years.

Treatment

Surgery AS is a mechanical obstruction and the only way to relieve this is with surgery. AVR is safe effective procedure (surgical mortality 1%, complication rate thereafter 1%/year cumulative).

Medical β-blockers reduce myocardial O_2 demand and may improve coronary blood flow. Loop diuretics may relieve preload and help with dyspnoea (avoid hypovolaemia). In CCF or dilated LV, digoxin may help with dyspnoea (particularly if patient in AF/flutter). In severe AS avoid drugs which reduce afterload (e.g. GTN, ACE-I) as these may worsen gradient and cause syncope.

Balloon aortic valvuloplasty Introduced as non-surgical alternative treatment for AS. Results not as good as anticipated because of procedural complications (~3% mortality and ~6% MI/severe AR/myocardial perforation) and because of restenosis rates. Use restricted to children/adolescents with non-calcified AS and in patients deemed unfit for AVR or who refuse surgery. Balloon aortic valve replacement is being developed with a stent mounted tissue valve that is deployed below the coronary ostia.

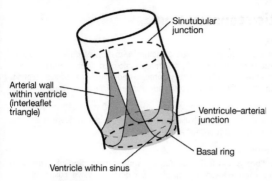

Fig. 2.4 A diagrammatic representation of the aortic root shows its considerable length. The leaflets are attached within the cylinder of the root in the form of coronet. Reproduced with permission from Anderson RH (2000). Clinical anatomy of the aortic root. *Heart* **84**: 670–673.

Aortic regurgitation

Causes

Valvular: rheumatic fever (often combined with AS), infective endocarditis, degenerative calcific (with AS), trauma. Aortic root disease. Aortic dissection, hyper-tension, Marfan's syndrome, osteogenesis imperfecta, syphilis, spondyloarthritides (ankylosing spondylitis, Reiter's, etc.)

Incidence

Less common than AS. Valvular causes becoming less frequent and aortic root causes now account for >50% cases.

Pathogenesis

Valvular fibrosis and fusion of cusps results in retraction of cusps such that they cannot appose properly. SBE destroys valve cusps directly. Aortic root disease Progressive dilatation of aortic root causes failure of coaptation of cusps and regurgitation.

Pathophysiology

As valve fails, more of LV stroke volume regurgitates into LV. Cardiac output is maintained by increase in stroke volume but at expense of increase in end-diastolic volume. Eventually with further LV dilatation myocyte function deteriorates and further LV dilatation occurs.

Symptoms

Dyspnoea/symptoms of CCF, angina, symptoms of aortic dissection.

Examination

Very wide pulse pressure with associated signs: collapsing (water-hammer) pulse, Corrigan's sign (visible carotid pulsation), De Musset's sign (head nodding with each pulse), Müller's sign (visible pulsation of uvula), Traube sign (also called 'pistol shot femorals'—loud noises heard with stethoscope over femoral artery), Quincke sign (visible capillary pulsation in nailbed), Duroziez sign (heard over femoral artery when artery is digitally compressed). Apex beat displaced inferolaterally and diffuse/hyperdynamic. May feel apical systolic thrill.

Auscultation: A2 may be normal (or louder) if AR is due to aortic root pathology, may be soft or absent if AR due to aortic valve pathology. S3 may be heard with dilated LV or with incipient failure. An ESM similar to AS may be audible (either due to mixed AR/AS or due to turbulent flow due to ↑stroke volume). Murmur of AR is high pitched murmur immediately following A2. Best heard with patient sitting up and leaning for-ward in expiration. Heard clearest along left sternal border (occasionally along right sternal border). Duration of murmur in diastole correlates with severity of AR.

Austin Flint murmur is a mid-diastolic murmur heard at apex due to antegrade flow across a mitral valve orifice which has been narrowed by a combination of rising LV pressure and jet of AR directed at anterior MV leaflet.

Investigation

ECG: LVH with strain; left axis deviation. *CXR:* In chronic AR get enlarged cardiac shadow. Dilated ascending aorta with aortic root pathology. *TTE:* Colour Doppler and CW Doppler confirm diagnosis and assess severity. M-mode measures aortic root and LV dimensions. *Cardiac catheterization:* to assess for concomitant coronary artery disease prior to aortic valve/root surgery. Aortogram in LAO projection shows aortic root and severity of AR.

Prognosis

Chronic AR can be well tolerated for many years and is associated with a good prognosis. 5 year survival ~75%, 10 year survival ~50%. Prognosis worsens as symptoms intervene (see box). Acute severe AR however is associated with a high mortality from LVF and early intervention is indicated.

Natural history of AR	
Asymptomatic patients with normal LV function	
Progression to symptoms/signs CCF	<6%/year
Progression to asymptomatic LV dysfunction	<3.5%/year
Sudden death	<0.2%/year
Asymptomatic patients with LV systolic dysfunction	
Progression to cardiac symptoms	>25%/year
Symptomatic patients	
Mortality rate	>10%/year

From ACC/AHA Guidelines for the management of patients with valvular heart disease (1998). *JACC* **32**: 1486.

Treatment

Medical Asymptomatic mild/moderate AR with normal LV—routine follow up (every 1–2 years) with echo. Asymptomatic severe AR with normal LV—frequent (6 monthly) follow up—or sooner if symptoms intervene. Symptoms of CCF respond to loop diuretics and digoxin while arrangements are made for surgery. Vasodilators (ACE-I, Ca^{++} channel blockers) offer good symptomatic relief and may improve haemodynamic profile. Anginal chest pain can be treated with nitrates but use beta-blockers with caution. Concomitant hypertension can worsen AR therefore treat in usual way.

Surgical Because of the relatively benign nature of asymptomatic AR with normal LV function, these patients should be kept under observation. Once symptoms intervene or evidence of significant LV dysfunction appears, referral for AVR/root re-placement should be considered. In borderline cases frequent (2–4 monthly) follow up is indicated.

Right heart valve lesions

Tricuspid stenosis

Causes Rheumatic fever (almost always associated with MS), congenital, carcinoid, pacemaker lead.

Symptoms fatigue, anorexia, peripheral oedema.

Examination Wasting, oedema, hepatomegaly, elevated JVP with prominent 'a' waves, rumbling mid-diastolic murmur heard best at LLSE in inspiration.

Investigation ECG: sinus rhythm with signs RA enlargement (↑'p' waves in II, V1—often coincides with signs LA enlargement because of MS) but no RVH. CXR: enlarged RA but normal PA size. TTE: 2-D image can show thickened restricted leaflets. CW Doppler is diagnostic. If diagnosis of TS is made, always look for co-existent MS.

Treatment Salt restriction and diuretics may markedly improve symptoms. If co-existent MS is being operated on then surgical valvuloplasty may help. TV replacement occasionally performed. Bioprosthetic valves give better results than mechanical valves. Recent evidence of usefulness of TV balloon valvuloplasty.

Tricuspid regurgitation

Causes Any cause of RV dilatation (MV disease, congenital heart disease, RV infarction, etc), endocarditis (particularly IV drug abuse), Marfan's syndrome, Ebstein anomaly, rheumatic fever, carcinoid.

Symptoms Usually minimal. As right heart failure develops, patients complain of oedema, ascites, nausea, anorexia, abdominal pain (tender, congested liver).

Examination Cachexia/wasting, jaundice, oedema, AF common, elevated JVP with systolic CV waves, tender pulsatile hepatomegaly. Auscultation— RV S3 often heard (↑on inspiration), PSM audible at LSE (↑on inspiration). Murmur loudest in TR secondary to pulmonary hypertension.

Investigation ECG: non-specific, may show evidence of underlying condition. CXR: cardiomegaly in patients with functional TR, occas distended azygos vein, pleural effusion. TTE: colour Doppler confirms diagnosis. CW Doppler of TR jet can assess PA systolic pressure. 2-D images can give idea of cause of TR (RV infarction, VSD, Ebstein, etc).

Treatment In absence of pulmonary hypertension, TR is well tolerated and may not require specific treatment (indeed in SBE of TV, valve excision is sometimes performed with good recovery). Symptoms of RV failure respond to diuretics and fluid/salt restriction. If co-existent MV disease is being operated on and TR is mild (with minimally elevated PA pressure), TR usually improves following surgery as PA pressure falls. In these patients with severe TR due to annular dilatation then TV annuloplasty may be sufficient. TR secondary to valve pathology (Ebstein, carcinoid) may require valve replacement, preferably with large bioprosthesis to minimize risk of thrombosis (but high operative mortality ~15%).

Pulmonary stenosis

Causes Congenital, carcinoid, rheumatic, extrinsic compression.

Symptoms Usually none. If severe stenosis—exertional dyspnoea, light-headedness. Latterly may get symptoms of RV failure (see previous).

Examination Prominent 'a' wave in JVP, RV heave, occasionally thrill in 2nd left intercostal space. Auscultation—widely split S2 (as PV closure becomes later), P2 becomes softer (unless stenosis is supravalvular), ESM at left edge upper sternum, heard best in inspiration.

Investigation ECG: RVH and RA overload. CXR: dilated pulmonary arteries, occasionally with calcification of valve, if severe then oligaemic lung fields. TTE: confirms diagnosis and can show level of stenosis (valvular, supravalvular or RV outflow tract). Will also show associated conditions (ASD, PDA, Fallot's, etc).

Cardiac catheterization: to assess severity of obstruction and haemodynamic effects.

Treatment In general, invasive intervention is recommended when gradient across valve is >50 mmHg at rest or when symptoms occur. *Medical*—supportive/symptomatic treatment of RV failure, diu-retics, fluid restriction. *Balloon Valvuloplasty*—treatment of choice for stenosis at valvular level. Highly effective, safe with good long term results. *Surgical*—valvotomy is very effective with minimal recurrence. Pulmonary regurgitation may occur requiring surgery. *Pulmonary Valve Replacement*—indicated if not suitable for above treatments or if develops severe PR following these treatments.

Pulmonary regurgitation

Causes Any cause of pulmonary ↑BP (causes dilatation of valve ring), infective endocarditis, connective tissue disease (e.g.' Marfan's), iatrogenic (following valvotomy or PA catheter placement), carcinoid.

Symptoms Often asymptomatic. Symptoms occur when pulmonary ↑BP or RV failure exist. Then get dyspnoea on exertion, lethargy, peripheral oedema, abdominal pain.

Examination RV heave, occasionally a thrill in pulmonary area. Auscultation—P2 may be delayed (large stroke volume), loud (if pulmonary ↑BP) or soft (if PV stenosis). Murmur of PR heard best in 3rd/4th intercostals space on left adjacent to sternum, ↑ during inspiration.

Investigation ECG: RVH (if pulmonary ↑ BP), RBBB/rsR pattern in V1. CXR: enlarged PA and RV. TTE: 2-D images may show RV dilatation/hypertrophy. Abnormal septal motion if RV volume overload. PR seen on colour and quantified with pulsed Doppler.

Treatment Usually supportive treatment suffices. Treat RV failure in usual way (diuretics, etc). If PR due to PV ring dilatation secondary to pulmonary hypertension, treating cause of pulmonary ↑ BP can relieve this and decrease the severity of PR (e.g. mitral valve surgery). If severe right heart failure then PV replacement can be considered.

Prosthetic heart valves

Types
Mechanical: ball and cage (Starr–Edwards) or tilting disc (single leaflet—Medtronic Hall, Bjork–Shiley; bileaflet—St Jude Medical, Carbomedics)
Bioprosthetic: porcine or bovine (Carpentier–Edwards)
Homograft: preserved human valve

Mechanical valves
Very durable (often last >20 years). Thrombogenic therefore requiring life-long warfarin therapy (± aspirin if high risk). Ball and cage valves are earlier models. Very durable but also very thrombogenic and require more intensive anticoagulation. More recent tilting disc valves are less thrombogenic (bileaflet valves less thrombogenic than single leaflet).

Tissue valves
(Bioprosthetic or homograft) have advantage of not requiring long term anticoagulation but are not as durable as mechanical valves (15 year failure rate of 10–20% for homografts and 20-30% for bioprostheses—higher in patients <40 yrs of age). Consequently, mechanical valves tend to be placed in younger patients or those with another reason for warfarin (AF, impaired LV) and bioprostheses implanted in older patients or those who refuse warfarin.

Valve haemodynamics
Different prosthetic valves have unique profiles and valve areas. For any given valve dimension the bioprosthetic valves and ball and cage valves have the smallest effective valve area and homografts have largest valve area (~native valve area).

Assessment of prosthetic valve function
Clinically: each prosthetic valve produces distinctive sound. Dysfunction may be indicated by new sounds, a change in sound or volume of sound or a new (or changing) murmur.

Imaging modality: fluoroscopy can be used to assess valve leaflet movement (in mechanical valves). Diminished motion in thrombosis, excessive movement of base ring if valve dehisced. TTE—limited use because of echo shadow caused by metal in valve. Can be used to look at valve ring motion (in mechanical valves), leaflet motion (in tissue valves) and regurgitation (with Doppler). TOE—better at assessing prosthetic mitral valve function but less good at prosthetic aortic valve assessment. MRI—safe in majority of modern mechanical valves. Expensive and time consuming therefore reserved for cases when TTE/TOE inconclusive.

Cardiac catheterization: can assess valve gradient (and therefore valve area). Can quantify degree of regurgitation. Risk of passing catheter across mechanical valves therefore used prior to reoperation or when non-invasive tests inconclusive.

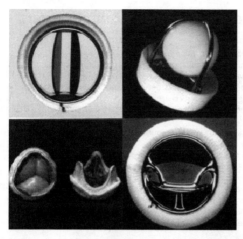

Fig. 2.5 Common types of heart valve prostheses (from top left clockwise): St Jude's Medical bileaflet, Starr–Edwards ball and cage, Bjork–Shiley tilting disk, stented porcine prosthesis. Reproduced with permission from Bloomfield P (2002). *Heart* **87**: 583–589.

Class I and II AHA/ACC recommendations for choice of prosthetic valve*	
Recommendations for valve replacement with a mechanical prosthesis	
Patients with expected long lifespan	I
Patients with a mechanical valve already in place in a different position than the valve being replaced	I
Patients with renal failure on haemodialysis or with hypercalcaemia	II
Patients requiring anticoagulation due to risk factors for thromboembolism†	IIa
Patients <65 years for AVR and < 70 years for MVR	IIa
Recommendations for valve replacement with a bioprosthesis	
Patients who cannot or will not take warfarin treatment	I
Patients >65 years needing AVR with no risk factors for thromboembolism†	I
Patients considered to have possible compliance problems with warfarin	IIa
Patients > 70 years needing MVR with no risk factors for thromboembolism†	IIa
Valve replacement for thrombosed mechanical valve	IIb

* Reproduced with permission from Bloomfield P (2002). *Heart* **87**: 583–589.

† Risk factors: atrial fibrillation, severe LV dysfunction, previous thromboembolism, hypercoagulable condition. AVR (aortic valve replacement); MVR (mitral valve replacement)

Prosthetic heart valves: complications

Valve thrombosis

Incidence: 0.1–5.7% per patient-year.

Risks: inadequate anticoagulation and mitral prostheses. Similar rates in bioprosthetic valves and mechanical valves receiving adequate anticoagulation. Also no difference in rates between different types of mechanical valves receiving adequate antico-agulation.

Clinical presentation: pulmonary oedema, systemic embolisation, sudden death.

Investigation: ↓intensity of valve sounds, ↓movement of leaflets on TTE or fluoroscopy (and ↑valve gradient on TTE).

Treatment: anticoagulation with heparin. If thrombus is <5 mm on TTE then anticoagulation may suffice. If > 5mm then will need further treatment (thrombolysis, thrombectomy or valve replacement).

Prognosis: valve replacement for valve thrombus has mortality rate of <15%, thrombolysis has mortality rate of <10% (with embolisation in <20%). Thrombolysis more effective for aortic valve thrombosis and in recent (<2 week) onset.

Embolisation

Most manifest as cerebral infarctions.

Incidence: in un-anticoagulated patients 4% per patient-year (causing death or neurological defect), 2% per patient-year on antithrombotic therapy and 1% per patient-year on warfarin.

Risks: AF, age >70 years, ↓LV function, mitral prostheses, ball and cage valves, >1 valve. Consider endocarditis in patients with prosthetic valves presenting with peripheral embolization. If cerebral embolization, withhold anticoagulation until CT scan excludes bleed (if bleed confirmed, seek specialist help).

Haemolysis

Low level of background haemolysis is common in patients with mechanical prostheses (even when functioning normally). Severe haemolysis is uncommon and is usually secondary to valve dysfunction (leakage, dehiscence, infection).

Investigation: ↓Hb, ↑LDH, ↓serum haptoglobin level, reticulocytosis.

Treatment: treat underlying problem (including further valve surgery), blood transfusion, folic acid, ferrous sulphate.

Endocarditis (see Chapter 5)

Prevalence: occurs at some time in 3–6% of patients with prosthetic valves. Early endocarditis cases occur within 60 days of valve surgery and late endocarditis occurs >60 days since surgery. Early prosthetic valve endocarditis (PVE) usually arise from skin/wound infections or from indwelling IV cannulae. Commonly due to *S. aureus*, *S. epidermidis*, gram-negative bacteria and fungi. Late PVE has similar organisms as native valve endocarditis (mainly streptococci). Similar risk for tissue and mechanical valves.

Out-patient review

⚠ Be very wary about discharging patients from routine follow-up.

General considerations

Valvular heart disease tends to worsen with time. Consequently, long-term follow up is the norm rather than the exception. Very minor lesions (e.g. mild mitral, aortic, or tricuspid regurgitation) with no symptoms are relatively benign and do not need regular review (but remember endocarditis prophylaxis).

Symptoms review

Has there been any progression since last review (NB—can be insidious and patients often don't notice—ask about specific activities and whether they can still do them as well as before). Are there any new symptoms (particularly chest pain, dyspnoea, palpitation, syncope). Are there any symptoms to suggest endocarditis (fevers, weight loss, malaise, joint, or back pains)? When did they last visit the dentist and are they aware of need for prophylaxis? Ask about medications (what are they on, has there been any additions or dose changes? If so, why?).

Examination

Look for peripheral stigmata of endocarditis (see Chapter 5), record pulse and BP. Assess JVP, apex beat and then auscultate all areas and remember to listen to lung bases and to check for pedal oedema.

Investigation

ECG, TTE (± CXR). Compare with previous results to look for progression of condition.

Specific conditions

With all conditions, patients should be advised to seek earlier review if symptoms change in intervening period.

Mitral stenosis: if mild with no symptoms, can be reviewed every 2 years. Moderate to severe (or with symptoms) should be seen at least annually.

Mitral regurgitation: patients with asymptomatic mild MR can be reassured and discharged. Moderate to severe or with symptoms should be seen at least annually. If LV dimensions start to enlarge, consider referral for surgery.

Aortic stenosis: asymptomatic patients with mild AS should be seen every 2–3 years. Anything greater than moderate AS or with symptoms should be seen annually. In severe AS or patients with moderate AS and symptoms, work up for AVR should be commenced.

Aortic regurgitation: asymptomatic patients with mild AR can be reassured and discharged. Patients with symptoms or moderate AR should be seen at least annually. If LV starts to dilate or severe AR, refer for consideration of AVR.

Prosthetic valves: see annually. After >8 years, review patients 6 monthly (↑ incidence of valvular failure). If new valvular dysfunction detected then investigate promptly (often requiring admission from out-patients) as can dramatically worsen very rapidly.

Infective endocarditis

Presentation

Clinical presentation of infective endocarditis (IE) is highly variable and dependent on a combination of intra-cardiac pathology, evolution of the infection, and possible extra cardiac involvement. Presentation can be insidious as in streptococcal infections or with striking constitutional symptoms as in *Staphylococcus aureus* infection. Presenting features can include:-

Symptoms and signs of the infection: this includes malaise, anorexia, weight loss, fever, rigors, and night sweats. Long standing infection produces anaemia, clubbing and splenomegaly.

Cardiac manifestations of the infection: congestive cardiac failure, palpitations, tachycardia, new murmur, pericarditis, or AV block.

Symptoms and signs due to immune complex deposition

Skin: petechiae (most common), splinter haemorrhages; Osler's nodes (small tender nodules (pulp infarcts) on hands and feet and persist hours to days); Janeway lesions (non-tender eryhthematous and/or haemorrhagic areas on the palms and soles).
Eye: Roth spots (oval retinal haemorrhages with a pale centre located near the optic disc), conjunctival splinter haemorrhages, retinal flame haemorrhages.
Renal: microscopic haematuria, glomerulonephritis & renal impairment.
Cerebral: toxic encephalopathy.
Musculoskeletal: arthralgia or arthritis.

Complications of the infection

Local effects:

• Valve destruction results in a new or changing murmur. This may result in progressive heart failure and pulmonary oedema.
• A new harsh pansystolic murmur and acute deterioration may be due to perforation of the interventricular septum or rupture of a sinus of Valsalva aneurysm into the right ventricle.
• High degree AV block (2–4% of IE) occurs with intra-cardiac extension of infection into the interventricular septum (e.g. from aortic valve).
• Intra-cardiac abscess may be seen with any valve infection (25–50% of aortic endocarditis, 1–5% of mitral but rarely with tricuspid) and is most common in prosthetic valve endocarditis.

Embolic events:

• Septic emboli are seen in 20–45% of patients and may involve any circulation (brain, limbs, coronary, kidney, or spleen; pulmonary emboli with tricuspid endocarditis (p104)).
• ~40% of patients who have had an embolic event will have another.
• The risk depends on the organism (most common with G-ve infections, *S. aureus* or candida) and the presence and size of vegetations (emboli in 30% of patients with no vegetation on ECHO, 40% with vegetations <5 mm and 65% with vegetations >5 mm).
• Ask specifically for a history of dental work, infections, surgery, IV drug use or instrumentation, which may have led to a bacteraemia.
• Examine for any potential sources of infection, e.g. teeth/skin lesions.
• Risk factors for endocarditis are shown in the table opposite.

Risk factors for infective endocarditis	
• **High risk**	Prosthetic valves
	Previous bacterial endocarditis
	Aortic valve disease
	Mitral regurgitation or mixed mitral disease
	Cyanotic congenital heart disease
	Patent ductus arteriosis
	Uncorrected L→R shunt
	Intracardiac and systemic-pulmonary shunts.
• **Moderate risk**	MVP with regurgitation or valve thickening
	Isolated mitral stenosis
	Tricuspid valve disease
	Pulmonary stenosis
	Hypertrophic cardiomyopathy
	Bicuspid aortic valve disease
	Degenerative valve disease in elderly
	Mural thrombus (e.g. post infarction).
• **Low risk**	MVP without regurgitation
	Tricuspid incompetence without structural abnormality
	Isolated ASD
	Surgically corrected L→R shunt with no residual shunt
	Calcification of MV annulus
	Ischaemic heart disease and/or previous CABG
	Permanent pacemaker
	Atrial myxoma.

Other predisposing factors

- Arterial prostheses or arteriovenous fistulae.
- Recurrent bacteraemia (e.g. IV drug-users, severe periodontal disease, colon carcinoma).
- Conditions predisposing to infections e.g. diabetes, renal failure, alcoholism, immunosuppression).
- Recent central line.

In many cases no obvious risk factor is identified

Diagnosis

Clinical features can be non-specific and diagnosis difficult. A high index of suspicion must be maintained if patients present with unexplained fever, a predisposing cardiac lesion, bacteraemia and embolic phenomena.

The *Duke* classification was developed in 1994 as a means of standardising the diagnosis of IE and is highly specific (99%) and sensitive (92%). It has been modified since then to improve it:

Definite endocarditis 2 major criteria, or 1 major and 3 minor criteria, or 5 minor criteria.

Possible endocarditis Findings which fall short of definite endocarditis but are not rejected.

Rejected diagnosis Firm alternative diagnosis, or sustained resolution of clinical features with <4 days of antibiotic therapy.

Major criteria

- **Positive blood culture**
  - Typical microorganism for IE from two separate blood cultures.[1]
  - Persistently positive blood culture.[2]
  - Single positive blood culture for *Coxiella Burnettii* or phase I antibody
  - titre to *C. Burnettii* > 1:800
- **Evidence of endocardial involvement**
  Positive echocardiogram.
  i)   Oscillating intracardiac mass (vegetation).
  ii) Abscess.
  iii) New partial dehiscence of prosthetic valve.
  iv) New valve regurgitation.

Minor criteria

- Predisposing condition or drug use.
- Fever >38° C.
- Vascular phenomena: arterial emboli, septic pulmonary infarcts, mycotic aneurysm, intracranial and conjunctival haemorrhage, Janeway lesions.
- Immunologic phenomena: glomerulonephritis, Osler's nodes, Roth spots, rheumatoid factor.
- Microbiological evidence: positive blood cultures but not meeting major criteria or serological evidence of organism consistent with IE.
- Echocardiogram: positive for IE but not meeting major criteria.

---

1 Strep viridans, strep bovis, HACEK group (HACEK = Haemophilus, Acintobacterium, Eikenella and Kingella sp), community acquired *Staphylococcus aureus* or enterococci in the absence of primary focus.

2 Blood cultures drawn 12 hours apart or 3 more cultures with first and last drawn 1 hour apart.

	Common organisms in IE
50–60%	Streptococci (esp. *Strep. viridans* group)
10%	Enterococci
25%	Staphylococci
	S. *aureus* = coagulase +ve
	S. *epidermidis* = coagulase –ve
5–10%	Culture negative
<1%	Gram negative bacilli
<1%	Multiple organisms
<1%	Diptheroids
<1%	Fungi

Investigations

- Blood cultures   Take 3–4 sets of cultures from different sites at least an hour apart and inoculate a minimum of 10 ml/bottle for the optimal pick-up rate. Both aerobic and anaerobic bottles must be used. Lab should be advised that IE is a possibility especially if unusual organisms are suspected. In stable patients on antibiotic therapy doses must be delayed to allow culture on successive days. Ask for prolonged (fungal) cultures in IV drug-users.

- FBC   May show normochromic, normocytic anaemia (exclude haematinic deficiency), neutrophil leukocytosis and perhaps thrombocytopenia.

- U&Es   May be deranged (this should be monitored throughout treatment).

- LFTs   May be deranged, especially with an increase in ALP and γ -GT.

- ESR/CRP   Acute phase reaction.

- Urinalysis   Microscopic haematuria ± proteinuria.

- Immunology   Polyclonal elevation in serum Igs, complement levels

- ECG   May have changes associated with any underlying cause. There may be AV block or conduction defects (especially aortic root abscess) and rarely (embolic) acute MI.

- CXR   May be normal. Look for pulmonary oedema or multiple infected or infarcted areas from septic emboli (tricuspid endocarditis).

- ECHO   Transthoracic echo may confirm the presence of valve lesions and/or demonstrate vegetations if >2 mm in size. TOE is more sensitive for aortic root and mitral leaflet involvement. A normal ECHO does not exclude the diagnosis.

- MRI   Useful in investigation of paravalvular extension, aortic root aneurysm and fistulas.

- Dentition   All patients should have an OPG (orthopentamogram—a panoramic dental x-ray) and a dental opinion.

- Swabs   Any potential sites of infection (skin lesions).

- V/Q scan   In cases where right sided endocarditis is suspected this may show multiple mismatched defects.

- Save serum for: *Aspergillus* precipitins; *Candida* antibodies (rise in titre); Q fever (coxiella *burnetti*) complement fixation test; *Chlamydia* complement fixation test; *Brucella* agglutinins; *Legionella* antibodies; *Bartonella* species

Antibiotics

⚠ Be guided by your local microbiologist and always follow local antibiotic prescription guidelines.

Once diagnosis is confirmed (or even suspected) explain to the patient the need for a prolonged parenteral (usually IV) course of antibiotics. Microbiology will determine sensitivities to, and minimum inhibitory concentration (MIC) of, appropriate antibiotics. If fully sensitive organism with 'low' MIC then shorter courses of antibiotics may suffice (and the latter part of the course may be completed on an out-patient basis). Evidence shows that combination therapy is more effective than single chemotherapeutic agents.

Strep viridans group

- Fully sensitive (MIC of penicillin <0.1 mg/L)—native valve endocarditis (NVE): benzylpenecillin 1.2 g/4h IV for 4 weeks, occasionally can successfully treat with 2 week course of benzylpenecillin and gentamicin. For prosthetic valve endocarditis (PVE): benzylpenecillin for 6 weeks (in combination with gentamicin for first 2 weeks).
- Mild penicillin resistance (MIC of penicillin >0.1–0.5 mg/L)—NVE: benzylpenecillin for 4 weeks with gentamicin for first 2. PVE: Benzylpenecillin for 6 weeks with gentamicin for first 4 weeks.
- Moderate penicillin resistance (MIC>0.5 mg/L)—NVE: benzylpenecillin (or amoxicillin) and gentamicin for 4–6 weeks. PVE: benzylpenecillin (or amoxicillin) and gentamicin for at least 6 weeks.
- NB: can use vancomycin if allergic to penicillin

Staphylococcal species

- Methicillin sensitive staphylococci—NVE: flucloxacillin 2g/6 hrs IV for 4–6 weeks with gentamicin for at least 1st week. PVE: flucloxacillin for 6 weeks + gentamicin for first 2 weeks + rifampicin 600mg bd PO for 6 weeks.
- Methicillin resistant staphylococci—NVE: IV vancomycin for 4–6 weeks ± gentamicin for 1st week. PVE: vancomycin + Rifampicin for 6 weeks + gentamicin for 2 weeks.

Enterococcus species

- As for streptococcus with moderate penicillin resistance (above)

HACEK species[1]

- NVE: IV cephalosporin (e.g. ceftriaxone) for 4 weeks, or 6 weeks for PVE.

Coxiella burnetii (Q fever)

- NVE & PVE: Requires prolonged (3–4 years) therapy with tetracycline (e.g. doxycycline) and second agent (co-trimoxazole, rifampicin, quinolone) with careful monitoring of IgG titres. Usually requires surgery.

---

1 (HACEK = Haemophilus, Acintobacillus, Cardiobacterium, Eikenella and Kingella sp).

'Blind' treatment

- Infective endocarditis is usually a clinical diagnosis and must be considered in any patient with a typical history, fever, and a murmur with no other explanation. Often antibiotics need to be started before the culture results are available. Be guided by the clinical setting (see table below[1]).

Presentation	Choice of antibiotic
Gradual onset (weeks)	Benzylpenicillin + Gentamicin
Acute onset (days) or history of skin trauma	Flucloxacillin + Gentamicin
Recent valve prosthesis (possible MRSA, diptheroid, *Kelbsiella*, corynebacterium or nosocomial staphylococci)	Vancomycin (or teicoplanin) + Gentamicin + Rifampicin
IV drug user	Vancomycin

Suggested antibiotic doses are

Benzylpenecillin	4MU (2.4g) q4h IV
Flucloxacillin	2g qds IV
Vancomycin	15mg/kg q12h IV over 60 min, guided by levels
Gentamicin	3mg/kg divided in 1–3 doses guided by levels
Rifampicin	300mg q12h po
Ciprofloxacin	300mg q12h iv for 1 week, then 750 mg q12h po for 3 weeks

- Identification of an organism is invaluable for further management and blood cultures should be taken before antibiotics with meticulous attention to detail.
- Antibiotics should be administered IV, preferably via a tunnelled central (Hickman) line.
- If an organism is isolated, antibiotic therapy may be modified when sensitivities are known.
- Suggested antibiotic combinations are shown above; however individual units may have specific policies; patients should be discussed with your local microbiologist.

1 Oakley CM (1995) *Eur Heart J* **16**(*suppl. B*): 90–93.

Duration of treatment

- This is controversial with a trend toward shorter courses.
  Microbiology and ID opinion is important especially in resistant and/or
  uncommon organisms. The table below shows one suggested protocol.
- The duration of treatment varies depending on the severity of infection
  and the infecting organism. IV therapy is usually for at least 2 weeks,
  and total antibiotic therapy for 4–6 weeks.
- If the patient is well following this period, antibiotic treatment may be
  stopped. Provided no surgery is indicated (p106) the patient may be
  discharged and followed up in out-patient clinic.
- Patients should be advised of the need for endocarditis prophylaxis in
  the future (see table on p108).
- Patients with valvular damage following infection should be followed
  long-term and patients with ventricular septal defects should be
  considered for closure.

- Viridans streptococci & *Streptococcus bovis* (penicillin sensitive)
      Benzyl-penicillin only (4 weeks)
      Vancomycin or teicoplanin (4 weeks)
      Penicillin + aminoglycoside (2 weeks)
      Ceftriaxone 2g (4 weeks)
- Group B, C, G streptococci, *Strep. pyogenes, Strep. pneumoniae*
      Penicillin (4 weeks) + aminoglycoside (2 weeks)
      Vancomycin (4 weeks) + aminoglycoside (2 weeks)
- Group A streptococci
      Penicillin (4 weeks)
      Vancomycin (4 weeks)
- Enterococci
      Penicillin + aminoglycoside (4–6 weeks)
      Vancomycin + aminoglycoside (4–6weeks)
- Extra-cardiac infection from septic emboli
      Penicillin (4 weeks) + aminoglycoside (2 weeks)
      Vancomycin (4 weeks) + aminoglycoside (2 weeks)
- *Staphylococcus aureus* and coagulase negative staphylococci
  - Left sided endocarditis:
      Flucloxacillin (4–6 weeks) + aminoglycoside (2 weeks)
      If MRSA—Vancomycin + rifampicin (6 weeks)
                                      ± aminoglycoside (2 weeks)
  - Right sided endocarditis:
      Flucloxacillin (2 weeks) + aminoglycoside (2 weeks)
      Ciprofloxacin (4 weeks) + rifampicin (3 weeks)
      If MRSA—Vancomycin (4 weeks) + rifampicin (4 weeks)
- Fungi
Amphotericin B IV to a total dose of 2.5–3 g.

Monitoring treatment

Patients need careful clinical monitoring both during and for several months after the infection. Reappearance of features suggestive of IE must be investigated thoroughly to rule out recurrent infection or resistance to treatment regime.

Clinical features

- Signs of continued infection, persistent pyrexia and the persistence of systemic symptoms.
- Persistent fever may be due to drug resistance, concomitant infection (central line, urine, chest, septic emboli to lungs or abdomen) or allergy (?eosinophilia, ?leukopenia, ?proteinuria: common with penicillin but may be due to any antibiotic—consider changing or stopping antibiotics for 2–3 days).
- Changes in any cardiac murmurs or signs of cardiac failure.
- The development of any new embolic phenomena.
- Inspect venous access sites daily. Change peripheral cannulae every 3–4 days.

ECHO

- Regular (weekly) transthoracic echocardiograms may identify clinically silent, but progressive, valve destruction and development of intra-cardiac abscesses or vegetations.
- The tips of long-standing central lines may develop sterile fibrinous 'fronds' which may be visible on TOE: change the line and send the tip for culture.
- 'Vegetations' need not be due to infection (see Table on p103).

ECG

- Looking specifically for AV block or conduction abnormalities suggesting intra-cardiac extension of the infection. A daily ECG must be performed.

Microbiology

- Repeated blood cultures (especially if there is continued fever).
- Regular aminoglycoside and vancomycin levels (ensuring the absence of toxic levels and the presence of therapeutic levels). Gentamicin ototoxicity may develop with prolonged use even in the absence of toxic levels.
- Back titration to ensure that minimum inhibitory and bactericidal concentrations are being achieved.

Laboratory indices

- Regular (daily) urinalysis.
- Regular U&Es and liver function tests.
- Regular CRP (ESR every 2 weeks).
- FBC—rising Hb and falling WCC suggests successful treatment; watch for beta-lactam associated neutropenia.
- Serum magnesium (if on gentamicin).

Culture negative endocarditis

- The commonest reason for persistently negative blood cultures is prior antibiotic therapy and affects up to 15% of patients with diagnosis of IE.
- If the clinical response to the antibiotics is good these should be continued.
- For a persisting fever:
  - Withhold antibiotics if not already started.
  - Consider other investigations for a 'PUO'.
  - If there the clinical suspicion of IE is high, it warrants further investigation.
  - Repeated physical examination for any new signs.
  - Regular ECHO and TOE. 'Vegetations' need not be due to infection (see table opposite).
  - Repeated blood cultures, especially when the temperature is raised. Discuss with microbiology about prolonged culturing times (4+ weeks) and special culturing and subculturing techniques. Most HACEK group organisms can be detected.
- Consider unusual causes of endocarditis:
- **Q-fever** *(Coxiella burnetii)*: complement fixation tests identify antibodies to phase 1 and 2 antigens. Phase 2 antigens raised in the acute illness, phase 1 antigens raised in chronic illnesses such as endocarditis. PCR can be performed on operative specimens. Treat with indefinite (life-long) oral doxycycline ± co-trimoxazole, rifampicin or quinolone.
- *Chlamydia psittaci:* commonly there is a history of exposure to birds and there may be an associated atypical pneumonia. Diagnosis is confirmed using complement fixation tests to detect raised antibody titres.
- **Brucellosis:** blood cultures may be positive though organisms may take up to 8 weeks to grow. Serology usually confirms the diagnosis.
- **Fungi:** candida is the most common species and may be cultured. The detection of antibodies may be helpful though levels may be raised in normals. The detection of a rising titre is of more use. Other fungal infections (e.g. histoplasmosis, aspergillosis) are rare but may be diagnosed with culture or serology, though these are commonly negative. Antigen assays may be positive, or the organism may be isolated from biopsy material. Fungal IE is more common in patients with prosthetic valves and IV drug users. Bulky vegetations are common. Treatment is with amphotericin B ± flucytosine. Prosthetic valves must be removed. Mortality is >50%.

Causes of culture negative endocarditis

- Previous antibiotic therapy
- Fastidious organism
  - Nutritionally deficient variants of *Strep. viridans*
    Brucella, Neisseria, Legionella
    Nocardia
  - Mycobacteria
  - The HACEK group of oropharyngeal flora
  - Cell wall deficient bacteria and anaerobes
- Cell dependent organisms
  - *Chlamydia*, rickettsiae *(Coxiella)*
- Fungi

(HACEK = *Haemophilus, Acintobacillus, Cardiobacterium, Eikenella* and *Kingella sp.*)

Causes of 'vegetations' on ECHO

- Infective endocarditis
- Sterile thrombotic vegetations
  - Libman Sacks endocarditis (SLE)
  - Primary anti-phospholipid syndrome
  - Marantic endocarditis (adenocarcinoma)
- Myxomatous degeneration of valve (commonly mitral)
- Ruptured mitral chordae
- Exuberant rheumatic vegetations (Black Africans)
- Thrombus ('pannus') on a prosthetic valve
- A stitch or residual calcium after valve replacement

Right-sided endocarditis

- Always consider this diagnosis in IV drug-users (or patients with venous access).
- Endocarditis on endocardial permanent pacemaker leads is rare but recognized cause.
- Patients most commonly have staphylococcal infection and are unwell, requiring immediate treatment and often early surgery.
- Lesions may be sterilised with IV antibiotics.
- Surgery may be required for:
  - Resistant organisms (*Staph. aureus*, *Pseudomonas*, *Candida* and infection with multiple organisms).
  - Increasing vegetation size in spite of therapy.
  - Infections on pacemaker leads (surgical removal of lead and repair or excision of tricuspid valve).
  - Recurrent mycotic emboli.

Prosthetic valve endocarditis (PVE)

Conventionally divided into early (<2 months post-operatively) and late (>2 months post-operatively).

Early prosthetic valve endocarditis

- Most commonly due to staphylococci, gram negative bacilli, diptheroids or fungi.
- Generally infection has begun either pre-operatively or in the immediate post-operative period.
- Often a highly destructive, fulminant infection with valve dehiscence, abscess formation and rapid haemodynamic deterioration.
- Discuss with the surgeons early. They commonly require reoperation. Mortality is high (45–75%).

Late prosthetic valve endocarditis

- The pathogenesis is different. Abnormal flow around the prosthetic valve ring produces microthrombi and non-bacterial thrombotic vegetations (NBTV), which may be infected during transient bacteraemia. The source is commonly dental or urological sepsis or from indwelling venous lines.
- Common organisms are coagulase negative staphylococci, *Staph. aureus*, *Strep. viridans* or enterococci.
- Frequently needs surgical intervention and this carries a high mortality, but less than for early PVE.

It may be possible to sterilise infections on bioprostheses with IV antibiotics only. Surgery (see p106) may then be deferred.

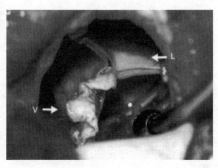

Fig. 3.1 Mobile vegetation (V) attached to the leaflet (L) of a prosthetic aortic valve in a man with infective endocarditis. Reproduced with permission from Tuna IÇ, Harrison MR (2001). Images in clinical medicine. *N Engl J Med* **344**(4): 275.

Surgery

Discuss early with the regional cardiothoracic centre: immediate intervention may be appropriate.

- Surgical intervention may be necessary either during active infection or later because of degree of valve destruction. Optimal timing depends on a number of factors:
  1. Haemodynamic tolerance of lesion.
  2. Outcome of the infection.
  3. Presence of complications.
- Choice of antimicrobial therapy should be modified depending on microbiological results from intraoperative specimens. Samples should be sent for culture, staining, immunological testing, and PCR depending on suspected organism.
- Duration of antimicrobial treatment is dependent on the clinical picture:
  1. Culture negative operative specimens: 2–3 week for valve infection and 3–4 weeks for abscess.
  2. Culture positive operative specimens: 3–4 weeks for valve infection and 4–6 weeks for abscess.
- Timing is dictated by clinical picture. Indications for urgent surgery are listed below. In patients with neurological injury, surgery should be delayed to avoid intracranial hemorrhage if cardiac function permits (embolic infarct—delay 10–14 days, haemorrhage 21–28 days and when ruptured mycotic aneurysms have been repaired).
- The table opposite summarizes the absolute and relative indications for surgery.

Haemodynamic tolerance

- If the patient is haemodynamically stable, surgery may be delayed until after antibiotic course is completed. The final management depends on the valve affected, the degree of destruction and its effect on ventricular function. Severe aortic and mitral regurgitation usually require surgery; tricuspid regurgitation, if well tolerated, is managed medically.
- Decompensation (severe congestive cardiac failure or low cardiac output syndrome with functional renal failure) may respond to surgery but the mortality is high.
- 'Metastable' patients who have been successfully treated after an episode of acute decompensation should be considered for early operation after 2–3 weeks antibiotic therapy.

Outcome of infection

- Persistence or relapse of infection (clinical and laboratory indices) despite appropriate antibiotics at an adequate dose may either be due to a resistant organism or an abscess (paravalvular, extra-cardiac). Consider valve replacement if no extra-cardiac focus found.
- The organism may influence the decision: consider early surgery for fungal endocarditis or prosthetic endocarditis with *E. coli* or *Staph. aureus*.

The presence of complications

- High degree AV block.
- Perforation of interventricular septum.
- Rupture of sinus of Valsalva aneurysm into RV.
- Intracardiac abscess.
- Recurrent septic emboli.
- Prosthetic endocarditis especially associated with an unstable prosthesis.

Indications for surgery in infective endocarditis

Absolute indications

- Moderate to severe heart failure secondary to valve regurgitation
- Unstable prosthesis
- Uncontrolled infection: persistent bacteraemia, ineffective antimicrobial therapy (IE secondary to fungi, *Brucella*, *Pseudomonas aeroginosa* (especially aortic and mitral valve))
- *Staph. aureus* prosthetic infection with an intracardiac complication

Relative indications

- Perivalvular extension of infection.
- Poor response to staph aureus native valve infection.
- Relapse after adequate treatment.
- Large (>10 mm) hypermobile vegetations.
- Persistent unexplained fever in culture negative endocarditis.
- Endocarditis secondary to antibiotic resistant enterococci.

Endocarditis prophylaxis[1]

Procedures that require antibiotic prophylaxis	
Dental	• All procedures
Upper respiratory tract	• Tonsillectomy, adenoidectomy
Gastrointestinal	• Oesophageal dilatation or laser therapy • Oesophageal surgery • Sclerosis of oesophageal varices • ERCP • Abdominal surgery • Barium enema • Sigmoidoscopy ± biopsy
Urological	• Instrumentation of ureter or kidney • Biopsy or surgery of prostate or bladder
Procedures for which the risk of IE is controversial	
Upper respiratory tract	• Bronchoscopy • Endotracheal intubation
Gastrointestinal	• Upper GI endoscopy ± biopsy
Genital	• Vaginal hysterectomy or delivery

- The table on p89 shows cardiac conditions at risk of IE. High and moderate risk requires prophylaxis; 'low' risk does not.
- The regimen may be modified depending on the 'degree of risk' (both patient and procedure related) as shown in the table below.

---

[1] This is one regime (after Leport C *et al* (1995) *Eur Heart J* **16** (*suppl. B*) 126–131). Refer to your local policy.

Antibiotic prophalaxis

Minimal regimen

	1h before	6h after
No penicillin allergy	Amoxycillin 3 g po	No 2nd dose
Allergy to penicillin	Clindamycin 300–600 mg po	No 2nd dose

Flexible modifications depending on the 'degree of risk'

- Additional doses after procedure
- Additional aminoglycosides
- Parenteral administration

Maximal regimen

	1h before	6h after
No penicillin allergy	Amoxycillin 2 g iv + Gentamicin 1.5 mg/kg im/iv	1–1.5 g po No 2nd dose
Allergy to penicillin	Vancomycin 1 g iv over 1 hr + Gentamicin 1.5 mg/kg im/iv	1 g iv at 12h No 2nd dose

Coronary artery disease

Atherosclerosis: pathophysiology

Atherosclerosis is a disease of the large and medium sized arteries. The term atherosclerosis is derived from Latin and means gruel-like ('athero') hardening ('sclerosis') of the arteries. The disease is characterized by a gradual build-up of fatty plaques within the arterial wall, which eventually results in a significant reduction of the vessel lumen impairing blood flow to the distal tissues. These plaques may also cause acute coronary syndromes by becoming unstable and triggering coronary thrombosis.

Pathophysiology

The atherogenic process is characterized by dysfunction of the endothelial lining of the vessel, associated with inflammation of the vascular wall leading to the build-up of lipids, cholesterol inflammatory cells, and cellular debris within the intima and sub-intimal layers of the vessel, resulting in plaque formation, and remodelling of the arterial wall.

The pathophysiology is complex, involving a series of interactions between endothelial and smooth muscle cells, leukocytes and platelets in the vascular wall. The mechanisms underlying this process are uncertain, but the most widely accepted theory is the 'response-to-injury' hypothesis defined by Ross in the 1970s.

Endothelial dysfunction

The initiating trigger of this disease process appears to be injury of arterial endothelial cells from exposure to stimuli such as tobacco toxins, oxidized LDL, advanced glycation end products, elevated homocysteine, or infectious agents. Endothelial cell injury initiates a cascade of events resulting in cellular dysfunction (see Fig. 4.1). The hallmark of endothelial dysfunction is a change in the balance of production of endothelium-derived vasoactive molecules. There is a *reduced bioavailability of endothelial nitric oxide (NO)*, which possesses important vasodilator, anti-thrombotic, and antiproliferative properties, in parallel with increased generation of the potent vasoconstrictor agents, endothelin-1 and angiotensin-II, which also promote cell migration and growth. Dysfunctional endothelial cells also express adhesion molecules and secrete chemokines promoting cell migration and adhesion. Furthermore, the local thrombotic balance is altered. Levels of plasminogen activator inhibitor and tissue factor are increased, tissue plasminogen activator and thrombomodulin are reduced, and low NO release results in increased platelet activation and adhesion.

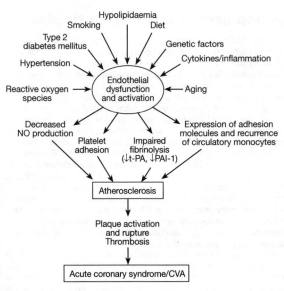

Fig. 4.1 Endothelial dysfunction is the underlying process in atherosclerosis, from lesion initiation, progression, through to acute cardiovascular events. Endothelial dysfunction is caused by a variety of genetic factors (and aging) as well as environmental factors that can be modified.

Development of atherosclerotic plaques

Endothelial dysfunction creates a local milieu which facilitates the initiation and development of the atherogenic process (see Fig. 4.2). Circulating leukocytes, predominantly monocytes, are attracted and bind to activated endothelial cells followed by migration into the sub-endothelial layer where they transform into macrophages. Here they act as local 'scavenger' cells with the capacity to take up modified LDL cholesterol, ultimately becoming the characteristic 'foam cells' of established atherosclerosis. The earliest lesions are known as 'fatty streaks' which consist predominantly of lipid accumulating macrophages and foam cells. These lesions may develop into fibrous plaques, as a consequence of further lipid accumulation accompanied by local migration, proliferation and fibrous transformation of smooth muscle cells. These cells are responsible for the deposition of extra-cellular connective tissue matrix leading to formation of a fibrous cap, which overlies a central core, consisting of foam cells, extra-cellular lipid, necrotic cellular debris, and a mixture of other inflammatory cells including T-lymphocytes. This process is facilitated by ongoing endothelial dysfunction, together with local generation of powerful mitogens such as PDGF, TGF-b, and IGF from endothelial cells, macrophages and activated platelets.

Further growth of the plaque initially causes outward remodeling of the vessel wall, thus minimizing the impact on the cross-sectional area of the lumen and the vessels ability to deliver blood. However, progressive plaque accumulation results in luminal narrowing and ultimately vessel obstruction.

Lesion initiation and progression tends to occur more predictably at certain locations of the vascular system. Blood flow through arteries causes local generation of fluid 'shear-stress', which influences the biology of the underlying endothelial cells. High laminar shear (from blood flowing quickly through a straight vessel) favours the generation of NO which helps maintain the functional integrity of the vessel. In contrast, low shear, or 'differential' shear caused by turbulent flow, causes dysfunction of the underlying endothelial cells which facilitates initiation and progression of atheroma. This helps explain why plaques are found more commonly at sites of vessel branching or curvature which experience more dramatic and abrupt changes and irregularities of direction and velocity of blood flow. These shear stress-mediated effects are most marked in vessels that carry a high (basal) blood flow, such as the coronary, carotid, renal and ilio-femoral arteries, in which the majority of clinically important atherosclerotic lesions develop.

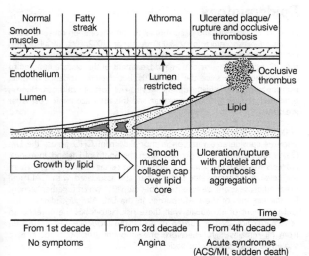

Fig. 4.2 Cellular interactions in the development and progression of atherosclerosis. VSMC, vascular smooth muscle cells. Reproduced with permission from Weissberg PL (2000). Atherogenesis: current understanding of the causes of atheroma. *Heart* **83**: 247–252.

Epidemiology

Diseases of the heart and circulation is the most common cause of death in the UK, responsible for 238,000 deaths in 2002, 39% of all deaths. Coronary artery disease (CAD) results in over 117,000 deaths a year in the UK. Advances in prevention and treatment of this disease have led to a fall in the death since the late 1970s, but the UK incidence of CAD remains amongst the highest in the world. The cost of healthcare alone is estimated at over £1.7 billion a year and the total economic cost is far greater.

Regional variation

There is considerable variation in mortality from CHD across the UK. Death rates are higher in Scotland than the South of England, in manual workers than in non-manual workers and in certain ethnic groups. There are several important risk factors that are associated with CAD and other atherosclerotic disease (see table on p121) which together account for the majority of the CAD burden in the UK. Although identification and treatment of individuals with these risk factors has the potential to reduce significantly the burden of CAD, the incidence and death rate from MI remains high. Therefore prevention of atherosclerotic disease should be a high priority for society.

The vulnerable plaque

Erosion or denudation of the endothelial layer, or rupture of the overlying fibrous cap of the plaque may expose the highly thrombogenic lipid-rich core of the plaque to circulating blood. Collagen, tissue factor, and other factors activate platelets and trigger the coagulation cascade. This leads to acute thrombosis, which may rapidly occlude the vessel, leading to myocardial infarction of this vascular territory, usually characterized by ST-segment elevation on the ECG. Coronary thrombosis is a dynamic process in-vivo, and may be reversed, at least in part, by activation of tissue plasminogen activator and proteins C and S of the intrinsic anti-thrombotic/fibrinolytic system. Acute, sub-total occlusion of the vessel typically causes acute symptomatic deterioration and non-ST-segment elevation MI or unstable angina.

Atheromatous plaques that have a thin fibrous cap, a large necrotic lipid core and containing a high proportion of inflammatory cells and mediators are particularly predisposed to destabilization or rupture, with consequent thrombosis. Conversely, plaques with a smaller lipid pool, thicker fibrous caps, and less inflammatory activity are more stable and less prone to rupture. Several studies have shown that well over half of all MIs are caused by acute destabilization of plaques that were previously not obstructing flow in the vessel, suggesting that the likelihood of an acute coronary event is more closely related to the stability of the plaque rather than the severity of the stenosis.

Assessment of atherosclerotic risk

Identification and treatment of risk factors is essential for the prevention of atherosclerotic disease both in individuals and society. When multiple risk factors such as dyslipidaemia, high blood pressure, and smoking coexist, as is commonly the case, the cardiovascular risk is greatly increased, suggesting a synergistic interaction between these factors. For example, the absolute risk of a cardiovascular event occurring in a patient with high blood pressure is greatly influenced by the age, sex, lipid profile, and other factors. Thus, modern approaches to risk management should involve a careful consideration of the combined impact of all important factors operating in the individual that contribute to their risk of atherosclerotic disease.

Global risk assessment

Several risk assessment systems are currently available, which are derived from large prospective population cohorts, most commonly the Framingham study. These systems allow the calculation of the 'absolute risk' of having a cardiovascular event (i.e., the probability of having a heart attack or stroke) within the next 10 years, which is derived from the patients' risk factor variables (age, sex, cholesterol, HDL, BP, smoking).

Current UK practice recommends use of the Joint British Societies risk assessment tables (see p119) or a computer program. Other commonly used methods include the Framingham risk scoring system, the Sheffield Tables, and the European SCORE charts. Subjects with stable angina have a 10-year event rate of approximately 20%, therefore subjects without clinical disease that have a predicted 10-year likelihood of suffering a cardiovascular event of ≥20% are considered to be at 'high-risk' and are candidates for aggressive risk factor management.

Although these conventional scoring systems have the potential to identify the majority of individuals in Western populations, a significant proportion of events occur in subjects calculated to be at intermediate and low risk. For example, risk is typically underestimated when using conventional methods in young subjects with multiple risk factors, subjects with a family history of premature cardiovascular disease, and in certain ethnic groups including individuals of South Asian racial origin living in the UK. Identification of subjects with intermediate (10–20%) conventional risk scores that are actually at 'high' risk remains a major challenge, as these individuals are also likely to benefit from preventive therapy. It has been proposed that measurement of C-reactive protein levels, ultrasound assessment of carotid arterial intima-media thickness, detection of coronary artery calcification with electron-beam CT scanning and a number of other tests, may improve risk assessment. These techniques are highly promising, and under intense investigation, but their clinical utility and cost have not yet been confirmed in large prospective clinical studies, and are not currently used in routine clinical practice in the UK. Use of stress-testing for routine CAD screening in asymptomatic subjects is also not currently recommended.

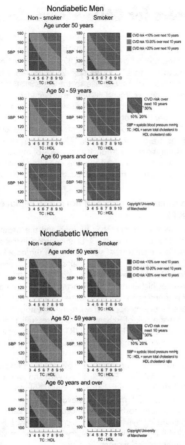

Fig. 4.3 2004 Joint British Societies Risk Prediction Tables © The University of Manchester.

- Calculation of risk is unnecessary in subjects who already have clinical atherosclerotic disease, as secondary prevention measures are mandatory in these individuals.
- Similarly, risk calculation is not required for subjects with diabetes mellitus, whose risk approaches that of subjects with established atherosclerosis.

Risk factors for CAD

Age

The UK population is aging. Between 1971 and 2002 the percentage of older people (aged 65 and over) in the UK, increased from 13% to 16%, and is projected to rise to 23% in the next 25 years. Aging is a major risk factor for atherosclerotic disease, due to the degenerative process associated with ageing per se together with the cumulative impact of the worsening risk factor profile that develops with increasing age. By the age of 70, 15% of men and 9% of women have symptomatic coronary artery disease increasing to 20% by the age of 80. Over 40,000 premature (<75years) deaths are caused by CAD, 22% of premature deaths in men and 13% of those in women. Although about 45% of myocardial infarction occurs in people under 65 years of age, this condition is more likely to be fatal in older individuals with 80% of deaths due to MI seen in those over 65.

Gender, menopausal Status and hormone replacement therapy (HRT)

CAD is more common in men than women and the onset tends to be earlier in men. The incidence of CHD in women increases rapidly at menopause, and is similar to that seen in men in the population over 65. Although less common, the disease remains one of the biggest killers of women; for example, the age-adjusted mortality rates from heart disease are four to six times higher than their mortality rates from breast cancer. Female sex hormones probably contribute to the lower risk of atherosclerotic disease in pre-menopausal women. Additionally, observational studies show that the risk of ischaemic heart disease is reduced by up to 40% in women using HRT. However, HRT users are typically healthier than non-users, suggesting that these results could be explained by selection bias.

Several large, randomized controlled trials of HRT in post-menopausal women (WHI, HERS/HERS II, ESPRIT, ERA) with and without atherosclerosis have now clearly shown that HRT does not reduce the risk of cardiovascular events. HRT may, in fact, even lead to a small but statistically significant increase morbidity and mortality from cardiovascular and other diseases including gynaecologic malignancy. Thus, HRT should not be recommended for primary or secondary prevention of atherosclerotic disease in post-menopausal women.

Family history of atherosclerotic disease

CAD is a multi-factorial, polygenic disorder, caused by interactions between lifestyle, the environment, and the effects of variations in the genetic sequence of a number of genes. The family history is considered to be significant when atherosclerotic disease presents in a first degree male relative before the age of 55, or before 65 in a female relative. A positive family history is associated with a 75% increase in risk in men, and an 84% increase in women. The risk is more than doubled if both parents are affected.

Risk factors for coronary heart disease

Non-modifiable risk factors	Modifiable risk factors
• Increasing age	• Smoking
• Male gender	• High blood pressure
• Family history	• Dyslipidaemia
• Ethnic origin	• Diabetes mellitus
	• Obesity and the metabolic syndrome
	• Psychological stress
	• High calorie high fat diet
	• Physical inactivity

Emerging risk factors

- *Inflammation*
- *Fibrinogen, and other factors involved in thromboregulation*
- *Homocysteine*
- *Oxidative stress*
- *Asymmetric dimethylarginine*

Ethnic origin

The age-standardised mortality from CAD is around 50% higher in individuals of South Asian racial origin living in the UK compared to Whites. Although an increased prevalence of risk factors, including high triglycerides, low HDL, insulin resistance and reduced physical activity explain much of this increased risk, genetic factors are thought to contribute significantly. In contrast, the observed incidence of CAD is lower in Black individuals of West Indian and African origin in the UK, although the incidence of stroke is greater than in the Caucasian population.

Smoking

Smoking increases the risk of CHD by approximately 50% with mortality from any cardiovascular disease around 60% higher in smokers (and 85% higher in heavy smokers) compared to non-smokers. In the UK today around 13 million adults (28% of men and 26% of women) smoke cigarettes. Although numbers of smokers have declined substantially over the past 50 years, this trend has slowed down in the young, and the numbers of teenage girls that smoke has recently increased. Over 30,000 cardiovascular deaths per year (14% in men and 12% in women, with an even higher proportion of premature deaths) attributable to smoking. Second-hand smoke (smoke that has been exhaled by a smoker) can also increase the risk of CHD by around 25%.

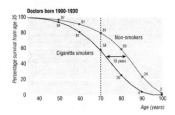

Fig. 4.4 Survival from age 35 for continuing cigarette smokers and lifelong non-smokers among UK male doctors born 1900–1930, with percentages alive at each decade of age (Adapted from ** with permission).

Stopping smoking carries almost immediate benefit and although the long-term benefits are greatest in those who stop smoking before the age of 40, stopping in middle age is also beneficial. For example, in those aged 30–59 who stop smoking after a myocardial infarction, the five year mortality is 10% compared with 14% in those who continue to smoke.

Individuals with and at increased risk of atherosclerosis should be advised to stop smoking. Evidence now exists that focused psychosocial support, nicotine replacement, and bupropion therapy are effective in helping individuals stop smoking. These services are delivered in an integrated fashion by smoking cessation clinics, which can deliver a four-fold increase in the likelihood that a smoker will quit, vs. use of willpower alone.

Obesity

Obesity increases the risk of CHD: between 25–49% of CHD in developed countries is attributable to increased body mass index (BMI). Overweight is defined as a BMI between 25 and 30 kg/m², and obesity as a BMI ≥30 kg/m². The prevalence of obesity is increasing rapidly worldwide. In the UK adult obesity has increased by over 50% in less than 10 years. Of particular concern is the dramatic increase in the prevalence of obesity in children, which has almost doubled in the UK in less than 10 years. This trend is likely to exacerbate the problem in adulthood, and undo many of the other recent improvements in cardiovascular health.

Central obesity, in which excess fat is concentrated mainly in the abdomen, can be identified by a high waist-to-hip ratio and confers a particularly high relative risk of CHD if the waist circumference is >102 cm (40 in.) in men and >88 cm (35 in.) in women. Associated metabolic abnormalities of central obesity include high triglycerides, low HDL, high blood pressure, low-grade systemic inflammation, insulin resistance, and type-II diabetes mellitus.

Overweight and obese individuals also tend to be less physically active and eat lower quality diets, which contributes further to their atherogenic risk. Diet and exercise should be considered as the first line of intervention in these individuals, together with careful surveillance for and aggressive treatment of diabetes, high blood pressure and dyslipidaemia when present.

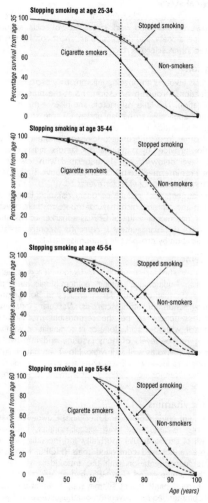

Fig. 4.5 Effects on survival of stopping smoking cigarettes at age 25–34 (effect from age 35), age 35–44 (effect from age 40), age 45–54 (effect from age 50), and age 55–64 (effect from age 60) (Adapted from ** with permission).

(**Doll R, Peto R, Boreham J, Sutherland I. (2004). Mortality in relation to smoking: 50 years' observations on male British doctors. *BMJ* **328**(7455): 1519.)

Psychological stress

The burden of risk attributable to psychological stress is more difficult to quantify. However, increased work stress, lack of social support, hostile personality type, anxiety, and depression are most consistently associated with increased atherosclerosis risk.

Inflammation

Atherosclerosis involves an ongoing inflammatory process from the time of lesion initiation, through progression and at the time of acute thrombotic complication. This links risk factors and disease mechanism in a way that is directly applicable to human patients. Large studies have shown that low-grade elevation in markers of inflammation, most notably CRP, predicts outcomes from atherosclerotic disease and may add to prognostic information provided by traditional risk factors. It has been suggested that a CRP level below 1 mg/L is associated with low risk, between 1–3 mg/L reflects intermediate risk and a level above 3 mg/L is associated with a high long-term risk of vascular events.

Certain treatments that reduce coronary risk also limit inflammation, such as statins and aspirin which may contribute to their clinical benefits. However, the incremental value of CRP as a marker of risk and target of therapy in global risk management is currently a controversial topic that requires clarification by prospective randomised trials.

Homocysteine

The genetic disease homocystinuria is associated with aggressive, premature atherosclerosis. Additionally, strong epidemiologic and mechanistic evidence suggests that even modest increases in homocysteine levels increase progression of atherosclerosis. Vascular inflammation and oxidative stress appear to be the responsible mechanisms. Dietary supplementation with folic acid, alone or in combination with vitamins B6 and B12, can reduce levels of homocysteine and improve aspects of vascular biology in-vivo as well as in-vitro. However, until results of large, outcome-driven, randomised clinical trials are available, folate ± B6/B12 supplementation cannot be routinely recommended for prevention of atherosclerotic disease.

Antioxidant vitamins

Despite excellent epidemiologic and mechanistic evidence that increased oxidative stress is associated with vascular injury, inflammation and increased risk of cardiovascular morbidity and mortality, it is disappointing that large randomised controlled trials (HOPE, HPS and GISSI-P) showed that supplementation with the antioxidant vitamin E (supplemented with vitamins A and C in HPS) had no effect on cardiovascular outcome. Currently, antioxidant vitamin supplementation should not be routinely recommended for prevention of atherosclerotic disease.

Dietary measures

Several dietary measures can reduce the risk of cardiovascular disease. Total fat intake should be reduced to below <30% of total calorie intake, intake of saturated fat and foods high in 'trans' fatty acids should be limited, and replaced with monounsaturated fat (canola and olive oil). Dietary salt intake should be reduced, and intake of fresh fruits and vegetables increased (≥5 portions per day). Fish consumption, especially oily fish, should be encouraged with evidence suggesting that at least 1 fish meal ideally 2–3 per week can reduce the incidence of heart attack and stroke.

Physical activity

The contribution of physical inactivity to CHD deaths is difficult to quantify, however people who are physically active appear to have a lower risk of CHD. This is mediated, at least in part by weight loss, a reduction in blood pressure and improvement of the lipid profile (particularly increased HDL). Regular, aerobic exercise of moderate intensity should be undertaken ≥3 times per week for at least 30 minutes, but greater frequency and duration of exercise is associated with increasing benefits.

Alcohol

Moderate alcohol consumption (one or two drinks per day) is associated with a reduced risk of CHD whereas higher levels of alcohol intake (in excess of 21 units/week for men or more than 14 units/week) in women, particularly in 'binges' is associated with an increased risk of CHD.

Hypertension

Definition

A continuous relationship exists between increasing blood pressure and cardiovascular risk; therefore it is impossible to define hypertension precisely. For practical purposes, levels of blood pressure above which the risk increases significantly and treatment can provide a clear-cut benefit are used as a working definition of hypertension (see table opposite). The average of two readings at each of a number of visits should be used to define the blood pressure.

Causes of hypertension

The majority of subjects (>95%) have essential (primary) hypertension, in which an underlying cause for the hypertension is not found.
There are many causes of secondary hypertension (see table opposite).

Symptoms and signs

Hypertension is usually asymptomatic, although a patient will occasionally complain of headache. A history of cardiac or neurologic symptoms should always be sought. The cardiovascular system should be examined in detail and fundoscopy should be performed to look for retinopathy (see table opposite).

Clinical signs of an underlying cause (radio-femoral delay or weak femoral pulses, renal enlargement or bruit, or cushingoid features) and evidence of end-organ damage (heart failure, retinopathy, aortic aneurysm, carotid or femoral bruit) should be sought.

Malignant hypertension is diagnosed when severe hypertension (SBP >200 ± DBP >130 mmHg) is identified together with grade III–IV retinopathy. The patient often has a headache and occasionally visual disturbance. Proteinuria and haematuria are often present. This is a medical emergency requiring immediate treatment to prevent rapid progression to renal failure, heart failure and/or stroke. Untreated, the 1 year mortality is approximately 90%.

Investigation

All patients presenting with hypertension should have an ECG, fasting glucose and a full lipid profile (Total, HDL and LDL cholesterol and triglycerides), U&E, creatinine and urinalysis for blood and protein.

If secondary hypertension is suspected, further investigation should focus on the possible underlying cause (e.g. urinary cortisol, plasma renin-aldosterone levels, renal ultrasound, MRA of renal arteries, MAG-3 renogram, and 24-hour urinary catecholamines or VMA).

Blood pressure classification

Category	SBP (mmHg)	DBP (mmHg)
Optimal BP	<120	<80
Normal BP	<130	<85
High–normal BP	130–139	85–89
Grade 1 Hypertension	140–159	90–99
Grade 2 Hypertension	160–179	100–109
Grade 3 Hypertension	≥180	≥110

(Adapted from British Hypertension Society 2004, http://www.bhs.co.uk).

Secondary hypertension (<5%)

Renal disease
- Diabetic nephropathy, renovascular disease, glomerulonephritis, vasculitides, chronic pyelonephritis, polycystic kidneys.

Endocrine disease
- Conn's and Cushing's syndromes, glucocorticoid remediable hypertension, phaeochromocytoma, acromegaly, hyperparathyroidism.

Other
- Aortic coarctation, pregnancy-induced hypertension and pre-eclampsia, obesity, excessive dietary salt or licquorice intake, drugs (NSAIDs, sympathomimetics, illicit stimulants e.g. amphetamine, MDMA, and cocaine.

Grading of hypertensive retinopathy

I. Tortuous arteries, with thickened bright walls ('silver wiring').
II. Arterio-venous nipping (narrowing in a vein where crossed by an artery).
III. Flame haemorrhages and cotton wool spots (small retinal bleeds and exudates).
IV. Papilloedema.

Treatment of high blood pressure

When to treat

Patients with malignant hypertension or with persistent BP >160/100 mmHg after lifestyle measures should receive drug treatment. Subjects with BP >140/90 mmHg after lifestyle measures who have evidence of end-organ damage (LVH on ECG, proteinuria or retinopathy) or a calculated 10-year risk of a cardiovascular event ≥20% should also receive drug treatment. Subjects who have clinical evidence of CAD, peripheral or cerebrovascular disease should also be treated with antihypertensive agents if BP >140/90 mmHg.

Blood pressure targets

Most patients should have their blood pressure lowered to target of <140/85mmHg. Patients with diabetes, have been shown to benefit from more aggressive BP reduction (UKPDS and HOT studies) and a target of <130/80mmHg is more appropriate in this group.

Lifestyle measures

- Minimize dietary salt intake(<100 mmol/day).
- Reduce alcohol to <21 (Men) and <14 units (women) per week.
- Take regular aerobic exercise if not contraindicated (at least 30 min, 3x/week).
- Achieve and maintain healthy BMI (20–25 kg/m^2).
- Consume at least 5 portions/day of fresh fruit and vegetables.
- Stop smoking, reduce dietary fat content, especially saturated and trans-fatty acids.

These measures should be followed in all individuals with raised blood pressure, whether or not the decision has been made to implement drug therapy. Uptake of these lifestyle measures is often difficult to sustain, and implementation is most successful in a multidisciplinary professional setting when supported by clear written information including individualized strategies and goals.

Choice of drug therapy

Large meta-analyses of studies of blood pressure lowering therapy have clearly shown that the degree of blood pressure lowering is the best determinant of risk reduction. Comparative studies, such as ALL-HAT, have typically shown that there is little evidence favouring one class of drug over another with respect to overall cardiovascular outcome.

Thiazide diuretics are effective and cheap and widely recommended as first line anti-hypertensive therapy.

Although calcium channel blockers may be less protective than other agents against the development of heart failure, their safety and effectiveness in preventing atherosclerotic events is now confirmed despite previous concerns.

Treatment with the angiotensin receptor blocker losartan demonstrated a small advantage, particularly in reducing stroke, compared to beta blocker therapy in high risk hypertensive patients with left ventricular hypertrophy (LIFE study).

Compelling indications for specific class of antihypertensive agents

Class of drug	Compelling indication
Alpha-blocker	Benign prostatic hypertrophy
ACE-inhibitor/ ARB*	Heart failure/LV-dysfunction
	Established CAD
	Type-I diabetic nephropathy, secondary stroke prevention
	ACE-inhibitor intolerant (ARB-indicated)
	Type-II diabetic nephropathy
	Hypertension + LVH
Beta-blocker	MI
	Angina
	Heart failure
Ca-channel blockers	Elderly
	Systolic hypertension
	Angina
Thiazide diuretics	Elderly
	Heart failure
	Systolic hypertension

* ARB = angiotensin receptor blocker.
(Table adapted from British Hypertension Society 2004, www.bhs.co.uk).

Combining antihypertensive drugs

Most hypertensives require more than one drug to control their blood pressure. Combining drugs at an earlier stage in the up-titration of therapy often results in better control with fewer side-effects than maximizing the dose of individual agents.

The British Hypertension Society has produced a practical algorithm that helps guide appropriate combination of antihypertensive drugs in clinical practice (see opposite). This is based on the A-B-C-D principle (A = ACE-inhibitor or ARB, B = β-blocker, C = calcium-channel antagonist, D = diuretic). A or B being effective first-line drugs in the young, who typically have high-renin hypertension that responds well to these drug classes, whereas C or D are more effective first line agents in the elderly and Black individuals who typically have lower levels of renin and are less responsive to these agents.

Drugs can be substituted or added in a stepwise fashion according to the response until blood pressure is controlled, with cautious reduction in therapy if blood pressure drops below the optimal level. Care should be taken if prescribing B+D together as this combination may slightly increase the incidence of type-2 diabetes, whereas ACE-inhibitor and ARB therapy can both reduce risk of developing this condition.

Other therapy

The lipid lowering arm of the ASCOT study was terminated early due to a sizeable reduction in major vascular events seen in patients with hypertension and 'average' cholesterol levels treated with atorvastatin 10 mg daily for less than 4 years.

It is recommended that aspirin 75 mg daily should be prescribed to hypertensive patients that have evidence of clinical atherosclerotic disease or ≥20% 10year cardiovascular event risk, after adequate blood pressure control is achieved (<150/90).

Statin therapy should also be initiated in these high-risk individuals regardless of baseline cholesterol levels. Target lipid levels are total-cholesterol <4.0 mmol/L, LDL-cholesterol <2.0 mmol/L, or a >25% or >30% reduction in total- or LDL- cholesterol respectively, whichever is the greater.

Combining antihypertensive drugs: (The BHS A-B-C-D Principle)

	<55 years and non-Black	>55 years or Black
STEP-1	A or B	C or D
STEP-2	A + C or D	
STEP-3	A (or B) + C + D	
STEP-4	Add α-blocker/spironolactone/or other diuretic	

Adapted from British Hypertension Society 2004, www.bhs.co.uk. Other drugs to consider include hydralizine, a-methyl dopa, clonidine, moxonidine, and minoxidil but it is advisable that use of these drugs is supervised by a specialist.

Lipid management in atherosclerosis

Dyslipidaemia and risk of atherosclerosis

Numerous epidemiologic studies have confirmed that a direct relationship exists between cholesterol level and risk of CHD, even with the normal range of cholesterol. Increasing LDL cholesterol levels appears to be the main driver of this pathologic relationship, but other atherogenic lipoprotein particles including VLDL, chylomicron remnants and Lp(a) also appear to play an important role. LDL, particularly modified LDL, is recognized by the scavenger receptor on the surface of macrophages in the arterial wall which take up these cholesterol rich particles and eventually become the foam cells that form the lipid-rich core of atherosclerotic plaques. Increasing levels of HDL, involved in reverse cholesterol transport from the peripheries to the liver, protect against the development of atherosclerosis. Increased triglyceride levels are now also established as an independent risk factor for CHD. Emerging studies suggest that in addition to the circulating lipid concentrations, the nature of the lipoprotein particles plays an important part in their atherogenic risk. For example, small dense LDL particles, as seen in subjects with diabetes, are more readily taken up be macrophages and appear to be more atherogenic than larger less dense LDL.

Lipids and risk assessment

It is critical to consider the lipid profile together in the context of the other risk factors present in the individual, by calculating 10-year cardiovascular risk. Although only total and HDL cholesterol are considered in most risk models, the levels of LDL and cholesterol and triglycerides should also be considered in the overall picture. Although blood should ideally be drawn for lipid analysis after a 12 hour fast, total and HDL-cholesterol levels are only minimally affected by eating and are still are still valid in a non-fasting sample, unlike triglycerides and calculated LDL cholesterol.

Measure a fasting lipid profile if the patient:
- Is over 50 years of age
- Has clinical atherosclerotic disease
- Has ≥other risk factors for atherosclerosis
- Has clinical signs of hyperlipidaemia (xanthomata, xanthelasmata or corneal arcus at age <50 years)
- Has a family history of premature coronary artery disease or hyperlipidaemia.

Most subjects at increased global risk of coronary artery disease have cholesterol levels between 4.0 and 6.5 mmol/dL, but a significant proportion of individuals have primary or secondary dyslipidaemic syndromes with characteristic abnormalities in the lipoprotein profile.

Normal ranges for plasma lipid levels

Total cholesterol	4.0–6.5 mmol/L	(150–250 mg/dL)
LDL cholesterol	<4.1 mmol/L	(<160 mg/dL)
HDL cholesterol	0.8–2.0 mmol/L	(30–75 mg/dL)
Triglycerides	0.8–2.0 mmol/L	(70–175 mg/dL)

Primary hyperlipidaemias

Chol = plasma cholesterol mmol/L
Trig = plasma triglyceride (mmol/L); **coloured numerals = WHO** phenotype

Familial hyperchylomicronaemia (lipoprotein lipase deficiency or apoCII deficiency)[i]	Chol <6.5 Trig 10–30 Chylomicrons ↑		Eruptive xanthomata; lipaemia retinalis; hepatosplenomegaly (HSM)
Familial hyperchol-esterolaemia[ii] (LDL receptor defects)	Chol 7.5–16 Trig <2.3	LDL↑	Tendon xanthoma; corneal arcus; xanthelasma
Familial defective apoprotein B-100[iia]	Chol 7.5–16 Trig <2.3	LDL↑	Tendon xanthoma; arcus; xanthelasma
Polygenic hyper-cholesterolaemia[iia]	Chol 6.5–9 Trig <2.3	LDL↑	*The commonest 1° lipidaemia* xanthelasma; corneal arcus
Familial combined hyperlipidaemia[iib, iv or v]	Chol 6.5–10 Trig 2.3–12	LDL↑VLDL↑ HDL↓	*Next commonest 1° lipidaemia* xanthelasma; arcus
Dysbetalipoproteinaemia (remnant particle disease)[iii]	Chol 9–14 Trig 9–14	IDL↑ HDL↓ LDL↓	Palmar striae; tuberoeruptive xanthoma
Familial hypertri-glyceridaemia[iv]	Chol 6.5–12	VLDL↑	
Type V hyperlipoproteinaemia	Trig 10–30; chylomicrons		Eruptive xanthoma; lipaemia retinalis; HSM

Primary HDL abnormalities

Hyperalphalipoproteinaemia ↑HDL chol >2

Hypoalphalipoproteinaemia (Tangier disease) ↓HDL chol <0.92

Primary LDL abnormalities

Abetalipoproteinaemia Trig<0.3, Chol<1.3, missing LDL, VLDL and chylomicrons, and fat malabsorption, retinopathy, and acanthocytosis

Hypobetalipoproteinaemia chol<1.5 LDL↓, HDL ↓. Increased longevity.

Abbreviations *IDL* = intermediate-density liproprotein (*HDL* and *LDL* denote high and low density, respectively); chol = cholesterol; trig = triglyceride. Reproduced with permission from Longmore M, Wilkinson I, Rajagopalan S (2004). *Oxford Handbook of Clinical Medicine.* 6th ed. Oxford: Oxford University Press.

Secondary causes of dyslipidaemia
- Renal failure*
- Nephrotic syndrome*
- Hypothyroidism*
- Type II diabetes and obesity**
- Cholestasis
- Alcohol abuse
- Drugs
  - Anti-retroviral protease-inhibitors
  - Thiazides
  - Oral contraceptive pill
  - Isotretinoin
  - Steroids

* Cholesterol elevation **Minor elevation in cholesterol, but greater increases in atherogenic VLDL, chylomicron remnants and triglycerides as well as a fall in HDL.

Lipid lowering therapy

Statins

e.g. atorvastatin, fluvastatin, pravastatin, rosuvastatin, simvastatin

Statins reduce cholesterol levels by inhibiting HMG CoA-reductase, the rate limiting enzyme in cholesterol synthesis. They also increase clearance of circulating LDL by up regulating LDL-receptor expression, further lowering cholesterol levels. These agents are extremely effective at lowering cholesterol levels; for example, the most potent statins, Atorvastatin and rosuvastatin can more than halve LDL cholesterol levels at higher doses. A small increase in HDL and decrease in triglycerides is also commonly observed.

A significant evidence-base has been built up over the past decade that strongly supports the widespread use of statins in the primary and secondary prevention settings, and confirmed the safety of the commonly used drugs in this class. Data from large randomized clinical trials has shown a consistent reduction (around 25–30%) in the relative risk of major cardiovascular events with the use of atorvastatin, pravastatin and simvastatin in both the primary (ASCOT, WOSCOPS, HPS, CARDS) and secondary prevention settings (MIRACL, CARE, LIPID, 4S,HPS). In the first outcome study comparing two statins, the PROVE-IT study recently showed that high dose atorvastatin (80 mg) was more effective than pravastatin (40 mg) at preventing further major cardiovascular events during the first 2–3 years after presentation with an acute coronary syndrome.

Typically recommended evidence-based doses are simvastatin 40 mg nocte, pravastatin 40 mg od, and atorvastatin 10–80 mg od. Statins should not be prescribed to individuals with porphyria or severe liver or muscle disease, and caution is advised with their use in milder liver dysfunction, renal impairment and in combination with fibrates.

Fibrates

e.g. bezafibrate, ciprofibrate, fenofibrate, gemfibrozil

Fibrates improve the lipid profile by activating PPAR-a, resulting in a mild lowering of total and LDL-cholesterol, and a more significant reduction in triglycerides and increase in HDL. Subjects with combined hyperlipidaemia or other reasons for a low HDL and/or high triglycerides respond well to fibrates. Although the VA-HIT study showed that gemfibrozil (600 mmg bd) reduced major cardiovascular events in subjects with average cholesterol and low HDL (<1.0 mmol/L) levels, subgroup analysis of HPS suggested that similar benefits were observed with simvastatin (40 mg) in such individuals. For the majority of patients with and at risk of atherosclerotic events, fibrates are typically recommended as second line agents for prevention in patients intolerant of statins, particularly if they have low HDL or high triglycerides. The likelihood of liver or muscle side effects is increased if a fibrate and statin are used in combination and careful monitoring is recommended. The risk is lower if the statin is combined with fenofibrate than with other fibrates.

Anion-exchange resins

The agents cholestyramine (4–8 g tds) and cholestipol (5–10 g tds) bind bile salts in the small bowel. This inhibits their reabsorption resulting in up-regulation of the LDL receptor on hepatocytes and increased plasma cholesterol clearance. Although these drugs effectively lower cholesterol levels, most subjects experience intolerable GI side effects, limiting their widespread use. These drugs are generally recommended as second or third line therapy in subjects with hypercholesterolaemia.

Inhibitors of intestinal cholesterol absorption

The novel agent ezetimibe (10 mg od) binds to an intestinal cholesterol transport protein which inhibits absorption. LDL cholesterol is reduced by 15–20%. Ezetimibe is most effectively employed together with statin therapy in those patients who do not achieve cholesterol targets at higher statin doses, and is effective as monotherapy in those intolerant of statins.

Dietary plant stanols (3 g/day) can reduce LDL cholesterol by up to 15%.

Niacin

Niacin (100–1000 mg tds, or 375–2000 mg modified-release preparation (niaspan) od) reduces hepatic VLDL synthesis and inhibits fatty acid release from adipocytes. HDL levels are significantly increased, and reduced hepatic synthesis results in a small reduction in LDL. Although particularly beneficial in mixed dyslipidaemias, use of the short-acting formulation has been limited by a high incidence of intolerable GI side effects and facial flushing. The modified release formulation is considerably more tolerable, and ongoing outcome studies should confirm the place of this agent in the preventive armamentarium.

Fish oils

Marine oil supplements containing high concentrations of omega-3 fatty acids are indicated for the treatment of severe hypertriglyceridaemia (Omacor 4 capsules/day, Maxepa 10 capsules/day). Omacor (1 mg od, GISSI-P study) has a license for secondary prevention post-MI, but the benefits observed with this dose do not seem to be due to lipid lowering effects. An extensive clinical trial program spanning a wide range of primary and secondary prevention settings should clarify the wider role of this drug in CAD prevention.

When to treat lipids

Therapeutic lifestyle changes (TLCs) are the first step in the treatment of dyslipidemia. Moderate weight reduction (10% of body weight) improves the lipid profile and CV risk. The composition of the optimal diet is controversial.

General dietary recommendations include
• Reduced cholesterol and saturated fats (especially trans fats)
• Increased plant stanols, sterols and soluble fiber
• Adoption of Mediterranean diet,
Exercise should also be taken regularly.

Statin therapy should be initiated in all patients with established clinical atherosclerotic disease, including CAD, cerebrovascular, renovascular and peripheral arterial disease. Current UK, European, and US guidelines also recommend statin therapy in subjects with diabetes (CARDS, and subgroup analyses of HPS, ASCOT and other major trials). These guidelines also recommend statin therapy in subjects with a CAD equivalent 10y CV risk of ≥20%. Although all of these patients should receive statins (unless contraindicated) regardless of the cholesterol level (HPS, ASCOT, CARDS), it is still important to measure lipid levels to ensure that subjects are responding appropriately to therapy and achieving targets for cholesterol <4.0 mmol/L and LDL <2.0 mmol/L. These targets are based on observations from clinical trials and cohort studies suggesting that 'lower is better' when it comes to cholesterol!

There is less outcome-based evidence informing us when to initiate drug therapy for isolated dyslipidaemia in the absence of other risk factors. Younger subjects without a family history of CAD or other risk factors should be considered for drug treatment if or LDL cholesterol >5.0 mmol/L (or total >7.0 mmol/L). Primary and familial hyperlipidaemias should be treated aggressively particularly if there is a family history of premature CAD.

Diabetes and atherosclerosis

Approximately 2 million people in the UK currently suffer from diabetes mellitus (DM), the vast majority of whom have type 2 diabetes (>90%). Although diabetes is more common in older individuals, the incidence is increasing at a dramatic rate in all age groups especially young adults, driven by the obesity 'epidemic'. The prevalence of type 2 DM is also greater in Blacks and South Asians in the UK. Macrovascular disease is the most common cause of death in DM (>75%).

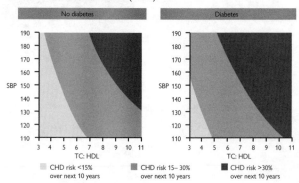

Fig. 4.6 The effect of type 2DM on CHD Risk (Non-smoker, age 60 years**)

** Adapted from the British Cardiac Society, British Hyperlipidaemia Society, British Hypertension Society, British Diabetic Association (1998). Heart **80** (suppl 2): S1–S29.

Mechanisms responsible for increased CV risk in DM

A complex mix of risk factors is typically present in diabetic patients. These include low HDL, high triglycerides (VLDL and remnant particles), increased small, dense LDL, moderate hypertension, low-grade inflammation, a procoagulant state (increased PAI-1, and platelet activation), increased oxidative stress and increased levels of harmful advanced glycation end products. Conventional risk factors only account for a relatively small proportion (≈25%) of the increased risk observed in diabetes.

Not only are diabetic subjects more likely to suffer a major vascular event, they are also more likely to die from this event than if they did not have diabetes. Furthermore the atherosclerotic process tends to be more diffuse in diabetics, often affecting multiple vascular territories, as well as making percutaneous and surgical revascularization more technically challenging and risky.

Outcome is better, when diabetics with multi-vessel coronary disease undergo CABG rather than percutaneous revascularization (RITA, BARI). However, data from large studies suggests that outcome after PCI in diabetics is improved by use of drug eluting stents as well as abciximab, a platelet glycoprotein IIb/IIIa antagonist. Visceral neuropathy is responsible for silent myocardial ischaemia, and reduced heart rate variability. Diabetic nephropathy further contributes to cardiac risk by increasing blood pressure and causing deterioration in the lipid profile.

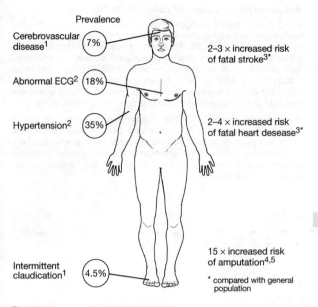

Fig. 4.7 Macrovascular disease in Type 2 DM.
1. Wingard DL *et al.* (1993). *Diabetes Care* **16**: 1022–25.
2. UKPDS 6.(1990). *Diabetes Res* **13**: 1–11.
3. Balkau B *et al.* (1997) *Lancet* **350**:1680.
4. King's Fund. Counting the Cost. BDA, 1996.
5. Most RS, Sinnock P (1983). *Diabetes Care* **6**: 67–91.

Recommendations for risk reduction in diabetes

Blood glucose should be aggressively controlled by means of diet and exercise coupled with appropriate intensity of hypoglycaemic drug therapy. Target HbA1c is ≤7%. However, intense blood sugar control is better at reducing progression of microvascular disease and neuropathy than prevention of macrovascular events (UKPDS study). Aggressive blood pressure (UKPDS, HOT studies) and lipid management (CARDS, ASCOT, HPS) has a greater impact on prevention of CAD and stroke than tight glucose control, and reduces progression of nephropathy.

As mentioned previously, CV risk in diabetes is similar to that seen in patients with established CAD, at least after the disease has been present for several years. Because of their rapid progression of arterial disease, it is recommended that patients with diabetes receive aggressive preventive therapy with statins, aspirin, and inhibition of the renin-angiotensin system (see table opposite).

Therapeutic recommendations for CV prevention in diabetes

Measure	Target
Aggressive lifestyle ± oral hypoglycaemic therapy	HbA1c ≤ 7%
Statin therapy (regardless of baseline lipid levels)	Chol. <4.0 mmol/L
	Or ↓>25%
	LDL <2.0 mmol/L
	Or ↓>30%
Aggressive blood pressure control	<130/<80 mmHg

ACE-inhibitor or ARB in most, especially if evidence of nephropathy.

The metabolic syndrome and insulin resistance

The metabolic syndrome is a term describing a frequently observed cluster of adverse factors within an individual. The syndrome is characterized by visceral obesity, insulin resistance, moderate hypertension, dyslipidaemia (low HDL and high triglycerides with average cholesterol levels) and low-grade inflammation. Several definitions of this syndrome have been proposed, but of these the American NCEP ATP-III diagnostic criteria (table) are the most practical and widely used, as well as being a robust predictor of vascular risk. The prevalence of this syndrome is increasing in parallel with the increase in numbers of obese and overweight individuals, and has been described in a high proportion of American children and adolescents. Thus, the metabolic syndrome is projected to contribute substantially to the burden of atherosclerotic disease in society in the next few decades. Unless effective interventions to reverse this trend are delivered at a population level, much of the progress we have made in the fight against CAD is likely to be reversed.

ATP-III criteria for diagnosis of the metabolic syndrome

Variable	Threshold	
Waist circumference	>102 cm	(>40") Men
	>88 cm	(>35") Women
Fasting glucose	>6.1 mmol/L (11 mg/dL)	
Blood pressure	>130/>85 mmHg	
HDL cholesterol	<1 mmol/L	(40 mg/dL) Men
	<1.3 mmol/L	(50 mg/dL) Women
Triglycerides	>1.7 mmol/L (>150 mg/dL)	

≥3 out of 5 criteria must be satisfied for firm diagnosis.

Mechanisms of increased risk

Visceral obesity causes insulin resistance, which is associated with increases in blood glucose, and adverse changes in blood lipids. Increased levels of inflammatory cytokines such as TNF-α, cause endothelial dysfunction which increases vascular tone and blood pressure, as well as promoting local proatherosclerotic changes in the vascular wall.

Increased leptin and reduced adiponectin levels influence insulin sensitivity, as well as some of the adverse metabolic consequences of obesity, but their incremental clinical value remains a subject of investigation. It has been proposed that the degree of insulin resistance is less important than the impact of other risk factors including lipids, blood pressure, inflammation and pro-thrombotic factors, but these issues also remain under investigation.

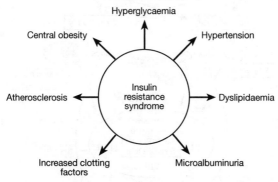

Fig. 4.8 Insulin resistance is an independent predictor of cardiovascular disease[1–4].

1. Haffner SM et al.(1992). *Diabetes* **41**: 715–722.
2. Haffner SM et al.(1997). *Am J Med* **103**: 152–162.
3. Reaven GM (1994). *J Int Med* **236** (Suppl 736): 13–22.
4. Abuaisha B et al.(1998). *Diabetes Res Clin Pract* **39**: 93–99.

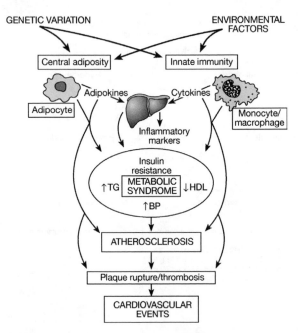

Fig. 4.9 Pathophysiology of atherosclerotic cardiovascular disease in the metabolic syndrome. Central adiposity and innate immunity play key roles in the development of insulin resistance, chronic inflammation, and metabolic syndrome features through the effects of adipokines (e.g. leptin, adiponectin, resistin) and cytokines (e.g. tumor necrosis factor-α, interleukin-6) on liver, skeletal muscle, and immune cells. In addition, monocyte/macrophage and adipocyte-derived factors may have direct atherothrombotic effects that promote the development of atherosclerotic cardiovascular events. Common genetic variants and environmental factors may impact the development of atherosclerosis at multiple levels through influences on central adiposity, innate immunity, glucose and lipoprotein metabolism, and vascular function. Reproduced with permission from Reilly MP, Rader J (2003). The metabolic syndrome: more than the sum of its parts. *Circulation* **108**: 1546–1551.

Metabolic syndrome: management

Weight loss and exercise are the cornerstones of management of the metabolic syndrome. Management of insulin resistance with insulin sensitising drugs (metformin, and thiazolidenediones) has theoretical benefits but is currently under investigation (see below) As far as management of the dyslipidaemia is concerned, treatment with statin is clearly indicated if 10y CV risk is ≥20%, or if LDL cholesterol is elevated (ATP-III recommend threshold of >3.3 mmol/l). The nature of the risk factor profile in the metabolic syndrome frequently results in the underestimation of 10y risk, but at present no studies are currently available to support use of specific evidence-based drug therapy in this syndrome.

Insulin sensitizers (thiazolidenediones, 'glitazones')

- The primary mode of action is to improve insulin sensitivity in muscle and adipose tissue (see Fig. opposite).[1,2]
- They are licensed as monotherapy, particularly in overweight patients with type 2 DM for whom metformin is not suitable
- They are associated with modest weight gain.[3]
- They maintain lasting glycaemic control and, by targeting insulin resistance, improve a range of cardiovascular risk factors.[4]
- There may be a role for this class of drugs in the prevention of DM: the TRIPOD study enrolled 266 Hispanic women, in S. California at high risk of developing DM, and randomized them to the thiazolidenedione, troglitazone, or placebo for 30 months. There was a 50% reduction in risk of developing DM with troglitazone use and the benefits sustained for >6 mo after discontinuing drug.[5]

1 Hallsten K et al. (2002). Diabetes **51**: 3479–3485.
2 Virtanen K et al. (2002). Diabetes **51**: (Suppl. 2): A145. Abs 585-P.
3 Carey DG et al. (2002). Obes Res **10**: 1008–1015.
4 St John Sutton M et al. (2002). Diabetes Care **25**: 2058–2064.
5 Buchanan et al. (2002). Diabetes **51**: 2796.

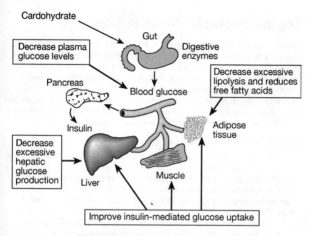

Fig. 4.10 Glitazones decrease insulin resistance at target tissues

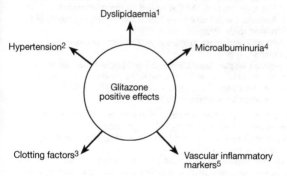

Fig. 4.11 Glitazones have positive effects on a range of cardiovascular risk factors.

1. Brunzell J et al. (2001) *Diabetes* **50** (Suppl 2): Abs 567-P.
2. Bakris GL et al. (2000) *Diabetes* **49** (Suppl 1): A96, Abs 388.
3. Freed M et al. (2000) *Diabetologia* **43** (Suppl 1): Abs 1024.
4. Bakris GL et al. (1999) *Diabetologia* **42** (Suppl 1): Abs 865 and poster.
5. Greenberg A et al. (2001) *Diabetologia* **44** (Suppl 1): A222, Abs 853.

Angina pectoris

Angina pectoris refers to the pain caused by myocardial ischaemia. Ischaemia is usually caused by coronary stenosis due to atheroma but may be caused by tachycardia, anaemia, aortic stenosis, left ventricular hypertrophy of other aetiologies, Syndrome X (chest pain with normal coronary arteries) and coronary artery spasm (Prinzmetal). These conditions may coexist and will be exacerbated by physical exertion or emotional stress, which increase cardiac workload and energy requirement. Coronary artery spasm, in contrast, normally occurs at rest.

History and examination

- Angina pectoris is characterized by a deep and diffusely-distributed central chest discomfort.
- Certain features of pain are of discriminative value. Patients will not be able to point to where the pain is coming from with one finger but will use an open palm or fist over the centre or left parasternal aspect of their chest.
  - The pain is not sharp, (some patients confuse 'sharp' with 'severe').
  - Pain lasts longer than a few seconds and rarely exceeds an hour without varying in severity. Most episodes will last 1–5 minutes.
  - The response to GTN, if at all, will be almost immediate. Responses which take more than 5 minutes are unlikely to be related to the drug.
- Chest wall tenderness suggests musculoskeletal pain and does not accompany angina.
- Dyspnoea, fatigue, nausea, and recurrent belching may also represent underlying ischaemia and can occur in the absence of the classical central chest pain. The clue to underlying IHD lies in their precipitation by exertion or emotional stress.

Angina is often classified according to its temporal pattern and its relation to exertion because this loosely reflects prognosis.
- Stable angina—characterized by pain occurring after a relatively constant level of exertion.
- Unstable angina—characterized by pain on minor exertion or at rest, which is either new onset or a dramatic worsening of existing angina.
- Crescendo angina—characterized by pain on ever-diminishing levels of exertion, usually over a period of days.
- Decubitus angina—provoked by lying flat.

The **Canadian Cardiovascular Society (CCS)** system provides a quantitative means to describe exertional capacity and is divided into 4 classes:
I. Minimal limitation of ordinary activity. Angina occurs with strenuous, rapid, or prolonged exertion at work or recreation.
II. Slight limitation of ordinary activity; angina occurs on walking or climbing stairs rapidly; walking in cold, in wind, or under emotional stress.

III. Marked limitation of ordinary physical activity; angina occurs on walking 50–100 m on level ground or climbing 1 flight of stairs at a normal pace in normal conditions.

IV. Inability to perform any physical activity without discomfort; angina symptoms may be present at rest.

Physical examination

- This rarely reveals any direct evidence of IHD but will help with risk stratification and to exclude co-existing disease.
- Measure the pulse rate. This may be slowed by inferior ischaemia due to AV node ischaemia. A resting tachycardia, if present, usually represents activation of the sympathetic nervous system but may be due to an arrhythmia precipitated by ischaemia.
- Blood pressure measurement is essential to look for evidence of hypertension (predisposing to atheroma), or hypotension (may reflect cardiac dysfunction or over-medication).
- Precordial examination should include palpation for left ventricular hypertrophy, cardiac enlargement or dyskinesis, and auscultation for added heart sounds (heart failure or acute ischaemia), aortic stenosis or mitral regurgitation (due to papillary muscle dysfunction).
- Examine for signs of heart failure by listening for fine, late-inspiratory crepitations at the lung bases, and looking for dependent pitting oedema (typically bilateral ankle ± leg oedema, but sacral oedema may be the only manifestation if the patient has been recumbent for some time).
- Look for evidence of peripheral vascular disease by palpating for aortic aneurysm, feeling the carotid and limb pulses, listening for carotid, renal or femoral artery bruits and assessing tissue integrity and capillary refill of the legs and feet.
- Examine for signs of hypercholesterolemia: the eyes for xanthelasmata and corneal arcus, and the skin and tendons (especially the Achilles) for xanthomata.

Differential diagnosis

- The differential diagnosis of anginal chest pain is wide and includes:
- Anxiety and hyperventilation
- Musculoskeletal chest wall pain
- Cervical or thoracic root pain
- Pneumothorax, pneumonia, or pulmonary embolus
- Oesophageal problem (inflammation/spasm)
- Other upper GI problem (gastritis, peptic ulcer, pancreatitis, cholecystitis)
- Pericarditis
- Aortic dissection
- Mitral valve prolapse
- Coronary emboli (LV mural thrombus, atrial myxoma).

Investigations

Further risk stratification will add to the diagnostic certainty achieved by history and examination. Measure FBC, U&E, a full fasting lipid profile (total, LDL and HDL cholesterol and triglyceride levels), and blood glucose. CXR is not mandatory, but should be performed if there is suspicion of heart failure, a pulmonary condition or an abnormality of the bony structures of the chest wall.

12-lead ECG

A resting ECG may not confirm the diagnosis but can point towards ischaemic heart disease. The presence of T wave inversion (2 mm) or Q-waves suggests previous myocardial injury. The presence of ST depression and to a lesser extent, T wave inversion during pain is a marker of ischaemia and patients with these signs should be further investigated. If ST segment deviation is observed at rest, an acute coronary syndrome must be excluded. 12-lead ECG can also help identify other causes of chest pain (LVH, arrhythmia, pericarditis).

Tests for inducible ischaemia

Tests such as exercise ECG, stress ECHO, or myocardial perfusion scanning are a useful adjunct to confirm the diagnosis and aid management.

Management

Lifestyle Stop smoking. Encourage daily aerobic exercise within limits of exercise capacity. Look at occupational needs and advise adjustment if symptom level not compatible. Advise healthy diet collaborating with dieticians if required.

Aspirin (75 mg/24hr) in all cases unless active peptic ulcer disease or bleeding diathesis. Those with past peptic ulcer disease may take a gastro-protective agent such as a H2 antagonist or proton pump inhibitor.

Anti-anginals

β-blockers: 1st line (e.g. atenolol 25–100 mg od or metoprolol 25–50 mg tds). Start on suspicion of IHD. Avoid only if contraindicated (asthma with confirmed β-agonist response (mortality improved in patients with angina and concomitant COPD if they can tolerate the reduced PEFR), uncontrolled severe LV dysfunction, bradycardia, coronary artery spasm).

Calcium antagonists: (e.g. amlodipine 5–10 mg od or diltiazem-MR 90–180 mg bd) If β-blocker contraindicated.

Nitrates: (e.g. GTN spray) Used for control of breakthrough angina. Long-acting nitrates (e.g. isosorbide mononitrate MR 60–120 mg od) are a useful addition to β-blockers for prevention of attacks.

Statins reduce mortality by approximately one third in all risk groups. However, the underlying risk of events must be taken into account when considering starting the drug because absolute risk reduction in young patients with low-risk IHD may be very small with a possible harm of myositis, hepatic failure, and reduced compliance with other medications.

Chest pain clinics

Rapid access or open access chest pain clinics have transformed the primary and secondary care interface for UK patients since their incorporation into the National Service Framework. They have facilitated the shift of care of stable angina from generalist to specialist and increased rates of angiography and revascularization. It is not known if this has an effect on mortality but it has certainly prioritized cardiac care and rates of diagnosis of IHD. The clinics usually involve a standardized referral form which can be used either by GP or hospital physician.

The emphasis is on early exclusion of non-cardiac disease and risk stratification for IHD. Thus in the first visit, the patient would see a specialist, perform an exercise test and have baseline risk factors estimated. At the end of the consultation, the patient will be reassured that there is a low likelihood of IHD or will begin the path of treatment of risk factors and symptoms, ultimately leading to revascularization if required.

Acute coronary syndromes

Acute coronary syndrome (ACS) is an operational term used to describe a constellation of symptoms resulting from acute myocardial ischaemia. An ACS resulting in myocardial injury is termed myocardial infarction (MI). ACS includes the diagnosis of unstable angina (UA), non-ST elevation myocardial infarction (NSTEMI) and ST elevation myocardial infarction (STEMI). The term ACS is initially generally, assigned by ancillary/triage personnel on initial contact with the patient. Guidelines for identification of ACS are summarized in the table on p197.

Definition

The current nomenclature divides ACS into two major groups, on the basis of delivered treatment modalities:(see Fig. 4.12 opposite).

ST elevation myocardial infarction (STEMI)—An ACS where patients present with chest discomfort and ST-segment elevation on ECG. This group of patients must undergo reperfusion therapy on presentation.

Non-ST elevation myocardial infarction (NSTEMI) and unstable angina (UA)—ACS where patients present with ischaemic chest discomfort associated with transient or permanent non-ST-elevation ischaemic ECG changes. If there is biochemical evidence of myocardial injury the condition is termed NSTEMI and in the absence if biochemical myocardial injury the condition is termed UA (see p192). This group of patients are not treated with thrombolysis.

Initial management of ACS

- All patients with suspected ACS should be placed in an environment with continuous ECG monitoring and defibrillation capacity.
- The referring doctor should be instructed to give aspirin (300 mg po if no contraindications) and **not** to give any im injections (causes a rise in total CK and risk of bleeding with thrombolysis/anticoagulation).

Immediate assessment should include

- **Rapid examination** to exclude hypotension, note the presence of murmurs and to identify and treat acute pulmonary oedema.
- Secure IV access.
- 12 lead ECG should be obtained and reported within 10 minutes.
- Give: *Oxygen* (initially only 28% if history of COPD)
          Diamorphine 2.5–10 mg IV prn for pain relief
          Metoclopramide 10 mg IV for nausea
          GTN spray 2 puffs/unless hypotensive
- Take blood for:
  - FBC/U&E   Supplement K+ to keep it at 4–5 mmol/L.
  - Glucose   May be ↑acutely post MI, even in non-diabetics, and reflects a stress-catecholamine response and may resolve without treatment.
  - Biochemical markers of cardiac injury (see p158).
  - Lipid profile   Total cholesterol, LDL, HDL, triglycerides
  - Serum cholesterol and HDL remain close to baseline for 24–48 hours but fall thereafter and take ≥8 weeks to return to baseline.

- Portable CXR to assess cardiac size, pulmonary oedema and exclude mediastinal enlargement.
- General examination should include peripheral pulses, fundoscopy, abdominal examination for organomegaly and aortic aneurysm.

Conditions mimicking pain in ACS

- Pericarditis
- Dissecting aortic aneurysm
- Pulmonary embolism
- Oesophageal reflux, spasm or rupture
- Biliary tract disease
- Perforated peptic ulcer
- Pancreatitis

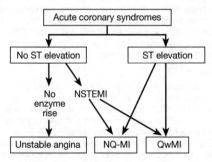

Fig. 4.12 Nomenclature of ACS: Patients with ACS may present with or without ST elevation on the ECG. The majority of patients with ST elevation (large arrows) ultimately develop Q-wave MI (QwMI) whereas a minority (small arrow) develop a non-Q-wave MI (NQ-MI). Patients without ST-elevation are experiencing either UA or an NSTEMI depending on the absence or presence of cardiac enzymes (e.g. troponin) detected in the blood. (Adapted with permission from Antman EM, Braunwald E (1997). Acute myocardial infarction. In Braunwald EB ed. *Heart Disease: a textbook of cardiovascular medicine*. Philadelphia, PA WB Saunders).

ST elevation myocardial infarction (STEMI)

Patients with an ACS who have ST-segment elevation/LBBB on their presenting ECG benefit significantly from immediate reperfusion and are treated as one group under the term ST elevation myocardial infarction (STEMI).

Presentation

- **Chest pain** usually similar in nature to angina, but of greater severity, longer duration and not relieved by SL GTN. Associated features: nausea and vomiting, sweating, breathlessness, and extreme distress.
- The pains may be **atypical** (e.g. epigastric), or radiate to the back.
- Diabetics, the elderly, and hypertensives may suffer **painless ('silent' infarcts) and/or atypical infarction**. Presenting features include breathlessness from acute pulmonary oedema, syncope or coma from dysrrhythmias, acute confusional states (mania/psychosis), diabetic hyperglycaemic crises, hypotension/cardiogenic shock, CNS manifestations resembling stroke secondary to sudden reduction in cardiac output and peripheral embolization.

Management

Diagnosis is normally made on presentation followed by rapid stablization to ensure institution of reperfusion therapy without delay. This is in contrast to NSTEMI/UA where diagnosis may evolve over period of 24–72 hours (see p192). The management principles of the various stages are outlined below and expanded subsequently.

- **Stabilizing measures** are generally similar for all ACS patients (p 162).
  - All patients with suspected STEMI should have continuous ECG monitoring in an area with full resuscitation facilities.
  - Patients should receive immediate aspirin 300 mg po (if no contraindications), analgesia and oxygen. Secure IV access.
  - Rapid examination to exclude hypotension, note the presence of murmurs and to identify and treat acute pulmonary oedema. RVF out of proportion to LVF suggests RV infarction (see p172).
  - Blood for FBC, biochemical profile, markers of cardiac injury, lipid profile , glucose and portable CXR.
- **Diagnosis** must be made on the basis of history, ECG (ST elevation/new LBBB), and biochemical markers of myocardial injury. (NB if ECG changes diagnostic, reperfusion must not be delayed to wait for biochemical markers).
- **Treatment:**   i)   General medical measures (p 162)
                     ii) Reperfusion (p 164–169).
- **All patients with STEMI should be admitted to CCU.**
- **Discharge and risk prevention.**

Factors associated with a poor prognosis

- Age >70 years
- Previous MI or chronic stable angina
- Anterior MI or right ventricular infarction
- Left ventricular failure at presentation
- Hypotension (and sinus tachycardia) at presentation
- Diabetes mellitus
- Mitral regurgitation (acute)
- Ventricular septal defect.

STEMI: diagnosis

This is based on a **combination of history, ECG, and biochemical markers of cardiac injury**. In practice, history and ECG changes are normally diagnostic resulting in immediate reperfusion/medical treatment. Biochemical markers of cardiac injury usually become available later and help reconfirm diagnosis as well as provide prognostic information (magnitude of rise).

ECG changes

- **ST segment elevation** occurs within minutes and may last for up to 2 weeks. ST elevation of ≥2 mm in adjacent chest leads and ≥1 mm in adjacent limb leads is necessary to fulfill thrombolysis criteria. Persisting ST elevation after 1 month suggests formation of LV aneurysm. Infarction site can be localized from ECG changes as indicated in the table opposite.
- **Pathological Q waves** indicate significant abnormal electrical conduction, but are not synonymous with irreversible myocardial damage. In the context of a 'transmural infarction' it may take hours or days to develop and usually remain indefinitely. In the standard leads the Q wave should be ≥25% of the R wave, 0.04s in duration, with negative T waves. In the precordial leads, Q waves in V4 should be >0.4 mV (4 small sq) and in V6 >0.2 mV (2 small sq), in the absence of LBBB (QRS width <0.1s or 3 small sq).
- **ST-segment depression (ischaemia at distance)** in a second territory (in patients with ST-segment elevation) is secondary to ischaemia in a territory other than the area of infarction (often indicative of multivessel disease), or reciprocal electrical phenomena. Overall it implies a poorer prognosis.
- **PR-segment elevation/depression** and alterations in the contour of the p wave are generally indicative of atrial infarction. Most patients will also have abnormal atrial rhythms such as AF/flutter, wandering atrial pacemaker and AV nodal rhythm.
- **T wave inversion** may be immediate or delayed and generally persists after the ST elevation has resolved.
- **Non-diagnostic changes**, but ones that may be ischaemic, include new LBBB or RBBB, tachyarrhythmias, transient tall peaked T waves or T wave inversion, axis shift (extreme left or right) or AV block.

Biochemical markers of cardiac injury

Serial measurements evaluating a temporal rise and fall should be obtained to allow a more accurate diagnosis. CK and CK-MB from a skeletal muscle source tend to remain elevated for a greater time period in comparison to a cardiac source.

Conditions that may mimic ECG changes of a STEMI

- Left or right ventricular hypertrophy
- LBBB or left anterior fasciculate block
- Wolff-Parkinson-White syndrome
- Pericarditis or myocarditis
- Cardiomyopathy (hypertrophic or dilated)
- Trauma to myocardium
- Cardiac tumours (primary and metastatic)
- Pulmonary embolus
- Pneumothorax
- Intra-cranial haemorrhage
- Hyperkalaemia
- Cardiac sarcoid or amyloid
- Pancreatitis.

Localization of infarcts from ECG changes

Anterior	ST elevation and/or Q waves in V1–V4/V5.
Anteroseptal	ST elevation and/or Q waves in V1–V3.
Anterolateral	ST elevation and/or Q waves in V1–V6 and I and aVL.
Lateral	ST elevation and/or Q waves in V5–V6 and T wave inversion/ST elevation/Q waves in I and aVL.
Inferolateral	ST elevation and/or Q waves in II, III, aVF and V5–V6 (sometimes I and aVL).
Inferior	ST elevation and/or Q waves in II, III and aVF.
Inferoseptal	ST elevation and/or Q waves in II, III, aVF, V1–V3.
True posterior	Tall R waves in V1–V2 with ST depression in V1–V3. T waves remain upright in V1–V2. This can be confirmed with an oesophageal lead if available (method similar to an NG tube). Usually occurs in conjunction with an inferior or lateral infarct.
RV infarction	ST segment elevation in the right precordial leads (V3R–V4R). Usually found in conjunction with inferior infarction. This may only be present in the early hours of infarction.

CK (creatinine phosphokinase)
- Levels twice upper-limit of normal are taken as being abnormal.
- Serum levels rise within 4–8 hours post STEMI and fall to normal within 3–4 days. The peak level occurs at about 24 hours but may be earlier (12 hours) and higher in patients who have had reperfusion (thrombolysis or PCI).
- False positive rates of ~15% occur in patients with alcohol intoxication, muscle disease or trauma, vigorous exercise, convulsions, im injections, hypothyroidism, PE and thoracic outlet syndrome.

CK-MB isoenzyme is more specific for myocardial disease. Levels may be elevated despite a normal total CK. However, CK-MB is also present in small quantities in other tissues (skeletal muscle, tongue, diaphragm, uterus, and prostate) and trauma or surgery may lead to false positive results. If there is doubt about myocardial injury with CK-MB levels obtained a cardiac troponin must be measured.

Cardiac troponins (TnT, TnI)
- Both TnT and TnI are highly sensitive and specific markers of cardiac injury.
- Serum levels start to rise by 3 hours post MI and elevation may persist up to 7–14 days. This is advantageous for diagnosis of late MI.
- In most STEMI cases the diagnosis can be made using a combination of the clinical picture and serial CK/CK-MB levels. In the event of normal CK-MB levels and suspected non-cardiac sources of CK, troponins can be used.
- Troponins can also be elevated in non-ischaemic myocyte damage such as myocarditis, cardiomyopathy, and pericarditis.

Other markers
There are multiple other markers, but with increasing clinical availability of troponins, measurements are not recommended. These include AST (rise 18–36 hours post MI) and LDH (rise 24–36 hours post MI).

The time course of the various markers is seen in Fig. 4.13.

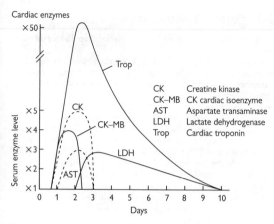

Fig. 4.13 Graph of the appearance of cardiac markers in the blood versus time of onset of symptoms.

<u>Peak A</u>: early release of myoglobin or CK-MB isoforms after AMI.

<u>Peak B</u>: Cardiac troponin after AMI.

<u>Peak C</u>: CK-MB after AMI.

<u>Peak D</u>: Cardiac troponin after unstable angina.

(Adapted with permission from Wu AH et al. (1999). Clin Chem **45**: 1104–1121).

STEMI: general measures

1. **Immediate stabilising measures** are as outlined on p 154 for all ACS.
2. **Control of cardiac pain**
- **Diamorphine** 2.5–10 mg IV is the drug of choice and may be repeated to ensure adequate pain relief, unless evidence of emerging toxicity (hypotension, respiratory depression). Nausea and vomiting should be treated with metoclopramide (10 mg IV) or a phenothiazine.
- **Oxygen** to be administered at 2–5 L/min for at least 2–3 hours. Hypoxaemia is frequently seen post-MI due to ventilation–perfusion abnormalities secondary to LVF. In patients with refractory pulmonary oedema, CPAP or via formal endotracheal intubation may be necessary. Beware of CO_2 retention in patients with COPD.
- **Nitrates** may lessen pain and can be given providing that patient is not hypotensive (sub-lingual or intravenous). They need to be used cautiously in inferior STEMI, especially with right ventricular infarction, as venodilation may impair RV filling and precipitate hypotension. Nitrate therapy has no effect on mortality (ISIS-4).

3. **Correction of electrolytes**
Both low potassium and magnesium may be arrhythmogenic and must be supplemented especially in the context of arrhythmias.

4. **Strategies to limit infarct size (β-blocade, ACE-I and reperfusion)**

β-blockade
- Early β-blockade in limiting infarct size, reducing mortality and early malignant arrhythmias. All patients (including primary PCI and thrombolysis patients) should have early β-blockade, but ones with the following features will benefit most:
  - Hyperdynamic state (sinus tachycardia, ↑BP)
  - Ongoing or recurrent pain/reinfarction
  - Tachyarrhythmias such as AF
- Absolute contraindications: HR<60, SBP<100 mmHg, moderate to severe heart failure, AV conduction defect, severe airways disease.
- Relative contraindications: asthma, current use of calcium channel blocker and/or β-blocker, severe peripheral vascular disease with critical limb ishaemia, large inferior MI involving the right ventricle.
- Use short acting agent IV initially (metoprolol 1–2 mg at a time repeated at 1–2 minute intervals to a maximum dose of 15–20 mg) under continuous ECG and BP monitoring. Aim for a PR 60 and SBP 100–110 mmHg. If haemodynamic stability continues 15–30 minutes after last IV dose start metoprolol 50 mg tds. Esmolol is an ultra-short-acting IV β-blocker, which may be tried if there is concern whether the patient will tolerate β-blockers.

ACE inhibitors

After receiving aspirin, β-blockade (if appropriate) and reperfusion, all patients with STEMI/LBBB infarction should receive an ACE inhibitor within the first 24 hours of presentation.

- Patients with high risk/large infarcts particularly with an anterior STEMI, a previous MI, elderly population, heart failure, and impaired LV function on imaging (ECHO) will benefit most.
- The effect of ACE-I appears to be a class effect: use the drug you are familiar with (e.g. ramipril 1.25 mg od).

STEMI: reperfusion therapy (thrombolysis)

Rapid reperfusion is the cornerstone of current management of STEMI and is marked by normalization of ST-segments on ECG. Primary PCI and thrombolysis are the main reperfusion modalities. The best long term outcome is achieved with primary PCI.

Reperfusion occurs in 50–70% of patients who receive thrombolysis within 4 hours of onset of pain (c.f. ~20% of controls). As with primary PCI, thrombolysis also results in reduced mortality, LV dysfunction, heart failure, cardiogenic shock, and arrhythmias. However, the magnitude of the benefits obtained, are smaller. Furthermore, patients must undergo cardiac catheterization to delineate their coronary anatomy before revascularization (achieved at the same time with primary PCI). Time is once again of paramount importance and thrombolysis should be administered as soon as possible.

Indications for thrombolysis

- Typical history of cardiac pain within previous 12 hours and ST elevation in 2 contiguous ECG leads (>1 mm in limb leads or >2 mm in V1–V6).
- Cardiac pain with new/presumed new LBBB on ECG.
- If ECG is equivocal on arrival, repeat at 15–30 minute intervals to monitor progression.
- Thrombolysis should not be given if the ECG is normal, there is isolated ST depression (must exclude true posterior infarct), or ST elevation with no preceding history of pain.

Timing of thrombolysis

- Greatest benefit is achieved with early thrombolysis (especially if given within 4 hours of onset of first pain).
- Patients presenting between 12–24 hours from onset of pain should be thrombolysed only with persisting symptoms and ST-segment elevation.
- Elderly patients (>65 years) presenting within the 12–24 hour time period with symptoms are best managed by primary PCI as thrombolysis has demonstrated increased cardiac rupture.
- Patients presenting within 12–24 hours from onset of pain whose clinical picture appears to have settled should be managed initially as an NSTEMI followed by early catheterization.

Choice of thrombolytic agent

- This is partly determined by local thrombolysis strategy.
- Allergic reactions and episodes of hypotension are greater with SK.
- Bolus agents are easier and quicker to administer with a decrease in drug errors in comparison to fist generation infusions.
- rtPA has a greater reperfusion capacity and a marginally higher 30 day survival benefit than streptokinase, but an increased risk of haemorrhage.

- More recent rPA derivatives have a higher 90 minute TIMI-III flow rate, but similar 30 day mortality benefit to rtPA.
- A rtPA derivative should be considered for any patient with:
  - Large anterior MI especially if within 4 hours of onset.
  - Previous SK therapy or recent streptococcal infection.
  - Hypotension (systolic BP< 100 mmHg).
  - Low risk of stroke (age <55 years, systolic BP <144 mmHg).
  - Reinfarction during hospitalization where immediate PCI facilities are not available.

The characteristics of the major thrombolytic agents are on p 167.

Patients with greatest benefit from thrombolysis

- Anterior infarct
- Marked ST elevation
- Age > 75 years
- Impaired LV function or LBBB, hypotensive
- Systolic BP <100 mmHg
- Patients presenting within 1 hour of onset of pain.

Complications of thrombolysis

- Bleeding is seen in up to 10% of patients. Most are minor at sites of vascular puncture. Local pressure is sufficient but occasionally transfusion may be required. In extreme cases, SK may be reversed by tranexamic acid (10 mg/kg slow IV infusion).
- Hypotension during the infusion is common with SK. Lay patient supine and slow/stop infusion until the blood pressure rises. Treatment with cautious (100–500 ml) fluid challenges may be required especially in inferior/RV infarction. Hypotension is not an allergic reaction and does not warrant treatment as such.
- Allergic reactions are common with SK and include a low-grade fever, rash, nausea, headaches, and flushing. Give hydrocortisone 100 mg IV with chlorpheniramine 10 mg IV
- Intracranial haemorrhage is seen in ~0.3% of patients treated with SK and ~0.6% with rt-PA.
- Reperfusion arrhythmias (most commonly a short, self-limiting run of idioventricular rhythm) may occur as the metabolites are washed out of the ischaemia tissue. See p184 for management.
- Systemic embolization may occur from lysis of thrombus within the left atrium, LV, or aortic aneurysm.

Absolute contraindications to thrombolysis

- Active internal bleeding
- Suspected aortic dissection
- Recent head trauma and/or intracranial neoplasm
- Previous haemorrhagic stroke at any time
- Previous ischaemic stroke within the past 1 year
- Previous allergic reaction to fibrinolytic agent
- Trauma and/or surgery within past 2 weeks at risk of bleeding.

Relative contraindications to thrombolysis
- Trauma and/or surgery more than two weeks previously
- Severe uncontrolled hypertension (BP >180/110)
- Non-haemorrhagic stroke over 1 year ago
- Known bleeding diathesis or current use of anticoagulation within therapeutic range (INR 2 or over)
- Significant liver or renal dysfunction
- Prolonged (>10 min) of cardiopulmonary resuscitation
- Prior exposure to SK (especially previous 6–9 months)
- Pregnancy or post partum
- Lumbar puncture within previous 1 month
- Menstrual bleeding or lactation
- History of chronic severe hypertension
- Noncompressible vascular punctures (e.g. subclavian central venous lines).

Doses and administration of thrombolytic agents

Streptokinase (SK)

- Give as 1.5 million units in 100 ml normal saline IV over 1 hour.
- There is no indication for routine heparinization after SK as there is no clear mortality benefit and there is a small increase in risk of haemorrhage.

Recombinant tissue-type plasminogen activator (rtPA, alteplase)

- The GUSTO trial suggested the 'front-loaded' or accelerated rtPA is the most effective dosage regimen.
- Give 15 mg bolus IV then 0.75 mg/kg over 30 min (not to exceed 50 mg), then 0.5 mg/kg over 60 min (not to exceed 35 mg).
- This should be followed by IV heparin (see text).

Reteplase

- Give two IV bolus doses of 10 units 10 minutes apart.

Tenectaplase

- Give as injection over 10 seconds at 30–50 mg according to body weight (500–600 µg/kg).
- Maximum dose is 50 mg.

APSAC (anistreplase)

- Give as an IV bolus of 30 mg over 2–5 minutes.

STEMI: reperfusion by primary PCI

Time is of the essence for reperfusion, and each institution should have its recommended protocol. It is imperative that there are no delays in both the decision-making and implementation processes for reperfusion. If primary PCI is chosen one telephone call should ensure a rapid response.

Primary PCI

- Primary PCI is the current gold standard reperfusion strategy for treatment of STEMI.
- Primary PCI requires significant co-ordination between the emergency services, community hospitals and invasive centers. It must only be performed if: i) a primary PCI programme is available ii) patient presents to an invasive centre and can undergo catheterization without delay.

Indication for primary PCI:

- All patients with chest pain and ST-segment elevation or new LBBB fulfill primary PCI criteria (compare with indications for thrombolysis).
- This will include a group of patients where ST-segment elevation may not fulfill thrombolysis criteria.
- In general patients in whom thrombolysis is contraindicated should be managed by primary PCI. Cases where there is significant risk of bleeding must be managed individually.

Outcome in primary PCI

- Data from over 10 large randomized trials demonstrate a superior outcome in patients with STEMI who are treated with primary PCI in comparison to thrombolysis.
- There is a significant short-term, as well as long-term reduction in mortality and major cardiac events (MACE) (death, non-fatal reinfarction and non-fatal stroke) in STEMI patients treated with primary PCI. Furthermore, primary PCI patients have overall better LV function, a higher vessel patency rate and less recurrent myocardial ischaemia.
- Multiple studies (including PRAGUE-2 and DANAMI-2) have also demonstrated that interhospital transportation for primary PCI (community hospital to invasive center) is safe and primary PCI continues to remain superior to thrombolysis despite the time delays involved.

Complications

- Include bleeding from arterial puncture site, stroke, recurrent infarction, need for emergency CABG and death, which are similar to high risk PCI cases (~1%).
- The best results are obtained from high volume centers with experience of primary PCI.

- Each primary PCI center will have its own policy for management of cases including the use of LMWH/UFH, anti-platelet agents (e.g. IIb/IIIa) etc. It is generally accepted that in the acute phase only the 'culprit' lesion(s)/vessel(s) will be treated. The pattern of disease in the remainder of the vessels will determine whether total revascularization should be performed as an inpatient or an elective case in the future.
- STEMI patients treated with primary PCI can be discharged safely within 72 hours of admission without the need for further risk stratification.
- Primary PCI is more cost effective in the long term with significant savings from fewer days in hospital, need for readmission and less heart failure.
- Post discharge care, secondary prevention and rehabilitation remains identical to other MI cases.

Rescue PCI

As an adjunct to thrombolysis, this should be reserved for patients who remain symptomatic post thrombolysis (failure to reperfuse), or develop cardiogenic shock (see p190). We recommend all patients who do not settle post-thrombolysis (ongoing symptoms and ongoing ST-elevation with/without symptoms) to be discussed with local cardiac centre for urgent catheterization and revascularization.

Surgery for acute STEMI

Emergency surgical revascularization (CABG) cannot be widely applied to patients who suffer a MI outside of the hospital. CABG in uncomplicated STEMI patients after 6 hours from presentation is contraindicated secondary to significant haemorrhage into areas of infarction. Unstable patients have a very high peri-operative mortality.

CABG in the context of an acute STEMI is of value in the following situations:
- Persistent or recurrent chest pain despite thrombolysis/primary PCI.
- High-risk coronary anatomy on catheterization (LMS, LAD ostial disease).
- Complicated STEMI (acute MR, VSD).
- Patients who have undergone successful thrombolysis but with surgical coronary anatomy on catheterization.
- Patients known to have surgical coronary anatomy on catheterization performed prior to admission with STEMI.

STEMI: additional measures

ACE-I
p163.

Low molecular weight and unfractionated heparin
- UFH
  - There is no indication for 'routine' IV heparin following SK.
  - IV heparin (4000 U/max IV bolus followed by 1000 U/hr max adjusted for an aPTT ratio of 1.5–2.0 times control) should be used routinely following rt-PA and its derivatives for 24–48 hours.
- LMWH
  - There is trial data for the use of LMWH and thrombolysis. (e.g. enoxaparin 30 mg iv bolus, then 1 mg/kg SC q12h).
  - LMWH can be used at a prophylactic dose to prevent thromboembolic events in patients slow to mobilize as an alternative to UFH.

Clopidogrel
- Should be administered to all patients undergoing primary PCI (loading dose 300 mg po followed by 75 mg od).
- If coronary stents are used, patients should remain on clopidogrel for at least 1 month in bare-metal stents and 12 months in coated stents.
- More data is required to see whether longer-term treatment may be of benefit following thrombolysis alone.

Glycoprotein IIb/IIIa inhibitors
- There are multiple ongoing trials to evaluate their role in combination with thrombolysis and/or LMWH.
- Are recommended routinely in the context of STEMI patients treated with primary PCI. Lower doses of LMWH/UFH should be used (consult manufacturers information sheet for individual agents).
- They can also be used in the context of rescue PCI subsequent to failed thrombolysis although there is a greater risk of bleeding. Each case must be judged on its merits.

Magnesium
- Earlier trials giving Mg^{2+} before or with thrombolytics showed some benefit in mortality. ISIS-4 showed no benefit from the routine use of IV magnesium post-MI. However Mg^{2+} was given late (6 hours) after thrombolysis by which time the protective effect of Mg^{2+} on reperfusion injury may have been lost. Trials are ongoing trials.
- Current accepted role for Mg^{2+} is confined to Mg^{2+} deplete patients and patients with reperfusion, supraventricular, and ventricular arrhythmias.
- Dose: 8 mmol in 20 ml 5% dextrose over 20 minutes followed by 65 mmol in 100 ml 5% dextrose over 24 hours. (Contraindications: serum Cr >300 μmol/l, 3° AV block.)

Calcium antagonists
- Best avoided, especially in the presence of LV impairment.
- Diltiazem and verapamil started after day 4–5 in post-MI patients with normal LV function have a small beneficial effect.
- Amlodipine is safe to be used in patients with poor LV post-MI.
- Nifedipine has been shown to increase mortality and should be avoided.

Right ventricular (RV) infarction

- RV infarction results in elevated right-sided pressures (RA, RVEDP) and low left sided pressures (BP, CO).
- It is common in inferior STEMI.

Diagnosis

- *Clinical*: signs of right heart failure (↑JVP, Kussmaul's sign, pulsus paradoxus) with absence of pulmonary oedema in the context of a low output state (↓BP, cold peripheries).
- *ECG*: in patients with inferior STEMI a 0.1 mV (>1 mm) ST segment elevation in any one of leads V4R–V6R is highly sensitive and specific for RV infarction. See Fig. 4.14 for different ECG patterns identified in right sided precordial leads. Changes may be transient and present in the early stages only.
- *ECHO*: looking for RV dilation and wall motion abnormalities.

Management

- Aim to maintain a high RV preload:
  - Initially give 1–2L of colloid rapidly.
  - Avoid use of nitrates and diuretics as they reduce pre-load and can worsen hypotension.
  - In patients requiring pacing AV synchrony must be maintained to ensure maximal CO (atrial and ventricular wires).
  - Cardiovert any arrhythmias (SVT, AF/flutter or ventricular rhythms).
- Reduce afterload:
  - This is particularly important if there is concomitant LV dysfunction.
  - Insert IABP
  - Arterial vasodilators can be used with caution (Na nitroprusside, hydralazine) or ACE inhibitors.
- Inotropic support should ideally be avoided and used if all other measures fail to restore haemodynamic status.
- Reperfusion of the RCA (PCI and thrombolysis) has been demonstrated to improve RV function and reduce mortality.

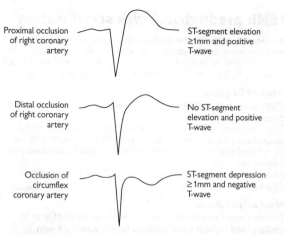

Proximal occlusion of right coronary artery — ST-segment elevation ≥1mm and positive T-wave

Distal occlusion of right coronary artery — No ST-segment elevation and positive T-wave

Occlusion of circumflex coronary artery — ST-segment depression ≥1mm and negative T-wave

Fig. 4.14 ST-elevation and T-wave configuration in lead V4R in inferoposterior AMI. Proximal occlusion of the RCA produces ST-elevation >1 mm and a positive T-wave. Distal occlusion is characterised by a positive T-wave but no ST-elevation. Occlusion of the circumflex artery produces a negative T-wave and ST-depression of at least 1 mm. Adapted with permission from Wellens HJ (1999). *N Engl J Med* **340**: 1383.

STEMI: predischarge risk stratification

It is important to identify the subgroup of patients who have a high risk of re-infarction or sudden death. They should undergo coronary angiography with view to revascularzation prior to discharge (if not treated with primary PCI) and/or electrophysiological investigations as necessary.

Primary PCI group

- STEMI patients treated with primary PCI are at a much lower risk of developing post MI complications.
- There is ongoing debate whether patients treated with primary PCI should have total revascularization as an inpatient or whether this can be achieved after functional testing on an outpatient basis. Follow your local policy.
- Patients who should have electrophysiological assessment prior to discharge are listed below.

Thrombolysis group

- Patients treated with thrombolysis should be risk stratified prior to discharge and high-risk patients should have in-patient (or early out-patient) angiography. High-risk patients include:
    - Significant post-infarct angina or unstable angina.
    - Positive exercise test (modified Bruce protocol) with angina, >1 mmST depression or fall in BP.
    - Cardiomegaly on CXR, poor LV function on ECHO (EF <40%).
    - Documented episodes of regular VEs and VT 24h post infarction.
    - Frequent episodes of silent ischaemia on Holter monitoring.

Electrophysiological study

All STEMI patients with i) non sustained VT and documented EF <40% or ii) sustained/pulse less VT/VF (regardless of EF) should undergo electrophysiological testing prior to discharge (MADIT and MUSTT trials) with view to defibrillator implantation.

Discharge and secondary prevention

- *Length of hospital stay in uncomplicated patients*: the thrombolysis group need to undergo risk stratification prior to discharge and tend to have a mean hospital stay of 5–7 days. The primary PCI group have shorter hospital stay between 3–4 days.
- Prior to discharge an agreed plan between patient (patient's family) and physician is necessary to address modifiable risk factors, beneficial medication, and rehabilitation programme.
- Modifiable risk factors include:
    - Management of lipids and use of statins.
    - Detection and treatment of diabetes.
    - Ensuring blood pressure is adequately controlled.
    - Counseling to discontinue smoking.
    - Advice on a healthy diet and weight loss.

- It is vital patients understand the medical regime and in particular the importance of long-term 'prognostic medication'. Unless there are contraindications all patients should be on a minimum of:
  - Aspirin 75 mg od (if true allergy, use clopidogrel 75 mg od).
  - ACE inhibitor at the recommended dosage.
  - Statin at the recommended dosage.
  - The role of long term formal anticoagulation is controversial.
- All patients must be plugged into a rehabilitation programme.

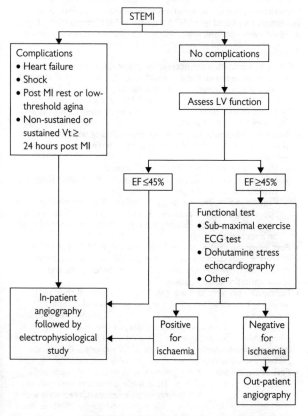

Fig. 4.15 Suggested stratergy post STEMI in patients who have undergone thrombolysis to determine the need for in-patient angiography/EPS. Adapted from Antman EM (2000) *Cardiovascular Therapeutics* 2nd edition. Saunders, Philadelphia.

STEMI: complications

Complications include:

- Continuing chest pain.
- Fever.
- A new systolic murmur—VSD, acute MR, or pericarditis.
- Dysrrhythmia (VT, AV block ectopics and bradycardia).
- Pump failure—hypotension, cardiac failure, and cardiogenic shock.

Complications are encountered more commonly in patients post STEMI, but can also be found in NSTEMI patients. In NSTEMI patients complications are more common where multiple cardiac events have occurred.

Further chest pain

- Chest pain post-MI is not necessarily angina. Careful history is needed to characterize pain. If there is doubt about the aetiology of pain in the absence of ECG changes, stress/thallium imaging may aid diagnosis.
- A bruised sensation and musculoskeletal pains are common in the first 24–48 hours, especially in patients who have received CPR or repeated DC shock. Use topical agents for skin burns.
- **Recurrent infarction** is an umbrella term including both extension of infarction in the original territory, or repeated infarct in a second territory.
  - Usually associated with recurrent ST elevation.
  - If cardiac enzymes not yet back to normal, a significant change is a twofold rise above the previous nadir.
  - Patients should ideally undergo immediate PCI. Thrombolysis is an alternative, but a less attractive approach. Standard thrombolysis criteria must be met. Bleeding is a risk (NB SK should not be used on a second occasion).
- **Post infarction angina** (angina developing within 10 days of MI) should be treated with standard medical therapy. All patients with angina prior to discharge should undergo cardiac catheterization and revascularization as an inpatient.
- **Pericarditis** presents as sharp, pleuritic, and positional chest pain, usually 1–3 days post infarct. It is more common with STEMI. A pericardial friction rub may be audible. ECG changes are rarely seen. Treat with high dose aspirin (600 mg qds po) covering with a proton pump inhibitor (eg lansoprazole 30 mg od po). Other NSAIDs have been associated with higher incidence of LV rupture and increased coronary vascular resistance and are probably best avoided.
- **Pericardial effusion** is more common with anterior MI especially if complicated by cardiac failure. Tamponade is rare and the result of ventricular rupture and/or haemorrhagic effusions. Detection is with a combination of clinical features and echocardiography. Most resolve gradually over a few months with no active intervention.

- **Pulmonary thromboembolism** can occur in patients with heart failure and prolonged bed rest. Routine use of prophylactic LMWH and UFH combined with early mobilization have reduced incidence of PE. Sources include lower limb veins and/or RV (see p638).

Fever

- Often seen and peaks 3–4 days post-MI.
- Associated with elevated WCC and raised CRP.
- Other causes of fever should be considered (infection, thrombophlebitis, venous thrombosis, drug reaction, pericarditis).

Ventricular septal defect post-MI

- Classically seen 24 hours (highest risk) to 10 days post-MI and affects 2–4% of cases.
- **Clinical features** include rapid deterioration with a harsh pan-systolic murmur (maximal at the lower left sternal edge), poor perfusion, and pulmonary oedema. The absence of a murmur in the context of a low output state does not rule out a VSD.
- **Diagnosis**
  - Echocardiography—the defect may be visualized on 2-D-ECHO and colour flow Doppler shows the presence of left-to-right shunt. Anterior infarction is associated with apical VSD and inferior MI with basal VSD. Failure to demonstrate a shunt on ECHO does not exclude a VSD.
  - PA catheter (especially in absence of ECHO or inconclusive ECHO results)—a step-up in oxygen saturation from RA to RV confirms the presence of a shunt, which may be calculated by:

$$Qp:Qs = \frac{(\text{Art sat} - \text{RA sat})}{(\text{Art sat} - \text{PA sat})} \text{ where } \begin{array}{l} Qp = \text{pulmonary blood flow} \\ Qs = \text{systemic blood flow} \end{array}$$

Management

Stabilization measures are all temporizing until definitive repair can take place. Hypotension and pulmonary oedema should be managed as described elsewhere. Important principles are:

- Invasive monitoring (PA catheter and arterial line) to dictate haemodynamic management. RA and PCWP dictate fluid administration or diuretic use. Cardiac output, mean arterial pressure and arterial resistance determine the need for vasodilator therapy.
- If SBP >100 mmHg, cautious use of vasodilator therapy, generally with nitroprusside, will lower the systemic vascular resistance and reduce the magnitude of the shunt. Nitrates will cause venodilatation and increase the shunt and should be avoided. Not be used with renal impairment.
- Inotropes if severely hypotensive (initially dobutamine but adrenaline may be required depending on haemodynamic response). Increasing systemic pressure will worsen shunt.
- In most cases intra-aortic balloon should be inserted rapidly for counter pulsation.
- Liaise with surgeons early for possible repair. Operative mortality is high (20–70%) especially in the context of peri-operative shock, infero-posterior MI and RV infarction. Current recommendations are for high-risk early surgical repair combined with CABG ± MV repair/replacement.
- If patient has been weaned off pharmacological and/or mechanical support it may be possible to postpone surgery for 2–4 weeks to allow for some level of infarct healing.

- Patients should ideally undergo catheterization prior to surgical repair to ensure culprit vessel(s) are grafted.
- Closure of the VSD with catheter placement of an umbrella-shaped device has been reported to stabilize critically ill patients until definitive repair is possible.

Acute mitral regurgitation post-MI

- MR due to ischaemic papillary muscle dysfunction or partial rupture is seen 2–10 days post MI. Complete rupture causes torrential MR and is usually fatal.
- More commonly associated with inferior MI (posteromedial papillary muscle) than anterior MI (anterolateral papillary muscle).
- 'Silent MR' is quite frequent and must be suspected in any post MI patient with unexplained haemodynamic deterioration.
- Diagnosis is by ECHO. In severe MR, PA catheterization will show a raised pressure with a large 'v' wave.

Management (p632)
- Treatment with vasodilators, generally nitroprusside, should be started as early as possible once haemodynamic monitoring is available.
- Mechanical ventilation may be necessary.
- Liaise with surgeons early for possible repair.

Pseudoaneurysm and free wall rupture

- Demonstrated in up to 6% of STEMI patients and leads to sudden death in 2/3.
- A proportion present subacutely with cardiogenic shock allowing time for intervention (see p190).
- Diagnosis of subacute cases can be made on a combination of clinical features of pericardial effusion, tamponade, and echocardiography.
- Patients who have undergone early thrombolysis have a lower chance of wall rupture.
- Stabilization of the patient follows similar lines to cardiogenic shock (p190). Case must be discussed with surgeons immediately, with view to repair.

Cocaine-induced MI

- The incidence of cocaine-induced MI, LV dysfunction, and arrhythmias are on the increase.
- It has been estimated that 14–25% of young patients presenting to urban emergency departments with non-traumatic chest pain may have detectable levels of cocaine and its metabolites in their circulation. Of this group 6% have enzymatic evidence of MI (figures are from USA).
- Most patients are young, non-white, male, cigarette smokers without other risk factors for ischaemic heart disease.

Diagnosis

- Can be difficult and must be suspected in any young individual with chest discomfort at low-risk of developing ischaemic heart disease.
- **Chest pain:** occurs most commonly within 12h of cocaine use. Effects can return up to 24–36h later secondary to long lasting active metabolites.
- **ECG:** is abnormal with multiple non-specific repolarization changes in up to 80% of cases and approximately 40% may have diagnostic changes of STEMI qualifying for reperfusion therapy (see p158).
- **Biochemical markers of cardiac injury:** can be misleading, as most patients will have elevated CK levels secondary to rhabdomyolysis. TnT and TnI are vital to confirm myocardial injury.

Management

General measures

- These are the same as for anyone presenting with an MI: Oxygen: high flow 5–10 L unless there is a contraindication; analgesia; aspirin 75 mg od.
- GTN: to be given at high doses as IV infusion (>10 mg/hr final levels) and dose titrated to symptoms and haemodynamic response (see STEMI).
- Benzodiazepines: to reduce anxiety.

Second line agents

- **Verapamil:** is given in high doses and has the dual function of reducing cardiac work load and hence restoring oxygen supply and demand, as well as reversing coronary vasoconstriction. Should be given cautiously as 1–2 mg IV bolus at a time (up to 10 mg total) with continuous haemodynamic monitoring. This should be followed by high dose oral preparation to cover the 24 hour period for at least 72 hours post last dose of cocaine (80–120 mg po tds).
- **Phentolamine:** is an α–adrenergic antagonist and readily reverses cocaine-induced vasoconstriction (2–5 mg IV and repeated if necessary). It can be used in conjunction with verapamil.
- **Labetalol:** has both α– and β–adrenergic activity and can be used after verapamil and phentolamine if patient remains hypertensive. It is effective in lowering cocaine-induced hypertension, but has no effect on coronary vasoconstriction.

- **Reperfusion therapy:** evidence for use of thrombolysis is limited and generally associated with poor outcome secondary to hypertension induced haemorrhagic complications. If patient fails to settle after implementing first line measures, verapamil, and phentolamine they should undergo immediate coronary angiography followed by PCI if appropriate (evidence of thrombus/vessel occlusion). In the event that angiography is not available thrombolytic therapy can be considered.
- **CAUTION: β-blockers must be avoided (e.g. propanolol).** They exacerbate coronary vasoconstriction by allowing unopposed action of the α–adrenergic receptors.

Teaching points: cocaine-induced MI

Pathogenesis
- The cause of myocardial injury is multifactorial including an increase in oxygen demand (↑HR, ↑BP, ↑contractility) in the context of decrease in supply caused by a combination of inappropriate vasoconstriction (in areas of minor atheroma), enhanced platelet aggregation, and thrombus formation.
- The effects can be delayed as the metabolites of cocaine are potent active vasoconstrictors and can remain in the circulation for up to 36 hours (or longer) resulting in recurrent wave of symptoms.

Other complications
- **Cocaine-induced myocardial dysfunction:** is multifactorial and includes MI, chronic damage secondary to repetitive sympathetic stimulation (as in pheochromocytoma), myocarditis secondary to cocaine impurities/infection, and unfavourable changes in myocardial/endothelial gene expression.
- **Cocaine-induced dysrrhythmias:** include both atrial and ventricular tachyarrhythmias, as well as asystole and heart block (see post-MI arrhythmias (p184–186) and cardiopulmonary resuscitation (p604)).
- **Aortic dissection** (see p660).

Ventricular tachyarrhythmias post-MI

1. **Accelerated idioventricular rhythm**
   - Common (up to 20%) in patients with early reperfusion in first 48h.
   - Usually self limiting and short lasting with no haemodynamic effects.
   - If symptomatic, accelerating sinus rate with atrial pacing or atropine may be of value. Suppressive anti-arrhythmic therapy (lignocaine, amiodarone) is only recommended with degeneration into malignant ventricular tachyarrhythmias.
2. **Ventricular premature beats (VPB)**
   - Common and not related to incidence of sustained VT/VF.
   - Generally treated conservatively and aim to correct acid-base and electrolyte abnormalities (aim K^+ >4.0 mmol/L and Mg^{2+}>1.0 mmol/L).
   - Peri-infarction β-blockade reduces VPB.
3. **Non-sustained and monomorphic ventricular tachycardia (VT)**
   - Are associated with a worse clinical outcome.
   - Correct reversible features such as electrolyte abnormalities and acid-base balance.
   - DC cardioversion for haemodynamic instability.
   - Non-sustained VT and haemodynamically stable VT (slow HR <100 bpm) can be treated with amiodarone (300 mg bolus IV over 30 min, followed by 1.2 g infusion over 24hr). Lignocaine is no longer recommended as first line. Procainamide is an effective alternative, but is arrhythmogenic.
   - For incessant VT on amiodarone consider overdrive pacing.
4. **Ventricular fibrillation and polymorphic VT**
   - A medical emergency and requires immediate defibrillation.
   - In refractory VF consider vasopressin 40U IV bolus.
   - Amiodarone 300 mg IV bolus to be continued as an infusion (see above) if output restored.

Atrial tachyarrhythmia post-MI

- Includes SVT, AF and atrial flutter.
- If patient is haemodynamically unstable must undergo immediate synchronized DC cardioversion.
- Haemodynamically stable patients can be treated with digoxin, β-blockers and/or calcium channel blockers (see p614).
- Amiodarone can be used to restore sinus rhythm. However, it is not very effective in controlling rate. Class I agents should generally be avoided as they increase mortality.
- In AF and flutter patients should undergo anticoagulation to reduce embolic complications if there are no contraindications.

Bradyarrhythmias and indications for pacing

Alternating or isolated RBBB/LBBB do not need pacing (unless haemodynamically unstable or progression to higher levels of block). New bifasicular block (RBBB with either LAD or RAD) or BBB with first degree AV block may require prophylactic pacing depending on the clinical picture. Indications for pacing should not delay reperfusion therapy. Venous access (femoral or internal jugular vein) should be obtained first and pacing wire inserted later. External temporary cardiac pacing, atropine (300 µg to 3 mg IV bolus) and isoprenaline can be used to buy time.

Bradyarrhythmias post-MI

1. **First degree AV block**
   - Common and no treatment required.
   - Significant PR prolongation (>0.20s) is a contraindication to β-blockade.
2. **Second degree AV block**
   This indicates a large infarction effecting conducting systems and mortality is generally increased in this group of patients.
   - Mobitz type I—is self limiting with no symptoms. Generally, requires no specific treatment. If symptomatic or progression to complete heart block will need temporary pacing.
   - Mobitz type II, 2:1, 3:1—should be treated with temporary pacing regardless of whether it progresses to complete heart block.
3. **Third degree AV block**
   - In the context of an inferior MI can be transient and does not require temporary pacing unless there is haemodynamic instability or an escape rhythm of <40 bpm.
   - Temporary pacing is required with anterior MI and unstable inferior MI.

Hypotension and shock post-MI

(see Cardiogenic shock p190)

The important principles in managing hypotensive patients with myocardial infarction are:
- If the patient is well perfused peripherally, no pharmacological intervention is required.
- Try to correct any arrhythmia, hypoxia, or acidosis.
- Arrange for an urgent ECHO to exclude a mechanical cause for hypotension (e.g. mitral regurgitation, VSD, ventricular aneurysm) that may require urgent surgery.

Patients may be divided into two subgroups:

1 Hypotension with pulmonary oedema.
- Secure central venous access—internal jugular lines are preferable if the patient may have received thrombolytic therapy.
- Commence **inotropes** (see p190, cardiogenic shock).
- Further invasive haemodynamic monitoring as available (PA pressures and wedge pressure monitoring, arterial line).
- Ensure optimal filling pressures, guided by physical signs and PA diastolic or wedge pressure. Significant mitral regurgitation will produce large v waves on the wedge trace and give high estimates of LVEDP.
- Ensure rapid coronary reperfusion (if not already done), either with thrombolytic therapy or primary PCI where available.
- Intra-aortic balloon counter pulsation (see p706) may allow stabilization until PCI can be performed.

2 Hypotension without pulmonary oedema.
- This may be either due to RV infarction or hypovolaemia.

Diagnosis
- Check the JVP and right atrial pressure. This will be low in hypovolaemia and high in RV infarction.
- RV infarction on ECG is seen in the setting of inferior MI and ST elevation in right-sided chest leads (V3R–V4R).

Management
- In either case cardiac output will be improved by cautious plasma expansion. Give 100–200 ml of colloid over 10 minutes and reassess.
- Repeat once if there is some improvement in blood pressure and the patient has not developed pulmonary oedema.
- Invasive haemodynamic monitoring with a PA catheter (Swan–Ganz) is necessary to ensure hypotension is not due to low left-sided filling pressures. Aim to keep PCWP 12–15 mmHg.
- Start inotropes if BP remains low despite adequate filling pressures.
- Use IV nitrates and diuretics with caution as venodilatation will compromise RV and LV filling and exacerbate hypotension.
- See p158 for management of RV infarction.

Cardiogenic shock

- Effects between 5–20% of patients and up to 15% of MI patients can present with cardiogenic shock.
- Management involves a complex interaction between many medical, surgical, intensive care teams with multiple invasive and non-invasive measures. Despite significant advances prognosis remains poor. Therefore, the absolute wishes of the patient with regard to such an invasive strategy should be respected from the onset.

Diagnosis

A combination of clinical and physiological measures:
- *Clinical:* marked, persistent (>30 min) hypotension with SBP <80–90 mmHg.
- *Physiological:* low cardiac index (<1.8 L/mm/m^2) with elevated LV filling pressure (PCWP >18 mmHg).

Management

- Complex and must be quick.
- Correct reversible factors including:
  - Arrhythmias and aim to restore sinus rhythm
  - Acid–base, electrolyte abnormalities
  - Ventilation abnormalities—intubate if necessary
- Rapid haemodynamic, echocardiographic, and angiographic evaluation:
  - *Haemodynamic:* to ensure adequate monitoring and access including central venous lines, Swan–Ganz, arterial line insertion, urinary catheter.
  - *Echocardiographic:* to assess ventricular systolic function and exclude mechanical lesions, which may need to dealt with, emergency cardiac surgery including mitral regurgitation (NB tall v waves on PCWP trace), VSD and ventricular aneurysm/psuedoanuerysm.
  - *Angiographic:* with view to PCI or CABG if appropriate.
- Aim to improve haemodynamic status achieving a SBP ≥90 mmHg guided by physical signs and LV filling pressures. As a general guide:
  PCWP <15 mmHg—cautious of IV fluids (colloids) in 100–200 ml aliquots.
  PCWP >15 mmHg—inotropic support ± diuretics (if pulmonary oedema).
- Inotropes should be avoided if at all possible in acutely ischaemic patients. The aim should be to rapidly restore/maximise coronary flow and off-load LV. Early revascularization is vital and has shown to decrease mortality. IABP will partially help achieve aforementioned goals.
- If haemodynamic status does not improve post-revascularization and IABP insertion, inotropes should be used. Choice of agent can be difficult and should partly be guided by local protocols and expertise. Generally accepted choices depend on the clinical picture and include:
  - If patient is hypotensive (± pulmonary oedema)—start with dopamine (up to 15 µg/kg/min) and if ineffective substitute to epinephrine and/or norepinephrine.

- If patient has adequate blood pressure (± pulmonary oedema)–
  dobutamine to increase cardiac output (starting at 2.5–5 µg/kg/min
  and increasing to 20 µg/kg/min) titrating to HR and haemodynamics.
  Phosphodiesterase inhibitors can be used as an alternative. If
  hypotension and tachycardia complicate dobutamine/PDI inhibitor
  treatment, (nor)epinephrine can be added to as a second agent to
  achieve desired haemodynamic effect.
- Use of diuretics, thrombolysis, GP IIb/IIIa antagonists, LMWH/UFH
  should follow normal principles and are based on the clinical
  picture.

Non-ST elevation myocardial infarction (NSTEMI)/unstable angina (UA)

UA and NSTEMI are closely related conditions with similar clinical presentation, treatment, and pathogenesis but of varying severity. If there is biochemical evidence of myocardial damage the condition is termed NSTEMI and, in the absence of damage, UA.

Unlike patients with a STEMI where diagnosis is generally made on presentation in the emergency department, diagnosis of NSTEMI/UA may not be definitive on presentation and evolves over the subsequent hours to days. Therefore, management of patients with NSTEMI/UA is a progression through a number of risk stratification processes dependent on history, clinical features, and investigative results; which in turn determine choice and timing of a number of medical and/or invasive treatment strategies.

The figure opposite is a summary of a recommended **integrated care pathway** illustrating a management plan for diagnosis and risk-directed treatment of a patient with STEMI/UA.

Clinical presentation

There are 3 distinct presentations:
- **Rest angina** (angina when patient is at rest).
- **New-onset severe angina.**
- **Increasing angina** (previously diagnosed angina which has become more frequent, longer in duration, or lower in threshold).

General examination (as indicated for all ACS (see p154) must be undertaken in particular to rule out pulmonary oedema, assess haemodynamic stability, cardiac valve abnormalities, and diaphoresis.

Integrated management plan

We recommend that all patients follow a local integrated care pathway on presentation. The various stages are broadly outlined below. See relevant pages for further information.
- **Initial stabilization** (see also ACS p154)
  - Transfer patient to area with continuous ECG monitoring and defibrillator facility.
  - Strict bed rest.
  - Give oxygen, aspirin 300 mg po, SL nitrate and mild sedation if required.
  - If pain persists give diamorphine 2.5–5 mg IV prn with metoclopramide 10 mg IV.
- **General investigations**—similar to STEMI patients (see p158) including blood for FBC, biochemical profile and markers of myocardial injury, lipid profile as well as CRP and TFT (if persistent tachycardia). Arrange portable CXR (rule out LVF, mediastinal abnormalities).
- **Confirm diagnosis** (see p194)
- **Risk stratification** (see p196) in order to determine appropriate medical and invasive treatment strategies. High risk patients should be admitted to CCU and low/intermediate patients to monitored beds in step-down unit.

- **Treatment** is based on patients risk and includes:
  - **Medical**
    i) anti-ischaemic (p200)
    ii) antiplatelet (p202)
    iii) anti-thrombic (p202)
  - Invasive strategies (p204).
- Secondary prevention and discharge

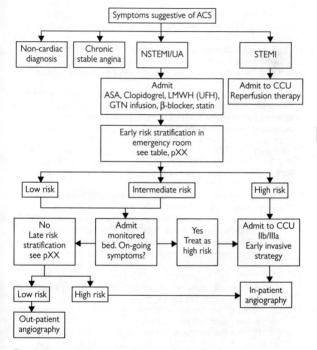

Fig. 4.16 NSTEM/VA—integrated care pathway.
Reproduced with permission from Ramrakha P and Moore K (2004). Oxford Handbook of Acute Medicine 2nd edition. Oxford University Press, Oxford.

NSTEMI/UA: diagnosis

Diagnosis in NSTEMI/UA is an evolving process and may not be clear on presentation. **A combination of history, serial changes in ECG and biochemical markers of myocardial injury** (usually over a 24–48 hour period) **determine the diagnosis**. Once a patient has been designated a diagnosis of ACS with probable/possible NSTEMI/UA (see p192) they will require:

1. **Serial ECGs:** changes can be transient and/or fixed especially if a diagnosis of NSTEMI is made. See p159 for localization of ischaemic areas.
   - ST-segment depression of ≥0.05 mV is highly specific of myocardial ischaemia (unless isolated in V1–V3 suggesting a posterior STEMI).
   - T wave inversion is sensitive but non-specific for acute ischaemia unless very deep (≥0.3 mV).
   - Rarely Q waves may evolve or there may be transient/new LBBB.
2. **Serial biochemical markers of cardiac injury are used to differentiate** between NSTEMI and UA, as well as determine prognosis. We recommend levels at 6, 12, 24, and 48 hours after last episode of pain. A positive biochemical marker (CK, CK-MB, or troponin) in the context of one or more of the aforementioned ECG changes is diagnostic of NSTEMI. If serial markers over a 24–72 hours period from the last episode of chest pain remain negative UA is diagnosed.
   - **Cardiac troponin T and I**—both are highly cardiac-specific and sensitive, can detect 'microinfarction' in presence of normal CK-MB, are not affected by skeletal muscle injury and convey prognostic information (worse prognosis if positive). Troponins can be raised in non-atherosclerotic myocardial damage (cardiomyopathy, myocarditis, pericarditis) and should therefore be interpreted in context of the clinical picture. Both TnT and TnI rise within 3 hours of infarction. TnT may persist upto 10–14 days and TnI up to 7–10 days. Results must be interpreted with caution in patients with chronic renal failure. See Fig.4.16 p193.
   - CK—levels do not always reach the diagnostic twice upper limit of normal and generally have little value in diagnosis of NSTEMI.
   - CK-MB—has low sensitivity and specificity—CK-MB isoforms improve sensitivity (CK-MB2>1 U/L or CK-MB2/CK-MB1 ratio >1.5), but isoform assays are not widely available clinically.
   - Myoglobin—is non-cardiac specific, but levels can be detected as early as 2 hours after onset of symptoms. A negative test is useful in ruling out myocardial necrosis.
3. **Continuous ECG monitoring** can detect episodes of silent ischaemia and arrhythmia. Both have been shown to be more prolonged with NSTEMI than in UA.

NSTEMI/UA: risk stratification

- NSTEMI/UA are a heterogeneous group of conditions with variable outcome. An assessment of risk for adverse outcome is vital to ensure formation of an adequate management plan.
- **Risk Stratification should begin on initial evaluation and continue throughout the hospital stay.** At each stage patients with a high chance of a poor outcome should be identified and managed appropriately.
- We recommend at least two formal risk stratification processes:
  1. **Early risk stratification:** (Fig.4.20, opposite) this should take place on presentation and forms part of the initial assessment used to make a diagnosis. It involves a combination of clinical features, ECG changes and biochemical markers of cardiac injury as demonstrated on p193. Patients are divided into high risk and intermediate/low risk.
  - **HIGH RISK** patients should be **admitted to CCU, follow an early invasive strategy**, and managed with a combination of:
    —ASA, clopidogrel, LMWH (UFH), IIb/IIIa.
    —anti-ischaemic therapy (first line β-blocker, GTN)
    —early invasive strategy (in-patient catheterization and PCI within 48 hours of admission).
  - **INTERMEDIATE/LOW RISK** patients should be admitted to a **monitored bed on a step-down unit and undergo a second in-patient risk stratification** once their symptoms have settled, to determine timing of invasive investigations. Initial management should include:
    —ASA, clopidogrel, LMWH (UFH).
    —anti-ischaemic therapy (first line β blocker, GTN).
    —undergo a **late risk stratification in 48–72 hours** from admission.
  2. **Late risk stratification:** (p198) involves a number of non-invasive tests to determine the optimal timing for invasive investigations in intermediate/low risk patients. It is generally performed if there have been no further episodes of pain/ischaemia at 24–48 hours after admission.
- Intermediate/low risk patients who develop recurrent pain and/or ischaemic ECG changes at any point during their admission, heart failure, haemodynamic instability in the absence of a non-cardiac cause should be managed as a high risk patient (IIb/IIIa and early invasive strategy).
- Fig.4.20 is a summary of a recommended integrated care pathway combining diagnosis, risk stratification and treatment.
- There are other risk stratification assessment scores including Braunwald and TIMI. As recommended above, high-risk patients from these assessments should also follow an early invasive strategy and intermediate/low risk patients a more conservative strategy.

Feature	High risk (At least 1 of the following features must be present)	Intermediate risk (No high-risk feature but must have 1 of the following)	Low risk (No high- or intermediate-risk feature) but may have any of the following features)
History	Accelerating tempo of ischaemic symptoms in preceding 48 hours	Prior MI, peripheral or cerebrovascular disease or CABG, prior aspirin use	
Character of pain	Prolonged ongoing (>20 minutes) rest pain	Prolonged (>20 minutes) rest angina now resolved, with moderate or high likelihood of CAD. Rest angina (<20 minutes) or relieved with rest or sublingual NTG	New-onset or progressive CCS Class III or IV angina the past 2 weeks without prolonged (>20 minutes) rest pain but with moderate or high likelihood of CAD
Clinical findings	Pulmonary oedema, most likely due to ischaemia. New or worsening MR murmur S_3 or new/ worsening rales. Hypotension, bradycardia, tachycardia. Age>75 years	Age>70 years	
ECG	Angina at rest with transient ST-segment changes >0/05 mV. Bundle-branch block, new or presumed new. Sustained ventricular tachycardia	T-wave inversions >0,2 mV. Pathological Q-waves	Normal or unchanged ECG during an episode of chest discomfort
Cardiac markers	Elevated (e.g. TnT or TnI >0/1 ng/mL)	Slightly elevated (e.g. TnT >0.01 but <0.1 ng/mL)	Normal

Fig. 4.17 Short-term risk of death non-fatal MI in patients with UA.
Adapted from Americal College of Cardiology Practice Guidelines.

NSTEMI/UA: late risk stratification

- The highest risk of adverse outcome in patients who are designated as intermediate/low risk on presentation is during the early phase of admission. Therefore, it is important that the second risk stratification process occurs within 24–48 hours of admission if the patient is stable.
- Late risk stratification is based on one of the following non-invasive investigations.
- A patient is regarded as being at high risk of adverse outcome if they fulfill one of the features listed below. These patients should have inpatient cardiac catheterization.

1. **Exercise ECG test**
- *Horizontal/down-sloping ST depression with:*
  - Onset at HR<120 bpm or <6.5 METS
  - Magnitude of >2.0 mm
  - Post exercise duration of changes >6 min
  - Depression in multiple leads reflecting multiple coronary distributions
- *Abnormal systolic BP response*
  - Sustained decrease of >10 mmHg or flat BP response with abnormal ECG
- *Other*
  - Exercise induced ST-segment elevation
  - VT
  - Prolonged elevation of HR

2. **Stress radionuclide myocardial perfusion imaging**
  - Abnormal tracer distribution in more than one territory
  - Cardiac enlargement

3. **LV imaging**
- *Stress echocardiography*
  - Rest EF <35%
  - Wall motion score index of >1
- *Stress radionuclide ventriculography*
  - Rest EF <35%
  - Fall in EF >10%

NSTEMI/UA: medical management

Anti-ischaemic therapy

All patients should be treated with a combination of the below agents to ensure adequate symptom control and a favourable haemodynamic status (SBP ≈ 100–110 mmhg, PR ≈ 60). *All patients should be treated with adequate analgesia, IV nitrates, β-blockers, and statins* (if no contraindications). Other agents can also be added depending on the clinical picture.

1. **Analgesia:** diamorphine 2.5–5 mg IV (with metoclopramide 10 mg IV). Acts as anxiolytic reduces pain and systolic blood pressure through venodilatation and reduction in sympathetic arteriolar constriction. Can result in hypotension (responsive to volume therapy) and respiratory depression (reversal with naloxone 400 µg to 2 mg IV).

2. **Nitrates:** GTN infusion (50 mg in 50 ml N saline at 1–10 ml/hr) titrated to pain and keeping SBP >100 mmHg. Tolerance to continuous infusion develops within 24 hours and the lowest efficacious dose should be used. Common side effects are headache and hypotension both of which are reversible on withdrawal of medication. *Absolute contraindication* is use of sildenafil (Viagra) in the previous 24 hours. This can result in exaggerated and prolonged hypotension.

3. **β-blockers:** should be started on presentation. Initially use a short acting agent (e.g. metoprolol 12.5–100 mg po tds), which if tolerated, may be converted to a longer acting agent (e.g. atenolol 25–1000 mg od). Rapid β-blockade may be achieved using short acting IV agents such as metoprolol. Aim for HR of ~50–60 beats/min.

   Mild LVF is not an absolute contraindication to β-blocker therapy. Pulmonary congestion may be secondary to ischaemic LV systolic dysfunction and/or reduced compliance. If there is overt heart failure β-blockade is contraindicated and a calcium antagonist (amlodipine 5–10 mg od) can be used. By reducing heart rate and blood pressure, β-blockers reduce myocardial oxygen demand and thus angina. When either used alone or in combination with nitrates and/or calcium antagonists, β-blockers are effective in reducing the frequency and duration of both symptomatic and silent ischaemic episodes.

4. **Calcium antagonists:** (diltiazem 60–360 mg po, verapamil 40–120 mg po tds) Aim to reduce HR and BP and are a useful adjunct to treatments 1–3 above. Amlodipine/felodipine 5–10 mg po od can be used with pulmonary oedema and in poor LV function. Calcium antagonists alone do not appear to reduce mortality or risk of MI in patients with UA. However when combined with nitrates and/or β-blockers they are effective in reducing symptomatic and silent ischaemic episodes, non-fatal MI and need for revascularization.

5. **Statins (HMG-CoA reductase inhibitors):** high dose statins (atorvastatin 80 mg od) have been shown to reduce mortality and recurrent MI in the acute setting. The role of statins in primary and secondary prevention of culture cardiovascular events is well documented.

6. **ACE inhibitors:** unlike patients with STEMI where early introduction of an ACE inhibitor has significant prognostic benefits, specific trials in the NSTEMI/UA setting are lacking. However, there is good evidence that patients both with low and high risk of cardiovascular disease will benefit from long-term ACE inhibition (HOPE and EUROPA Trials).

Antiplatelet therapy

All patients should be given aspirin and clopidogrel (unless contraindications)—IIb/IIIa antagonists to high-risk patients only.

1. **Aspirin:** (75–300 mg po) should be administered immediately in the emergency department and continued indefinitely (unless contraindications). It has been shown to consistently reduce mortality and recurrent ischaemic events in many trials. In patients with aspirin hypersensitivity or major gastrointestinal intolerance clopidogrel 75 mg od should be used.

2. **Thienopyidines:** clopidogrel (75 mg od) should be given on admission to all patients with proven NSTEMI/UA, regardless of risk, and continued for at least 1 month and ideally for 9 months. Clopidogrel, should be withheld in patients requiring CABG for 5–7 days to reduce haemorrhagic complications. Clopidogrel is preferred over ticlopidine because of its rapid onset of action and better safety profile.

3. **Glycoprotein IIb/IIIa antagonists:** there are multiple short- and long-acting commercially available molecules. These agents should be used in conjunction with aspirin, clopidogrel, and LMWH (or UFH). Eptifibatide and tirofiban should be used in high-risk patients with ongoing ischaemia and elevated troponin in whom an early invasive management strategy is not planned/available (<24 hours). In patients with an early invasive strategy all IIb/IIIa antagonists can be used. Infusion is generally continued for 12 hours post PCI. Taken as a group these agents protect NSTEMI/UA patients from death and nonfatal MI during the acute phase of their presentation and 24 hours post intervention. See table opposite for doses and administration regime.

Antithrombotic therapy

All patients should be given a LMWH (UFH).

1. **Low molecular weight heparins (LMWH):** have been shown to be as good as, or superior to, UFH in short term reduction of death, MI and revascularization in patients with NSTEMI/UA. They should be used in conjunction with aspirin and clopidogrel in all patients on presentation and continued for 2–5 days after last episode of pain and ischaemic ECG changes. Other advantages over UFH include subcutaneous administration, lack of monitoring, reduced resistance and thrombocytopaenia. The table opposite lists the doses of various agents in use for NSTEMI/UA.

2. **Unfractionated heparin (UFH):** multiple trials have demonstrated reduction of risk of death and MI in patients with UA/NSTEMI. UFH should be started on presentation as an alternative to LMWH in conjunction with aspirin and clopidogrel. Infusion should be continued for 2–5 days subsequent to last episode of pain and/or ischaemic ECG changes. Initial bolus of 60–70 U/kg (maximum 5000 U) should be followed by an infusion of 12–15 U/kg/h (≈1000 U/h). The infusion rate should be altered to achieve an aPTT value of 1.5–2.0 times control. Coagulation should be checked initially every 6 hours followed by once every 24 hours after two consistent values have been obtained.

Thrombolysis

There is no evidence to suggest that combing thrombolytic agents with aspirin, LMWH and conventional anti-ischaemic therapy is of benefit. In the TIMI IIIB trial the rtPA group had a worse outcome at 6 weeks and risk of bleeding was also greater with the thrombolyis group.

Doses of LMWH IIb/IIIa antagonists licensed for NSTEMI/UA

- LMWH
  - *dalteparin*   120 U/kg bd (max 10,000 U twice daily)
  - *enoxaparin*   1 mg/kg bd (100 U/kg twice daily)
- IIb/IIIa antagonists
  - *abciximab* (*Reopro*®)
    Bolus 250 mcg/kg over 1 minute followed by IV infusion
    125 ng/kg/min
  - *tirofiban* (*Aggrastat*®)
    400 ng/kg/min for 30 minutes followed by IV infusion
    100 ng/kg/min
  - *eptifibatide* (*Integrilin*®)
    Bolus 180 mcg/kg followed by IV infusion 2 mcgg/kg/min

NSTEMI: invasive vs. non-invasive strategies

The current evidence supports early angiography and revascularization in patients who present with either high-risk features or intermediate/low-risk features with ongoing symptoms. Furthermore, low- and intermediate-risk patients who settle on medical therapy should undergo symptom-limited non-invasive stress testing to identify a cohort of patients with an increased risk of adverse outcome. This second group will also benefit from an early invasive management.

Patients managed with an early conservative strategy tend to have an increased need for anti-anginal therapy, rehospitalistaion for angina, and many undergo coronary angiography within the year.

The following groups are recommended to benefit from an early invasive strategy (inpatient cardiac catheterization and PCI):

- **Patients with high risk features of NSTEMI/UA.**
  - Recurrent angina/ischaemic ECG changes despite optimal medical therapy.
  - Elevated troponin.
  - New/presumed new ST-segment depression.
  - Chest pain with clinical features of heart failure (pulmonary oedema, new/worsening MR, S3 gallop).
  - Haemodynamic instability.
  - Sustained ventricular tachycardia.
- **Poor LV systolic function (EF <40%).**
- **Patients allocated to low/medium-risk in whom, subsequent non-invasive testing demonstrates high-risk features.**
- **PCI in previous 6 months.**
- **Previous CABG.**
- **Patients with other comorbidities** (e.g. malignancy, liver failure, renal disease) in whom risks of revascularization are not likely to outweigh benefits.

Discharge and secondary prevention

- **Length of hospital stay** will be determined by symptoms and the rate of progression through the NSTEMI/UA pathway. Generally patients are hospitalized for 3–7 days.
- **Secondary prevention** remains of paramount importance and is similar in principle to STEMI patients.

Cardiac catheterization and intervention

Radiation protection in the catheter laboratory

All practitioners delivering ionizing radiation during medical procedures must attend a radiation protection course (IRMER Ionising Radiation Medical Exposure Regulations 2000). Furthermore staff working in the catheterization laboratory should be issued with radiation monitoring badges, for the body and neck, which should always be worn whilst in the catheter lab. These badges should be checked monthly to assess doses of radiation received by individual members of staff. No unnecessary staff should be within the catheter lab during a procedure, and all staff that needs to be in the lab should be as far from the tube as practical.

Minimizing patient dose
- Minimize screening time and minimize acquisition time.
- Keep distance between x-ray tube and image intensifier to a minimum.
- Use collimation and cones to minimize the irradiated area.
- Use lower magnifications when possible.
- Use lowest number of frames/second to allow adequate imaging.
- For prolonged procedures, the intensifier should be moved regularly a few degrees to try to minimize the possibility of skin burns.

Minimizing operator dose
- Lead aprons and lead collars should be worn.
- Additional screening should be used where available
  - Lead apron below table.
  - Mobile lead screen to go between operator and source.
- As above, minimize x-ray exposure by reducing screening and acquisition time.
- Some projections (e.g. LAO) give much higher scatter of x-ray, and operators should be aware of this.

The dose for an interventional cardiologist has been calculated as 60 mSv (based upon 150 working days per year and 4 interventions per day). The calculated effective dose if the operator wears the correct lead apron and thyroid collar is less than 5 mSv/yr. The maximum allowed dose is 20 mSv/yr.

Vascular access: the femoral artery

Procedure for femoral artery access

- The standard approach for left heart catheterization is the right common femoral artery.
- The artery is located by palpating below the inguinal ligament, the ideal position for puncture being approximately 3 cm below the inguinal ligament and slightly lateral to the position of the vessel.
- The area should be anaesthetized generously with of local anaesthetic (usually 10 ml of 2% or 20 ml of 1% lignocaine). Warn the patient of 'pins and needles' or transient numbness in the leg that may be caused by the effects of lignocaine on the femoral nerve.
- A small incision (3–5 mm) made in the overlying skin. The tissue underlying this incision may then be dilated; commonly this is done by using curved 'mosquito' forceps.
- The procedure used to puncture the artery is known as the 'Seldinger technique'. A hollow needle is introduced slowly; it is often possible to feel the pulsations of the artery via the needle before the vessel is punctured. When the needle is introduced into the vessel, pulsatile flow confirms its position in the arterial lumen. At this point a 0.035" wire can be advanced into the vessel and towards the heart; this should be performed under fluoroscopic guidance.
- The needle is then withdrawn and a haemostatic sheath (usually 5Fr–8Fr diameter) is introduced over the wire, the haemostatic sheath allows the introduction of a guide wire and catheter into the femoral artery, whilst preventing excess bleeding from the femoral puncture site.

Sheath removal (see p212)

- This can be performed immediately after diagnostic angiography, or after an interval of 4–6 hours if heparin has been administered.
- Haemostasis can be achieved by manual compression or by using a compression device (e.g. Femstop™).
- Vascular closure devices (e.g. angioseal™ or perclose™) allow earlier removal of sheaths in anti-coagulated patients and may reduce bleeding complications.

Complications

- Femoral artery dissection.
- Femoral artery pseudoaneurysm.
- Distal embolization.
- Haematoma.
- Retroperitoneal haemorrhage/haematoma (particularly with high punctures of the femoral artery above the inguinal ligament).

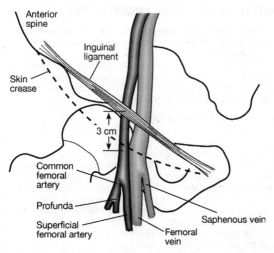

Fig. 5.1 Anatomy of the inguinal canal: the femoral vein lies medial to the femoral artery. The arterial puncture should be made ~3 cm below the inguinal ligament.

Vascular access: the radial artery

The radial approach for coronary angiography is now widely accepted. There are several advantages including a reduction in vascular complications, and the ability to mobilize patients immediately following their procedure. Patient selection for radial access should include palpation of the radial artery to confirm pulsations are present and then an Allen's test (see table opposite). In the absence of robust supply via the ulnar artery the radial approach should not be used.

Procedure for radial artery approach

- Consent patient.
- Perform Allen's Test.
- Remove all jewellery from arm, shave area, and disinfect.
- Local anaesthesia: Use 1–2 ml of 2% lignocaine instilled via a 25 gauge needle (i.e. enough to anaesthetize, but not to distort the anatomy).
- The artery should be palpated with the index and middle fingers, the index finger lifted, and the artery punctured at 45 degrees. The artery should be punctured as proximally as possible, and care should be take to avoid the flexor retinaculum.
- Once pulsatile flow is obtained, a guidewire can then be advanced through the needle and into the vessel.
- It is usual to make a small incision in the skin to allow passage of an arterial sheath. Care should be taken not to damage the radial artery whilst making this incision. Thus the blade should be used to incise in the longitudinal plane rather than transversely to reduce the risk of completely transecting the artery.
- A variety of long and short sheaths are commercially available. The advantage of long sheaths is that they minimize trauma to the radial artery.

Complications

- Radial artery spasm.
  This is the commonest complication of radial artery puncture and sheath introduction. There are various techniques to try and prevent radial artery spasm from occurring, these include:
  - Careful patient selection, avoiding small and difficult to palpate radial arteries.
  - Adequate patient sedation if required—pain provokes spasm.
  - The use of a 'cocktail' of drugs introduced directly into the radial artery. A variety of different regimens have been described. We use 1 mg ISDN, 2.5 mg verapamil and 2500 U heparin made up to 10 ml with normal saline. Repeated doses of nitrates or verapamil (up to 5 mg) given directly into the sheath or in the catheter may be required.
  - Shorter sheaths may be better tolerated.
  - Some sheaths have a hydrophilic coating to try to reduce spasm and for less discomfort on removal.
  - Always use guide wire to straighten catheters prior to removal from the aortic arch through the radial shoath.

The Allen's Test

Manual compression

- Compress radial and ulnar arteries.
- Ask patient to open and close their fingers making a fist (this will cause the hand to blanche).
- Release ulnar artery.
- Allen's test is POSITIVE if the colour of the palm of the hand re-turns to normal within 10 seconds (confirming that the ulnar circulation is intact).

Plethysmography

- Attach plethysmography probe (pulse oximetry).
- Compress both the radial and ulnar arteries (the plethysmography trace will flatten).
- Release ulnar artery.
- The test is POSITIVE if the plethysmograph curve is seen to return to normal (confirming that the ulnar circulation is intact).

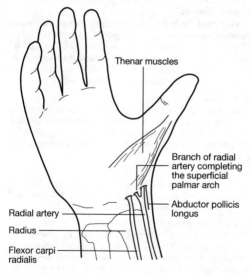

Fig. 5.2 Radial artery anatomy.

Vascular access site management

Femoral sheath removal

Femoral sheaths should only be removed by fully-trained members of staff. After diagnostic coronary angiography, when no or little heparin is given, the sheath may be removed immediately. Direct pressure should be applied just proximal to the site of the skin puncture for 5 to 10 minutes. After angioplasty, it is routine to wait for between 4 to 6 hours, an ACT <150 seconds suggests that the effect of systemic heparinization is wearing off, and it is acceptable for the sheath to be removed. Femoral clamps (FemoStop ®, RADI Medical Systems) can be used to reduce bleeding complications in patients.

Radial sheath removal

Radial sheaths are removed immediately after both diagnostic angiograms and angioplasty, as the position of the artery renders compression more simple. Compression bands (RadiStop®, RadiMedical Systems USA, TR-Band™, Terumo).

Vascular closure devices

Until recently mechanical compression was the only method for controlling bleeding from vascular access sites in the groin. Larger sheaths and the advent of the more widespread use of IIb/IIIa inhibitors have increased the risk of bleeding, and made homeostasis more difficult. Recently various closure devices have been introduced, the aim of these is to increase patient comfort, and reduce puncture related complications.

Suture based closure devices

Perclose® (Abbot Vascular, USA): This delivers a suture to the arterial puncture site. The device is sheath like in nature; needles are positioned above the sheath in the handle, and are deployed by a plunger. A 'clincher' that performs a knot-tying function completes a sliding surgical knot (see Fig. 5.3 opposite).

Collagen based closure devices

Devices that utilize a bioresorbable collagen plug that is deposited at the site of arteriotomy via a sheath, such devices include the VasoSeal® (Datascope Corp, USA) and Angio-Seal® (St Jude Medical, USA).

Other mechanical closure devices

StarClose® features an Nitinol® clip that is designed to promote the primary healing process to achieve a secure closure of femoral artery access sites following diagnostic or interventional vascular procedures. This clip provides 360 degree tissue apposition for rapid healing and hemostasis.

Drug-based closure devices

Clo-Sur® P.A.D (Medtronic, USA) this device contains a naturally occurring biopolymer Polyprolate acetate. This polymer has a coagulant property when brought into contact with heparinised blood. The device is placed over the puncture and the haemostatic sheath is removed. Direct continuous pressure is applied until haeomstasis is achieved.

o

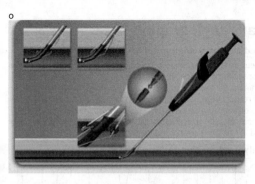

Fig. 5.3 Perclose™ vascular closure device.

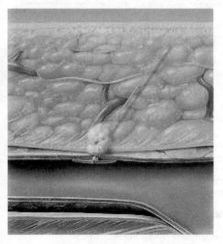

Fig. 5.4 Angioseal™ vascular closure devices.

Coronary angiography

Pre-shaped coronary angiographic catheters

The catheters used in diagnostic coronary angiography come in a wide variety of pre-formed shapes. In the UK the most commonly used pre-shaped catheters are the Judkins Left 4 and Judkins Right 4 (known as the JL4 and JR4 respectively), used to image the left and right coronary arteries, and the pigtail catheter used for left ventriculography. The diameter of catheters is measured in French gauge (Fr); catheters between 4Fr (0.053") and 8Fr (0.105") are commonly used.

Commonly used cardiac catheter shapes

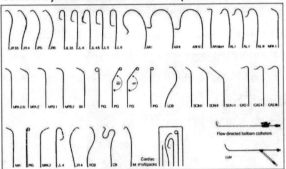

Catheter advancement and manifold usage

A 'J' tipped 0.035" guide wire is placed within the flushed catheter, which is then passed into the haemostatic sheath. The guide wire is advanced ahead of the catheter under fluoroscopic guidance, until it reaches the aortic root, just above the aortic valve. The catheter is then advanced to this position and the guiding wire is removed. To ensure that no air or clot is within the catheter a small volume of blood (5 ml) is aspirated from the catheter directly into a syringe and discarded. The catheter is then carefully connected to a 2-way manifold which allows pressure monitoring, saline flushing, and contrast injection through a closed system.

Contrast injection

Great care must be taken at all times to ensure that air is not injected into the coronary arterial tree. The injection syringe should be filled with contrast from the reservoir, and then the syringe held with the plunger elevated such that any air bubbles rise to the top of the syringe Contrast should then be injected at a continuous rate, aiming to full opacify the coronary vessel of interest. Care should be taken that the pressure trace prior to injection is normal—damping suggests an ostial stenosis, excessively deep intubation, or selective intubation of a branch.

Coronary angiography/left ventriculography

Left coronary artery
- The 50° left anterior oblique (LAO 50) is the best projection for cannulation of both the left and right coronary ostia.
- In reality however the left coronary ostium is often cannulated with the tower in the antero-posterior (AP) position.
- The JL4 catheter will almost invariably cannulate the left coronary ostium without manipulation.
- In patients with large aortic roots (large, hypertensive patients) the JL5 (with a larger curve) may be needed, and conversely a smaller root may need a smaller catheter curve, the JL3.5.

Right coronary artery
- The LAO 50 projection is best used for cannulation of the right coronary ostium.
- The JR4 catheter is introduced to the aortic root, until it lies 1–2 cm above the aortic valve.
- The catheter is then rotated ('torqued') in a clockwise direction such that the catheter tip rotates towards the right coronary ostium. It may be necessary to reduce the torque to prevent the catheter from over-shooting.
- There is often a noticeable lateral movement as the catheter enters the artery.
- Before contrast is injected it must be ensured that the pressure tracing transduced from the tip of the catheter is not damped.
- NB: Damping can suggest that the catheter has selectively intubated the conus branch of the right coronary artery, and injection of contrast into this vessel can induce ventricular arrhythmias.

Left ventriculography
- Position pigtail catheter a few centimeters above the aortic valve and pull wire back 5–10 cm to make catheter tip soft, and push gently (the catheter may cross at this point).
- If catheter does not cross, apply torque as it is gently withdrawn.
- If this technique is not successful, use a straight soft-tipped guide wire and catheters that allow that guide wire to be 'pointed' at the valve (e.g. AL1 or JR4). This may improve the chances of crossing the valve.
- Once the catheter has been placed in a stable (free of ectopics) position in the mid-LV cavity, connect to manifold and measure pressure.
- Disconnect manifold catheter connected to a power injector and expel all air.
- Set injection rate: typically 25–30 ml of contrast at a rate of 10 ml/s. Warn patient about hot flush and the feeling of extra systoles.
- When the left ventriculogram has been performed the catheter is reconnected to the manifold to allow pressure recording as the catheter is withdrawn across the aortic valve (the pullback pressure).

Interpreting the coronary angiogram

LCA angiographic views

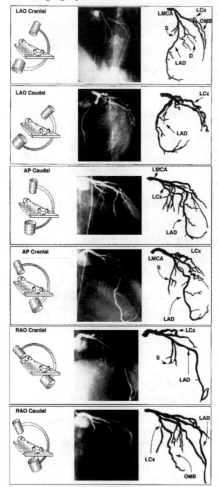

Fig. 5.6 Reproduced with permission from Braunwald E (ed) (2001). *Heart Disease: A Textbook of Cardiovascular Medicine.* 5th ed. WB Saunders: Philadelphia.

RCA angiographic views

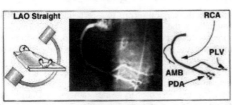

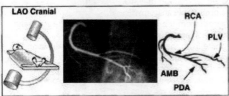

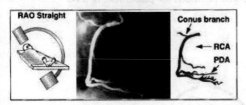

Fig. 5.7 Reproduced with permission from Braunwald E (ed) (2001). *Heart Disease: A Textbook of Cardiovascular Medicine*. 5th ed. WB Saunders: Philadelphia.

Angiographic study of grafts

It is important to study the surgical record to ascertain how many grafts were placed at the time of the operation. Sometimes, useful information (often from a surgeon's diagram) can be obtained as to the position in the ascending aorta that the grafts arise from. As a rule leftwards facing grafts are best cannulated from the RAO 50 projection, and rightwards pointing grafts are best cannulated in the LAO 50 projection. It may be necessary to perform an aortogram to visualize the position of grafts. Specialist catheters (e.g. the left coronary bypass catheter or LCB) have been designed to aid cannulation of grafts.

There is usually a predictable anatomy:

- PDA grafts originate from the right anterior aspect of the aorta and run vertically to the inferior surface of the heart.
- OM grafts originate from the left anterior aspect of the aorta and arc towards the posterolateral surface of the heart.
- LAD and diagonal grafts originate from an intermediate position and run laterally towards the anterior interventricular groove.

Common aortic positions for placement of SVG

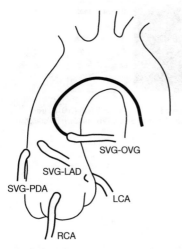

Fig. 5.8 Reproduced with permission from Braunwald E (ed) (2001). *Heart Disease: A Textbook of Cardiovascular Medicine.* 5th ed. WB Saunders: Philadelphia.

Complications of angiography

Peripheral vascular complications

Haematoma

The incidence of haematoma formation is related to the following factors:

- Length of time sheath is left in place.
- Gauge (size) of sheath.
- Anticoagulation.
- Risk factors e.g. hypertension, obesity, and pre-existing peripheral vascular disease.
- Technique of sheath removal.

Features that suggest a haematoma may require further investigation are an overlying bruit, expansile mass, and a large tense swelling.

Pseudoaneurysm

A pseudoaneurysm represents a rupture of the femoral arterial wall at the site of puncture, with the formation of a false aneurysm involving the media and adventitia. They are best visualized on ultrasound examination. Small pseudoaneurysms can often be managed by direct compression; however large pseudoaneurysms may require thrombin injection, or surgical intervention.

Haemorrhage

If prolonged then direct pressure (either manually or using a clamping device) may be needed. Heparin anticoagulation can be reversed using protamine.

Limb ischaemia

Rare, and usually occurs in patients with pre-existing limb ischaemia. If limb ischaemia is suspected then urgent vascular surgical team review should be sought.

Contrast reactions

Mild contrast reactions such as rash, urticaria, blurred vision and rigors are relatively common. These symptoms may settle spontaneously, but are often treated with a combination of IV chlorpheniramine 10 mg and IV hydrocortisone 100–200 mg. Anaphylactic reactions are rare, these should be treated with chlorpheniramine and hydrocortisone, but also plasma expanders and IM adrenaline.

Vasovagal reactions

These are common both during angiography and at the time of sheath removal and characterized by hypotension and bradycardia. They are treated with IV atropine and volume expanders.

Arrhythmia

Brief episodes of SVT are common and often transient. During catheter manipulation (esp. in the LV) salvoes of VT are common. VF may occur during coronary artery injection, and should be treated with rapid defibrillation.

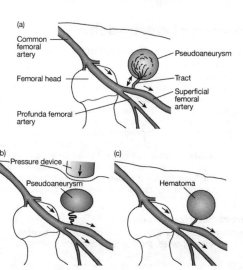

Fig. 5.9 Anatomy of a pseudoaneurysm. Panel A: Bleeding along a small tract allows blood to collect within the extra-vascular tissues. Manual compression fails to obliterate the tract (Panel B) and allows the haematoma to persist. Failure of thrombosis of the haematoma produces an extra-vascular collection with persistent connection and flow from the main artery (panel C). This can be visualized on USS (see below).

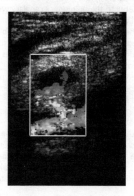

Fig. 5.10 USS of femoral pseudoaneurysm demonstrating flow (colour) in the aneurysm above the femoral artery.

Right heart catheterization

Indications for right heart catheterization include:

- Evaluation of cardiac shunts.
- Evaluation of valvular heart disease.
- Dyspnoea not explained by non-invasive investigation.

The acute settings in which right heart catheterization can be helpful (e.g. intensive drug therapy in cardiogenic shock) will not be discussed here.

Access to the right heart is usually achieved via the right femoral vein (RFV). The right femoral vein is located 0.5 cm to 1 cm medial to the femoral arterial pulsation (Fig. 5.1 p209). An 18-gauge needle, attached to a syringe partially filled with saline, can be used to locate the position of the vein, followed by the larger bore needle. When venous blood is freely aspirated a 0.035" guide wire is passed in to the vein, using a technique similar to femoral artery cannulation and a haemostatic sheath introduced.

Right heart catheterization protocol

- A 'multipurpose' catheter or balloon-tipped catheter may be used.
- Ensure that catheter is flushed, and that the transducer is correctly zeroed.
- Advance catheter to IVC, and further to the right atrium. Record the phasic and mean pressures.
- It is customary to then advance the catheter to the pulmonary artery wedge position. Advance into the RV. A combination of rotation of the catheter and gentle traction will allow the catheter to flick upwards into the RVOT. It can then be advanced into the main PA and out to the periphery. Occasionally the guide wire is necessary to achieve this.
- Advance the catheter to the pulmonary capillary wedge position, and record phasic and mean pressures.
- With a pigtail catheter in the LV measure and record the LV pressures. Record simultaneous PCWP and LV pressures ensuring that the scale allows interpretation of the end diastolic pressures with accurately (to assess for MV gradient).
- Withdraw the wedge catheter slightly and record pulmonary artery phasic and mean pressure. Obtain oxygen saturations from the main PA (also RPA and LPA if a PDA is suspected).
- Withdraw the pulmonary catheter to the RV. Measure and record simultaneous RV and LV pressures.
- Withdraw the catheter to the RA and measure the pressures again.
- The LV catheter should be pulled back to the ascending aorta while the pressure is being monitored to record any pull-back gradient. Aortic saturations should be measured to allow calculation of cardiac output (see opposite) and to compare with saturations from the R side if a shunt is suspected.
- For shunts a full saturation run should be performed (SVC, high-mid-and low-RA, IVC, RV, MPA, RPA, LPA, etc).

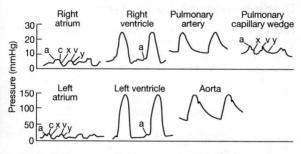

Fig. 5.11 Cardiac catheterization—normal pressure waveforms.

Cardiac output and LV Function

Cardiac output is most often measured using the thermodilution method with a pulmonary flotation catheter.

Cardiac output can also be measured using the Fick principle, which assesses the difference between the pulmonary arterial and aortic O_2 saturation.

$$\text{Cardiac output (l/min)} = \frac{\text{oxygen consumption (ml/min)}}{(\text{Ao SaO}_2 - \text{PA SaO}_2) \times \text{Hb} \times 1.34}$$

Systemic and pulmonary vascular resistance

Pulmonary vascular resistance is an important prognostic factor in patients with valvular heart disease, heart failure and cor pulmonale. The measurement of PVR and SVR is especially important in patients being assessed for cardiac transplantation.

PVR and SVR are measured Woods units (mmHg/l/min) or dyness cm^{-5}, with 80 dynes cm^{-5} = 1 wood unit.

$$\text{Cardiac output} = \frac{\text{mean aortic pressure} - \text{mean right atrial pressure}}{\text{systemic vascular resistance}}$$

$$\text{Cardiac output} = \frac{\text{mean PA pressure} - \text{mean left atrial pressure}}{\text{pulmonary vascular resistance}}$$

Cardiac catheterization in valve disease

Valve stenosis

Several parameters can be assessed during cardiac catheterization.

• **Peak-to-peak gradient**

Aortic and LV pressures are recorded during withdrawal of the pigtail catheter across the aortic valve. The gradient is the difference between peak aortic and peak LV pressure.

• **Peak instantaneous gradient**

More accurate and measured using a double lumen pigtail catheter.

• **Mean gradient**

The mean pressure gradient measured using planimetry of the area by aortic and LV pressure traces. This can be used to calculate valve area using the Gorlin equation, and a similar method can be used to assess the mitral valve area.

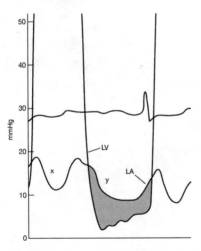

Fig. 5.12 Simultaneous LV and PCWP tracing in mitral stenosis. Reproduced with permission from Braunwald E (ed) (2001). *Heart Disease: A Textbook of Cardiovascular Medicine.* 5th ed. WB Saunders: Philadelphia.

Valve regurgitation

• The severity of aortic regurgitation can be estimated by performing an aortogram. In severe aortic regurgitation the LV is seen to opacify within one or two beats after contrast injection.

• Mitral regurgitation may be assessed by left ventriculography, with contrast seen to opacify the left atrium and pulmonary veins in severe regurgitation. In addition mitral regurgitation may be associated with a prominent 'V' wave in the pulmonary capillary wedge tracing.

Intravascular ultrasound

Intravascular ultrasound (IVUS) is a technology that allows direct visualization of atherosclerotic plaque and the vessel lumen, with recent advances allowing the echogenic characteristics of an IVUS image to give insights into the underlying histology. Ultrasound images are produced by passing an electrical current through a piezoelectric crystal that expands and contracts to produce sound waves when electrically stimulated. These sound waves are reflected from tissues, and return to the transducer where they are detected, converted to an electrical impulse which can be presented graphically. A phased array of crystals (usually 64) is used and these are sequentially activated to produce circumferential imaging. The equipment required to perform an IVUS examination involves a miniaturized ultrasound transducer mounted on a catheter (usually 2.6–3.5 Fr gauge), and computer interface that carries out image reconstruction.

Examination technique

- Intra-coronary ISDN and IV heparin should be administered.
- The IVUS catheter should be carefully advanced distal to the area of interest.
- A motorized pullback device is then used to draw the IVUS catheter proximally at a fixed speed.
- Landmarks such as side branches can be useful, and positions may also be recorded angiographically.

Advantages of ultrasound

- Full circumference of vessel wall is seen, not just two surfaces as in angiography, and is thus the method of choice to determine vessel luminal area.
- Useful in imaging ambiguous lesions such as:
  - Intermediate lesions of unknown severity.
  - Ostial stenosis.
  - Left main stem disease.
  - Disease at bifurcation sites.
- Images the plaque, not just the lumen.
- Allows optimal results during angioplasty and stenting.

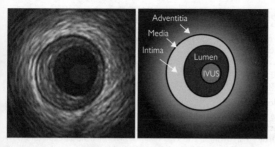

Fig. 5.13 Example of image obtained by IVUS.

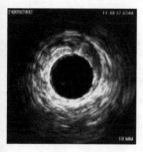

Fig. 5.14 IVUS image of a coronary stent.

Angioplasty and coronary stenting

- Currently coronary stents are implanted in >85% of revascularization procedures in the U.K.
- NICE guidelines state that 'stents should be used routinely for people with either stable or unstable angina or with acute myocardial infarction undergoing percutaneous intervention'

Angioplasty

Before stents became widely used in the mid to late 1990s, balloon angioplasty alone was the commonest percutaneous treatment for coronary artery narrowings. The two main designs of balloon catheters now commonly used are over-the-wire and rapid exchange systems, both types of catheter consists of three parts.
- The shaft: there are two main varieties
  - the hypotube, the advantage of which is a better balance between pushabillity and flexibility.
  - the corewire design which is superior in terms of flexibility.
- The lumen: coaxial design (a tube within a tube) is the most common.
- The balloon: these are constructed from varying plastics (e.g polyethylene, nylon) the mix of which affects the balloons compliance. The design of the tip is important, as tapered tips are less traumatic when crossing narrowings. The balloon may also have a hydrophilic coating to render it more lubricious.

'Plain old balloon angioplasty' (POBA) remains indicated in the treatment of some coronary artery narrowings, particularly small vessels, vein grafts, and bifurcation side branches, in which the benefit of stenting has not been clearly demonstrated.

Coronary stenting

The primary function of a stent is to act as a scaffold to maintain vessel patency, and thus much of the success of stents is primarily due to their mechanical ability to produce large acute gains in lumen dimensions. Stents can be made of stainless steel, cobalt based alloy, tantalum, nitinol, or polymer, however the majority of stents used today are stainless steel and balloon mounted. Many designs have been experimented with, in an attempt to obtain an ideal balance of flexibility and radial strength, with flexibility allowing the stent to be positioned easily, and radial strength necessary for the scaffold function of the stent.

Angioplasty procedure

- Consent the patient.
- Cannulate artery with chosen guiding catheter. Ideally the guiding catheter should be coaxial with the coronary ostium (thus allowing maximum support, and minimizing trauma to the vessel).
- A steerable 0.014" guidewire is introduced to the catheter via the haemostatic valve. The tip of the guidewire may be pre-shaped, however many operators prefer to take a straight guide wire and shape the tip by hand.
- Using x-ray screening, and contrast to delineate the coronary anatomy, the guidewire is advanced along the vessel, beyond the narrowing and placed as distally as possible in the vessel.
- An appropriately sized balloon is then chosen, the guiding catheter can be used as a reference when sizing the vessel. For calcific lesions and in-stent restenosis, shorter balloons with higher rated burst pressure may be better.
- The balloon is now advanced along the guidewire to the correct position. In some situations it will prove difficult to pass the balloon to the desired position and in these instances deeper insertion of the guide catheter, or a more supportive guide catheter may be needed.
- Radio-opaque markers are used to position the balloon accurately. Inflation should be undertaken under x-ray screening, to ensure that the balloon does not move.

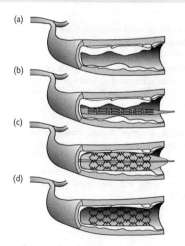

Fig 5.15 Coronary Stenting: A guide wire is introduced across the stastic segment of artery (a) and is used to position the stent (b). The stent is deployed by inflating the balloon (c). The balloon and guide wire are removed leaving the stent in place (d).

Restenosis following PTCA

Pathophysiology

The restenotic process consists of a series of complex events:

- Vessel injury leads to platelet activation and **local thrombosis.**
- An **inflammatory reaction** is invoked, with neutrophil, monocyte, and lymphocyte migration to the site of injury.
- **Smooth muscle proliferation** is driven by activated platelets and inflammatory mediators.
- Finally negative remodeling can occur.
- These processes occur at different rates, and may occur to different degrees depending upon the nature of vessel injury, and individual patient characteristics.

The Problem

Large randomized trials have established that following percutaneous intervention restenosis rates in the treated vessel are between 30 and 60% (following angioplasty) and 15–30% (following stent implantation), and higher still in selected high risk patients (e.g. diabetics). This relatively high incidence of **angiographic** restenosis however translates into revascularization in about 10% of patients, in whom **clinical** restenosis is said to have occurred.

Prevention of restenosis

Mechanical

Stent implantation

- Stent implantation reduces restenosis rates by increasing the mean luminal diameter after angioplasty, and preventing elastic recoil and adventitial constriction.

Optimization of stent deployment by IVUS guidance

- Using intravascular ultrasound to establish whether a stent has been adequately deployed improves the results of percutaneous intervention.

Pharmacological

Studies examining pharmacological interventions for reduction of restenosis have been disappointing.

Anti-thrombotic and anti-platelet treatment

Early aggressive anti-thrombotic and antiplatelet therapy using heparin, aspirin, IIb/IIa antagonists and clopidogrel reduce the incidence of acute stent thrombosis.

Drug eluting stents

- Similarities between tumor growth and benign neointimal proliferation introduced the concept that immunosuppressant and cytotoxic agents might be beneficial for preventing ISR.
- Incorporating these agents into stent coatings using a number of techniques has now enabled delivery of the active agent directly to its site of action, while limiting systemic side effects.
- Crucially the coatings allow sustained release of the agent, such that the therapy is present at the time that the target mechanism is physiologically active.
- The commonly used agents are sirolimus which has a cytostatic action and pacliataxel which is cytotoxic.

Drug eluting stents

Implantation of stents has to a great extent overcome the problem of elastic recoil and negative remodelling following PTCA. It is thus evident that neointimal proliferation, resulting in stent restenosis, remains the major limiting factor for stenting procedures. Much research has focussed on the role of anti-proliferative agents in the reduction of restenosis, and recently drug eluting stents have emerged as the preeminent solution to this problem. Drug eluting stents are coated stents, capable of releasing bioactive components into the local tissue and bloodstream. The advent of stents as a platform for the delivery of drugs, with subsequent reduction in rates of stent restenosis, is radically changing the treatment of patients with coronary artery disease. The number of CABG procedures performed worldwide is falling, with increasing numbers of patients, who previously would only have been candidates for CABG, being treated by PCI. Increasingly the favourable results obtained with DES mean that PCI is performed in 'complex' cases such as LMCA stenosis, diffuse disease, and bifurcation anatomy. The publication of several large RCT, which have demonstrated both the safety and efficacy of these stents, have supported the introduction of DES into routine clinical practice.

Sirolimus eluting stents

The drug sirolimus has potent anti-fungal, immunosuppressive, and anti-mitotic properties. Discovered during an expedition to Easter Island (Rapa Nui, and hence the original drug name of rapamycin), this agent was approved for rejection prophylaxis in renal transplantation in 1999, with trials of a sirolimus coated coronary stent following soon after.

- First in man experience of a sirolimus coated stent (45 patients) illustrated a virtual absence of neoinitimal proliferation at follow-up.
- The seminal RAVEL study enrolled 238 patients, randomly allocated to BX velocity stent, or sirolimus eluting BX velocity stent (the Cypher™ Stent). Reported 0% restenosis in the group treated with DES.
- The large scale SIRIUS study (n=1100) confirmed the potent anti-restenosis effects of Cypher™ stents.

Paclitaxel eluting stents

Paclitaxel has potent anti-tumour activity via its action as a microtubule stabilizing agent, the active agent was originally isolated from the bark of the Pacific yew tree (*Taxus brevifolia*). Coronary stents eluting paclitaxel have been extensively investigated.

- TAXUS I studied 61 patients randomly assigned to paclitaxel coated stent or bare metal stent, this study both established the safety of the stent, but also showed a MACE rate in the DES arm of 3%, compared with 10% in the BMS arm at one year follow-up.
- TAXUS II compared slow and moderate release formulations of paclitaxel with bare metal stenting, and found significantly lower MACE rates in both slow and moderate release DES (2.3%/4.7%), when compared to BMS treated control groups (20.2%).

SIRIUS and TAXUS, and each of their subsequent follow-up studies and registries, have established that Cypher™ and Taxus™ stents have similar, low rates of TLR (between 3–8%). However Cypher™ stents have been shown to have a greater reduction in binary angiographic restenosis and late lumen loss (LLL) compared to Taxus™ stents. LLL is known to be a strong predictor of both clinical and angiographic restenosis when DES have historically been compared to BMS. It remains to be seen whether the reduced LLL seen with Cypher™ stents translates to improved clinical outcomes. A direct comparison of Cypher™ and Taxus™ stents has recently been reported (the REALITY trial).

NICE recommends the use of a DES in PCI for patients with symptomatic CAD in whom the target artery is less than 3 mm in calibre or the lesion is longer than 15 mm. In real world practice this translates to coronary artery lesions in approximately 60–70% of patients undergoing PCI.

Physiological assessment of coronary flow

The shortcomings of coronary angiography in the *physiological* assessment of coronary stenosis are clear. Intravascular ultrasound can provide information on the size of the lumen and the composition of plaque, but again gives no information as the effect that an atheromatous plaque may have on coronary flow. The knowledge as to whether a narrowing seen on angiography is the 'culprit' causing haemodynamic effects, and thus anginal symptoms, is valuable when guiding percutaneous intervention.

The fractional flow reserve (FFR) correlates distal coronary pressure to myocardial blood flow during maximum hyperemia (induced by infusion of adenosine, or papaverine). FFR is defined as maximum myocardial blood flow in the presence of a stenosis divided by the theoretical maximum flow in the absence of a stenosis (see Figure opposite).

Thus the information derived from FFR allows an 'on-the-spot' diagnosis as to what extent a given stenosis contributes to myocardial ischaemia (and angina), and can guide decisions regarding revascularization. At present the best established indication for coronary FFR estimation is as a diagnostic tool to assess 'severe' coronary narrowings, and for this it is extremely sensitive when used with a cut-off point of 0.75. The technique has also been used to optimize the results of stent implantation.

Two technologies are currently available that provide haemodynamic information derived from FFR calculations; these are pressure wires (which consist of a pressure transducer mounted on a 0.014" guide wire), and Doppler flow wires (which examine coronary flow velocities using spectral analysis).

Pressure wire e.g. The PressureWire™ (Radi Medical Systems)
- The pressure transducer is located at the transition between the radiopaque wire tip, and the non-radiopaque stem.
- The analyzer shows simultaneous aortic and intracoronary pressure, as well as instantaneous FFR.

Doppler wire e.g. FlowWire™ (Endosonics)
- Obtains information on coronary flow velocity in the central area of the arterial lumen.
- Combining flow and ECG information it calculates systolic and diastolic components of flow velocity at baseline.
- Following induction of hyperaemia the machine can calculate the coronary flow velocity reserve.

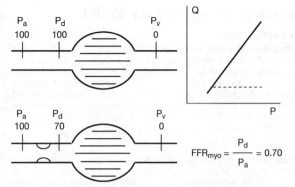

Fig. 5.16 During maximal arteriolar vasodilatation, the resistance of the myocardium is minimal, and so maximum myocardial blood flow is proportional to hyperaemic perfusion pressure. This equals P_d–P_v. As there is no decline in pressure along a normal coronary artery, and neglecting P_v, this implies that in a normal epicardial artery, perfusion pressure at hyperaemia equals P_a. In the presence of a stenosis, hyperaemic perfusion pressure decreases to P_d (after the stenosis). Thus the maximum flow in the presence of a stenosis as a ratio (fraction) of normal maximum flow is represented by the ratio of perfusion pressures: P_d/P_a. This fraction of normal maximum flow, which is maintained despite the stenosis, is called the fractional flow reserve (FFR). Reproduced with permission from Pijls NH (2004). Optimum guidance of complex PCI by coronary pressure measurement. *Heart* **90**: 1085–1093.

Primary angioplasty for STEMI

Pathophysiology

In the context of cardiac chest pain, ST segment elevation on the 12 lead ECG usually signifies complete occlusion of a proximal epicardial coronary artery. This occurs as a result of rupture or erosion of a vulnerable atheromatous plaque, which leads to platelet activation and adhesion, formation of platelet rich (white) thrombus, fibrin deposition, and red cell entrapment (forming red thrombus). If untreated myocardial necrosis commences within 30 minutes, affecting full myocardial thickness within 6 hours. 40% of patients die before reaching hospital.

Treatment

Urgent restoration of coronary blood flow (reperfusion) prevents further LV damage and improves prognosis. The amount of myocardium that can be salvaged falls exponentially with time, with the greatest benefit within 3 hours following symptom onset, and little benefit after 12 hours.

Primary angioplasty is the preferred reperfusion strategy, where angiography can be performed within 90 minutes of presentation (see p168).

Patients can be transferred safely (by a trained ambulance crew with an ALS trained escort) from a district hospital to a cardiac centre for primary angioplasty.

Options for reperfusion

- **Primary angioplasty**
  Immediate coronary arteriography and 'culprit' vessel angioplasty and stent implantation *without antecedent fibrinolysis*
  Achieves full arterial patency (TIMI grade 3 flow) in 90–95%
  Treats the occlusive thrombus and the culprit plaque
- **Intravenous fibrinolysis**
  Immediate administration of a fibrinolytic agent (also called thrombolysis) without planned coronary arteriography
  Achieves full arterial patency (TIMI grade 3 flow) in 50–60%
  Contraindicated in up to 30% of patients
  Does not treat the culprit plaque
- **Rescue angioplasty**
  Urgent coronary arteriography 'culprit' vessel angioplasty and stent implantation performed when fibrinolysis has failed to achieve reperfusion (Persistent ST segment Elevation ± pain at 60–90mins)
- **Facilitated angioplasty**
  Fibrinolysis prior to immediate coronary arteriography and 'culprit' vessel angioplasty and stent implantation

Primary angioplasty: procedure

Indications
- Cardiac chest pain <12 hours
- ST Elevation ≥1 mm in 2 contiguous leads
- Cardiogenic shock
- Able to consent
- NB:LBBB and 'true posterior' MI are not clear indications for primary angioplasty, though in practice some centres do include these patients. Discuss immediately with Cardiology registrar.

Contraindications
- Suspected aortic dissection

Relative contraindications
- Active bleeding (anti-platelet therapy may have to be avoided, but may compromise outcome. These cases should be discussed directly with the operator).

Pre-procedure (work quickly—minutes matter)
- Consent.
- The risk is higher than that of elective PCI. A procedural event rate of 5% (death, MI, stroke) should be quoted.
- FBC, clotting, Group and Save, U+E, CK, troponin.
- Analgesia + anti-emetic (diamorphine 5 mg; metoclopramide 10 mg).
- Oxygen if saturations <94%.
- Aspirin 300 mg (chewed).
- Clopidogrel 300–600 mg.
- Platelet glycoprotein GpIIb/IIIa receptor antagonist (abciximab) if no contraindication.
- The role of thrombolysis is undetermined (see below).

Procedure
- Access—Femoral or radial. The femoral region should always be prepared in case of a need for transvenous pacing or intra aortic balloon pump (IABP) insertion.
- A stent should be implanted where possible. Direct stenting without pre-dilatation may reduce the risk of distal embolization.
- The role of drug eluting stents in STEMI is undetermined.
- Platelet glycoprotein GpIIb/IIIa receptor antagonist if not already given.

Additional considerations
- Culprit vessel PCI is prognostic. Other vessels may be treated to provide complete revascularization. However, complex non-culprit PCI should be avoided in most cases.
- Procedural success is defined by TIMI grade 2 or 3 flow with residual stenosis <20%.

(a)　　　　　　　　　　　(b)

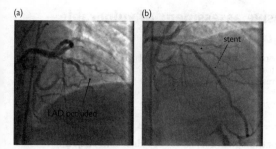

Fig. 5.17 Angiographic images from a 54 year old male presenting with chest pain and anterior ST elevation. (a) The left anterior descending (LAD) artery is occluded mid vessel (arrow). (b) The same artery now widely patent following primary angioplasty; A 3.5 x 24 mm bare metal stent has been implanted (arrow). The patient sustained minimal left ventricular damage, and was discharged 48 hours later.

1. Keeley EC, Boura JA, Grines CL (2003). Primary angioplasty vs. intravenous thrombolytic therapy for acute myocardial infarction: a quantitative review of 23 randomized trials. *Lancet* **361**: 13–20.

2. Andersen HR, Nielsen TT, Rasmussen K *et al.* (2003). A comparison of coronary angioplasty with fibrinolytic therapy in acute myocardial infarction. *N Engl J Med* **349**: 733–742.

3. Widimsky P, Budesinsky T, Vorac D, *et al.* (2003). Long distance transport for primary angioplasty vs immediate thrombolysis in acute myocardial infarction. Final results of the randomized national multicentre trial-PRAGUE-2. *Eur Heart J* **24**: 94–104.

Invasive assessment of vulnerable plaque

It has become apparent from intravascular ultrasound studies that non-obstructive and haemodynamically insignificant atherosclerotic plaques can be responsible for sudden death due to myocardial infarction. These high risk, or 'vulnerable' plaques are left untreated as it is unclear which will progress to rupture. Angiography does not help differentiate between benign and hazardous plaques, and thus new technologies have been developed to assist in the identification of these plaques.

Histopathological correlates of vulnerable plaque

• Lipid rich core.
• Thin fibrous cap.
• Necrotic core.
• High degree of macrophage infiltration.

Intravascular ultrasound

• Able to discriminate plaques with low (lipid) and high (fibrous) echodensity.
• Able to identify the capsule.
• Able to identify areas of rupture within the plaque.
• In combination with image analysis, information regarding the tissue types imaged can be derived, to provide a histological 'map' of the plaque.

Thermography catheters

• These catheters are able to detect the subtle temperature difference caused by inflammation that are present between stable and potentially unstable plaques.

Optical coherence tomography (OCT)

• This is similar in principle to intravascular ultrasound, but uses light instead of sound waves.
• The system has high axial resolution, down to 20 µm.
• At present useful anatomical information can be obtained by this technique, but this is yet to be correlated with functional data.

Intravascular elastography

• This technology uses sound waves in a similar way to IVUS.
• Images are based on radial strain, and the system is therefore able to help differentiate soft from hard material.
• It is known that plaque rupture is often seen to occur in areas of increased strain, such as at the edge of plaques.

Complex coronary angioplasty

Chronic total occlusion

Chronic total occlusion is defined as a completely occluded coronary artery, with the occlusion being known to have been present for >3 months. The age and length of the occlusion are the main determinants of success of PCI. The objectives in treating CTOs percutaneously are:

- Perforation of the total occlusion with a guide wire and advancement of this wire into the distal vessel (inability to cross with the guide wire is the reason for failure in 50% of attempts at CTO disobliteration).
- Dilatation of the underlying occlusion.
- Preservation of the newly recanalized lumen by the implantation of a stent and pharmacological means.

Techniques that may improve success include

- Aggressive guide catheter support, including deep cannulation of the coronary artery.
- Over the wire balloon to support the guide wire as it is advanced against the CTO.
- Stiffer guide wires that require greater forces to deflect the tip, and may be more successful in penetrating the 'cap' of the CTO. Great care must be taken with guide wires of this nature, as there is risk of perforation of the target vessel.

Unfortunately if the lumen is recanalized the rates of reocclusion are high, even when the CTO is stented. Drug eluting stents show some promise in reducing the restenosis and re-occlusion rate in these lesions.

Bifurcation lesions

- A simple definition of bifurcation lesions can be the involvement of a side branch with a reference diameter greater than 2 mm in the stenosis. IVUS studies show that plaque in the main vessel almost invariably extends some distance into side branches that arise within the plaque. Furthermore angioplasty to a plaque will often cause plaque-shift (the so-called 'snowplough' effect) into the daughter vessel.
- Unless flow in the side branch was severely impaired, or the ostium severely narrowed, during the treatment of the main vessel, a single stent technique is preferable to the use of two stents. This is the so-called '*provisional T-stenting*' technique.
- Dilating with a balloon through the stents of a strut carries the risk of deforming the distal parts of the stent and failure of adequate apposition of stent to vessel wall. This carries high risk of thrombosis and restenosis and thus a final 'kissing' balloon should be employed.
- Recent data regarding the use of a sirolimus coated stent in the treatment of bifurcations suggests that implantation of SES reduces the restenosis and reintervention rates after bifurcation lesion treatment.

What makes angioplasty complex?

- Increased risk of procedural failure.
- Suboptimal result likely.
- Complication rate higher.
- Worse long-term outcome (death, MI, repeat procedure).

Patient characteristics
- Clinical presentation—acute vs. stable.
- Diabetes.
- Body habitus.
- Significant co-morbidity.
- Access problems—Peripheral vascular disease.

Lesion characteristics
- Lesion characteristics e.g. long, calcified, bifurcation, left main stem, chronic total occlusions.
- Difficult anatomy.

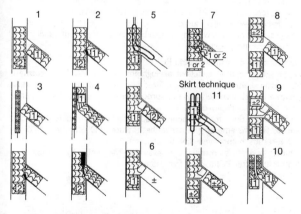

Fig. 5.18 Methods of treating bifurcation lesions. The numbering refers to the order in which the stents are deployed. All these methods have been tried, but recent data suggests that the 'provisional stent' technique (part 5) produces the best results. Adapted from Louvard Y, Lefèvre T, Morice M-C (2004). Percutaneous coronary intervention for bifurcation coronary disease. *Heart* **90**: 713–722, with permission.

Left main stem angioplasty

NICE guidelines had suggested that patients with stenosis of the left main coronary artery should be offered bypass graft surgery. However the emergence of registry data for both bare-metal stents and more recently drug eluting stents has suggested that PCI to the left main stem (LMS) in patients with suitable LMS anatomy achieves acceptable results with low rates of procedural complication, and long term vessel patency. The advent of drug eluting stents, and the reality of lower rates of in-stent restenosis compared to PCI with BMS, has further changed the approach of many interventional cardiologists to this previously taboo subset. In patients treated electively for LMS stenosis reference vessel size and left ventricular function appear to be the strongest predictors of favourable outcome.

Patient groups in whom LMS PCI may be appropriate

- Emergency LMS PCI.
  - Bailout PCI after complications involving the LMS.
- Elective LMS PCI.
  - Patients refused CABG, but with continuing angina.
  - Patients who refuse surgery.
  - Younger patients with favourable LMS anatomy (i.e. not ostial disease, not short LMS).

Optimization of results of LMS PCI

Nothing less than an excellent angiographic result should be accepted. Intravascular ultrasound may be utilized both pre-procedure to ascertain the true vessel diameter, and post-procedure to ensure that stents have been adequately deployed.

LMS bifurcations may be approached using the techniques described before. There is emerging evidence that the use of DES in the LMS bifurcation results in improved clinical outcomes.

Most operators routinely re-examine the LMS by angiography 2–4 months after PCI to look for restenosis.

Adjunctive therapy for angioplasty and stenting

Aspirin

The beneficial effect of aspirin during PCI has been shown in the Montreal Heart Study, in which the treatment with aspirin and dipyridamole was superior to placebo in the prevention of peri-procedural Q-wave MI. Subsequent studies showed that dipyridamole added nothing to the beneficial effects provided by aspirin. Low dose aspirin (usually 75 mg once daily), initiated at least 24 hr prior to procedure, is recommended in patients undergoing PCI.

Thienopyridines

Clopidogrel and ticlopidine are thienopyridine derivatives which inhibit platelet function independent of aspirin by interference with the platelet ADP receptor. Early studies showed that a dual anti-platelet therapy with aspirin and ticlopidine was superior to aspirin alone. The use of ticlopidine was limited by potentially severe neutropenia. Clopidogrel, a newer thienopyridine, with a safer side effect profile, has thus become the agent of choice. The PCI-CURE study showed that pre-treatment with clopidogrel (300 mg loading dose, followed by 75 mg daily) in addition to aspirin for a median of 10 days before percutaneous coronary intervention, compared with aspirin alone, reduced the composite of cardiovascular death, myocardial infarction or urgent target vessel revascularisation by 30% after 1 month. Most centres have adopted the policy of high loading dose clopidogrel (600 mg 2–4 hours pre-PCI) if the patient has not been pre-loaded.

Heparin

Although there is general agreement that patients undergoing PCI should receive heparin before the intervention, there remains controversy regarding the issue of optimal heparin dosage. An inverse relation between the level of anticoagulation (measured by activated clotting time (ACT)) and the occurrence of acute ischaemic complications has been observed, however longer ACTs are associated with higher bleeding risks. At present an ACT >300 seconds is recommended for patients undergoing PCI. Low molecular weight heparin (enoxaparin) has been shown to be effective in PCI, however it has not as yet replaced unfractionated heparin in routine use.

Glycoprotein IIb/IIa inhibitors

The final common pathway for platelet aggregation is mediated by the platelet glycoprotein IIb/IIIa receptor. Trials in both diabetics and non-diabetics undergoing percutaneous transluminal coronary angioplasty have found that the combination of stent and a glycoprotein IIb/IIIa inhibitor reduces cardiovascular morbidity and mortality compared with stent plus placebo.

Bivalirudin

Bivalirudin is a direct thrombin inhibitor that exerts its activity by specifically and reversibly interacting with circulating (inactive) and clot-bound (active) thrombin. Clinical trials of bivalirudin in PCI have demonstrated similar benefits to the combination of abciximab and heparin, with a reduced risk of clinically significant blood loss.

Nice guidelines on use of gp iib/iiia inhibitors

'...it is recommended that a GP IIb/IIIa inhibitor is considered an adjunct to PCI to all patients with diabetes undergoing elective PCI, and for those patients undergoing complex procedures.'

'If PCI is indicated as part of the early management of unstable angina or NSTEMI, but is delayed beyond the early management phase, then the use of a IIb/IIIa inhibitor is recommended as an adjunct to PCI...'

Embolic protection devices

The distal embolization of particulate matter which lodges in the microcirculation (e.g. plaque debris, thrombus, and fibrin) during balloon inflation and stent deployment is becoming increasingly recognized as a cause of suboptimal results after PCI. Vein grafts, and thrombotic lesions are now recognized as being particularly prone to complications arising from distal embolization, such as the 'no-reflow' phenomenon, which is seen in up to 30% of vein grafts which contain thrombus at the time of PCI. Hence the use of distal protection devices should be considered in these angioplasty subsets.

Devices for distal protection

Devices can be broadly split into those that occlude the conduit distally and then allow aspiration of debris, or distal filters that capture debris downstream

- Balloon occlusion devices
  - PercuSurge GuardWire. This consists of three parts 1. The GuardWire temporary occlusion catheter, which is place distally in the vessel to allow occlusion. 2. The MicroSeal adapter that allows control over the inflation and deflation of the balloon. 3. The Export aspiration catheter, which allows collected debris to be aspirated into a 20 ml syringe.
  - One of the main disadvantages of this system is that the target vessel is temporarily occluded, and thus the distal myocardium may be rendered ischaemic.
- Filter devices
  - AngioGuard. This device consists of an angioplasty guide wire with an expandable filter at the distal tip. The filter can be expanded once the target lesion has been crossed. Anterograde blood flow in the vessel is maintained, and displaced debris should theoretically be collected in the filter. The filter is then collapsed and withdrawn into retrieving catheter.
  - FilterWireEX. This device consists of a 'fishmouth' opening distal filter, mounted on an angioplasty guidewire. The 'mouth' of the filter in theory expands to fill the entire lumen of the vessel. The filter is deployed by withdrawing a delivery sheath, and collected into a retrieval sheath.

Limitations of distal protection devices

- Crossing profile may cause distal embolisation.
- Incomplete filter apposition, or incomplete conduit occlusion.
- Lack of protection of side branches.
- Distal ischaemia in balloon occlusion devices.

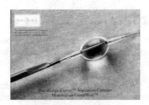

Fig. 5.19 Balloon occlusion device for distal protection.

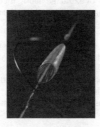

Fig. 5.20 Filterwire. Reproduced with permission from Boston scientific.

Thrombectomy

In the context of the limitations of distal protection devices as described before, devices that can aspirate particulate debris and thrombus proximally have been developed.

- The X-Sizer
  - The X-SIZER™ consists of a helical rotational cutter (1.5 or 2.0 mm in diameter) housed within the distal tip of the catheter. It is activated by a hand-held battery driven motor module.
    The catheter has two lumens, one for over-the-wire use and the other for aspiration of extracted debris. It comes as an independent, single use, disposable unit and is compatible with standard coronary guidewires and 6 F or 8 F guide catheters.
- The Transluminal extraction catheter (TEC)
  - Another rotational cutting device, however the blades are not protected and this limits use in native coronary arteries.
- The Angiojet
  - This device relies on the Venturi effect produced from backwardly directed fluid jets. These jets create vortices and areas of low pressure which cause debris distal to the catheter to be drawn in and aspirated.

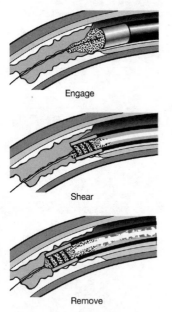

Engage

Shear

Remove

Fig. 5.21 The X-SIZER™.

Mitral valvuloplasty

In carefully selected patients with mitral stenosis percutaneous balloon mitral valvuloplasty (PMV) is now the treatment of choice. In fact the American Heart Association and American College of Cardiology state

'In centers with skilled, experienced operators, PMV should be considered the initial procedure of choice for symptomatic patients with moderate to severe mitral stenosis who have favourable valve morphology in the absence of significant mitral regurgitation or left atrial thrombus. In asymptomatic patients with favourable valve morphology, PMV may be considered if there is evidence of a haemodynamic effect on left atrial pressure (new-onset atrial fibrillation) or pulmonary circulation (pulmonary artery pressure >50 mmHg at rest or 60 mmHg with exercise)'

Case selection

Careful case selection is paramount. The factors that must be considered include

Age

- Older patients seem to have poorer outcomes in PMV. However this is likely to be related to valve morphology in this group as opposed to age *per se*. Patients in whom surgery to the mitral valve is contraindicated e.g. extreme age, and significant co-morbidity), adequate results can be obtained even in the presence of sub-optimal valve morphology.

Valve morphology

- A valve scoring system (echo based) is used to assess the valves suitability for PMV. Studies have shown that patients with a valve score of less than or equal to eight consistently achieve superior and more sustained results from the procedure than patients with scores greater than eight.

Mitral regurgitation

- The presence of significant mitral regurgitation is a contraindication to PMV.

Left atrial thrombus

- This is a contraindication to PMV. Patients in AF should have been fully anticoagulated for a period of 4–6 weeks prior to the procedure.

Pregnancy

- PMV can be performed in pregnancy. Radiation risk to the foetus is reduced after 14 weeks.

Complications of mitral valvuloplasty

- Mitral regurgitation.
- Pericardial tamponade.
- Thromboembolic events.
- Iatrogenic ASD.

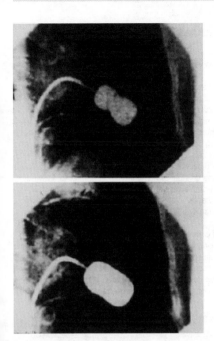

Fig. 5.22 Balloon mitral valvuloplasty: the upper panel shows the balloon partly inflated across the mitral valve demonstrating the typical dumb-bell shape. As the inflation pressure and volume are increased, the stenosed valve dilates (lower panel). Adapted with permission from Braunwald E (ed) (2001). *Heart Disease: A Textbook of Cardiovascular Medicine*. 5th ed. WB Saunders: Philadelphia.

Glossary of terms and abbreviations

- **Bifurcation**

A bifurcation lesion involving a main vessel and a side branch or a main vessel.

- **Binary angiographic restenosis (BAR)**

Greater than 50% luminal narrowing on follow-up angiogram

- **Canadian Cardiovascular Society (CCS) Angina Classification**

1. No chest pain. No limitation of physical activity by pain. Ordinary physical activity, such as walking and climbing stairs, does not cause angina. Angina with strenuous, rapid, or prolonged exertion at work or recreation.
2. Slight limitation of ordinary activity. Walking or climbing stairs rapidly, walking up hill, walking or stair climbing after meals, in cold, in wind, or when under emotional stress or during the first few hours after awakening may cause pain. Walking more than 2 blocks on the level and climbing more than one flight of stairs at a normal pace and in normal conditions.
3. Marked limitation of ordinary physical activity. Walking 1–2 blocks on a level and climbing one flight of stairs at normal pace results in angina.
4. Inability to carry on any physical activity without discomfort. Anginal syndrome may be present at rest.

- **Culprit (target) lesion revascularization (CLR/TLR)**

Repeat revascularization of a culprit lesion in the target vessel.

- **Chronic occlusion**

An occlusion presumed to have been present for at least one month prior to the procedure.

- **Total occlusion:**

An occlusion with no ante grade filling of contrast to the distal segment (TIMI grade 0).

- **Sub-total occlusion:**

TIMI grade I, and with collateral filling of the distal segment.

- **In-Stent**

The portion of coronary artery located within the margins of the stent.

- **In-Segment**

The portion of coronary artery located either within the margins of the stent or 5 mm proximal or distal to the stent.

- **IVUS**

Intravascular ultrasound

- **Late lumen loss**

Post-procedural minimum lumen diameter minus follow up minimum lumen diameter.

- **Minimum luminal diameter (MLD)**

The average of two orthogonal views (when possible) of the narrowest point within the area of assessment—in lesion, in-stent-or in-segment.

- **National Heart Lung and Blood Institute (NHLBI) Dissection Classification System**

A Minor radiolucencies within the lumen during contrast injection with no persistence after dye clearance.

B Parallel tracts or double lumen separated by a radiolucent area during contrast injection with no persistence after dye clearance.

C Extra luminal cap with persistence of contrast after dye clearance from the lumen.

D Spiral luminal filling defects.

E New persistent filling defects.

F Non-A-E types that lead to impaired flow or total occlusion.

- **Percutaneous coronary intervention (PCI)**

Refers to all interventional cardiology methods for treatment of coronary artery disease.

- **Reference vessel diameter (RVD)**

The mean of two angiographic measurements that are derived by interpolation at the target lesion.

- **Target lesion revascularization (TLR)**

Repeat PCI or CABG to the target lesion (culprit lesion).

- **Target vessel revascularization (TVR)**

Repeat PCI or CABG to the target vessel (culprit vessel), inclusive of target lesion.

- **TIMI flow grade**

0 No contrast flow through the stenosis.

1 A small amount of contrast flows through the stenosis but fails to fully opacify the vessel beyond.

2 Contrast material flows through the stenosis to opacify the terminal vessel segment. However, contrast enters the terminal segment perceptibly more slowly than more proximal segments.

3 Antegrade flow into the terminal coronary vessel segment through a stenosis is as prompt as antegrade flow into a comparable segment proximal to the stenosis.

- **QCA**

Quantitative coronary analysis

- **QIVUS**

Quantitative intravascular ultrasound

Heart failure

Introduction

Definition

Heart failure can be defined as a clinical syndrome characterized by dyspnoea and/or fatigue on exertion (and occasionally at rest) and evidence of fluid retention which may lead to peripheral oedema or pulmonary congestion. These symptoms and signs should be in the context of a structural or functional cardiac disorder that impairs its ability to fill and pump blood (at rest). A clinical response to treatment directed at heart failure *alone* (e.g. diuretic use) is not usually sufficient for diagnosis.

Epidemiology and prognosis

Unlike most cardiovascular diseases, CHF is becoming more common. There are currently around 6.5 million sufferers in Europe, 5 million in the USA. and 2.4 million in Japan. Nearly 1 million new cases are diagnosed annually worldwide. The prevalence increases with age, with the mean age of the heart failure population being in their mid 70 s. Prognosis is poor with three quarters of all patients hospitalized for the first time with heart failure dying within 5 years. Patients with heart failure can die suddenly (as the result of ventricular tachyarrhythmias) or with worsening heart failure symptoms and fluid overload.

Pathophysiology

The origin of symptoms in heart failure is poorly understood. An initial event (infarction, inflammation, pressure/volume overload) causes myocardial damage resulting in an increase in myocardial wall stress. This is followed by the activation of multiple neuroendocrine systems including the rennin–angiotensin–aldosterone system, the sympathetic nervous system, and the release of cytokines such as TNF. Neuroendocrine activation is also accompanied by structural and metabolic changes in the peripheral skeletal muscle and by abnormalities in cardiopulmonary reflex function such as the baroreflex and chemoreflex. These produce further wall stress perpetuating this vicious cycle (see Fig. 6.1)

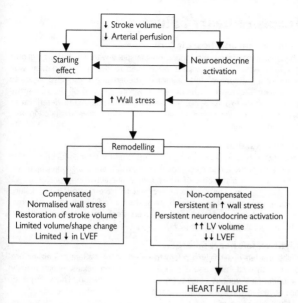

Fig. 6.1 Pathophysiology of heart failure.

Forms of heart failure

Acute vs. chronic heart failure

The clinical manifestations depend on the speed with which the syndrome develops. Acute heart failure is often used to describe the patient with acute onset dyspnoea and pulmonary oedema, but can also apply to cardiogenic shock where the patient is hypotensive and oliguric. Compensatory mechanisms have not yet become operative. Acute deterioration may be a consequence of MI, arrhythmia, acute valve dysfunction (e.g. endocarditis). See p620.

Systolic vs. diastolic heart failure

Most patients with heart failure have impaired LV systolic function: there is a failure of the LV to eject blood. However, there is a group of patients with signs and symptoms of heart failure but apparently preserved LV systolic function. These patients are said to have diastolic heart failure: there is an abnormality in the ability of the LV to fill in diastole. This may be transient (e.g. acute ischaemia) or persistent (restrictive or infiltrative cardiomyopathy, LVH) (see p294).

Right vs. left heart failure

Right and left heart failure refers to whether the patient has either predominantly systemic venous congestion (swollen ankles, hepatomegaly) or pulmonary venous congestion (pulmonary oedema). These terms do not necessarily indicate which ventricle is most seriously affected.

Fluid retention in heart failure is due to a combination of factors: reduced GFR, activation of the rennin–angiotensin–aldosterone system and sympathetic system. However, remember there are causes for swollen ankles other than heart failure (gravitational disorder e.g. immobility, venous thrombosis or obstruction, varicose veins, hypoproteinaemia e.g. nephrotic syndrome or liver disease, lymphatic obstruction).

High-output vs. low-output heart failure

A variety of high-output states may lead to heart failure e.g. thyrotoxicosis, Paget's disease, beriberi, and anaemia. This is characterized by warm extremities and normal or widened pulse pressure. In contrast, low-output states are characterized by cool pale extremities, cyanosis due to systemic vasoconstriction, and low pulse volume. The arterial-mixed venous oxygen saturation (a marker of the ability of the heart to deliver oxygen to the metabolizing tissues) is typically abnormally high in low-output states, but normal or even low in high-output states.

Causes and precipitants

In all patients with heart failure it is important to carefully consider the underlying aetiology, as there may be specific exacerbating factors or other diseases that influence the patients' management. A non-exhaustive list is given below.

Aetiology of heart failure

- Ischaemic heart disease (the commonest cause in the developed world).
- Dilated cardiomyopathy (no obvious underlying cause).
- Post viral.
- Alcohol.
- Hypothyroidism.
- Hypertension.
- Haemachromatosis.
- Familial.
- Infiltration (amyloid/sarcoid).
- Valve disease.
- Post–partum.
- Chemotherapy.
- Radiotherapy.
- Infections (Chagas's disease).
- Nutritional (Beri-Beri).

Patients with compensated heart failure have a high rate of readmission to hospital with acute exacerbations. A number of studies have demonstrated that a precipitating cause for emergency admission to hospital with heart failure can be identified in up to two thirds of patients.

- *Inappropriate reduction in therapy:* self discontinuation or iatrogenic withdrawal of diuretics, ACE-I, digoxin, as well as dietary excess of salt are recognized precipitants. Education of patient/family is important.
- *Cardiac arrhythmias:* most commonly AF, but any tachyarrhythmia will further reduce LV filling and stroke volume, and may exacerbate ischaemia. Marked bradycardia reduces cardiac output especially if stroke volume cannot increase any further.
- *Myocardial ischaemia or infarction:* exacerbates LV dysfunction, and may worsen mitral regurgitation due to ischaemia of papillary muscles.
- *Infection:* respiratory infections are more common, but any systemic sepsis can precipitate heart failure due to a combination of factors such as direct myocardial depression from inflammatory cytokines, sinus tachycardia, fever etc.
- *Anaemia:* this causes a high-output state that may precipitate acute heart failure, and may exacerbate underlying ischaemia.
- *Concomitant drug therapy:* drugs that directly depress myocardial function (e.g. calcium antagonists–verapamil, diltiazem; many antiarrhythmics, anaesthetics, over-enthusiastic initiation of β-blockers, etc) as well as drugs causing salt and water retention (e.g. NSAIDs, oestrogens, steroids, COX-2 antagonists) may precipitate heart failure.
- *Alcohol:* this is directly toxic and in excess can depress myocardial function as well as predispose to arrhythmias.
- *Pulmonary embolism:* the risk increases in the immobile patient with low-output state and atrial fibrillation.

It is very important to look for precipitating causes in all patients with heart failure. Once the precipitant has been identified and treated, appropriate measures (patient and family/education, adjustment of therapy, etc) should be put into place to prevent recurrence.

Population attributable risk of heart failure related to various risk factors*

Risk factor	Attributable risk (%)
Coronary disease	61.6
Cigarette smoking	17.1
Hypertension	10.1
Physical inactivity	9.2
Male sex	8.9
< High school education	8.9
Overweight	8.0
Diabetes	3.1
Valvular heart disease	2.2

*He, J, Ogden LG, Bazzano LA et al Risk factors for congestive heart failure in US men and women: NHANES 1 Epidemiologic Follow-up study. *Arch Intern Med* **161**: 996, (2001).

Conditions mimicking heart failure

- Obesity.
- Chest disease—including lung, diaphragm or chest wall.
- Venous insufficiency in lower limbs.
- Drug-induced ankle swelling (e.g. dihydropyridine calcium blockers).
- Drug-induced fluid retention (e.g. NSAIDs).
- Hypoalbuminaemia.
- Intrinsic renal disease.
- Intrinsic hepatic disease.
- Pulmonary embolic disease.
- Depression and/or anxiety disorders.
- Severe anaemia.
- Thyroid disease.
- Bilateral renal artery stenosis.

Signs and symptoms

- Dyspnoea (exertion or at rest)
- Fatigue
- Paroxysmal nocturnal dyspnoea
- Orthopnoea
- Palpitations
- Raised JVP
- 3rd heart sound

- Hepatomegaly
- Peripheral oedema
- Chest pain
- Gout
- Cachexia
- Sleep apnoea.

Many of these signs can be difficult to elicit particularly in a noisy A&E or outpatient clinic. Even in study conditions, the reproducibility and inter-observer agreement of the presence of signs is low. Despite this, a clinical diagnosis of heart failure can be made with some certainty when multiple signs are present in the same patient. (See table opposite.)

Symptoms alone can be used to classify the severity of CHF and to monitor the effect of treatment although the link between symptoms and degree of LV dysfunction is weak. The New York Heart Association classification (NYHA) is widely used.

NYHA classification of heart failure	
Class I	No limitation of physical activity.
Class II	Slight limitation of physical activity—symptoms with ordinary levels of exertion (e.g. walking up stairs).
Class III	Marked limitation of physical activity—symptoms with minimal levels of exertion (e.g. dressing).
Class IV	Symptoms at rest.

Framingham criteria for diagnosis of heart failure*

Major criteria

- Paroxysmal nocturnal dyspnoea
- Raised JVP; distended neck veins
- Crepitations in lung fields
- Cardiomegaly on CXR
- Acute pulmonary oedema
- S3 gallop rhythm
- Hepatojugular reflux
- Weight loss > 4.5kg in 5 days in response to treatment of heart failure.

Minor criteria

- Bilateral ankle oedema
- Nocturnal cough
- Dyspnoea on ordinary exertion
- Hepatomegaly
- Pleural effusion
- Tachycardia rate > 120/min
- Decrease in vital capacity by one third.

* From Ho, KL et al The epidemiology of heart failure: The Framingham Study. J Am Coll Cardiol 22(Suppl A): 6A, (1993). In this study the diagnosis of heart failure required 2 major or one major and 2 minor criteria. Minor criteria were only acceptable if they could not be attributed to another medical disorder.

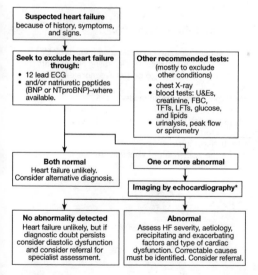

Fig. 6.2 Algorithm summarizing recommendations for the diagnosis of heart failure.

Alternative methods of imaging the heart should be considered when a poor image is produced by transthoracic Doppler 2D-echocardiography—alternatives include transoesophageal echocardiography, radionuclide imaging or cardiac magnetic resonance imaging.

BNP = B-type natriuretic peptide; ECG = Electrocardiogram; FBC = Full blood count; LFTs = Liver function tests; NTproBNP = N-terminal pro-B-type natriuretic peptide; TFTs = Thyroid function tests; U&Es= Urea & electrolytes.

Investigations

Investigations for all patients with heart failure

- *ECG:* although there are no specific changes in CHF, a completely normal ECG should encourage you to reconsider the diagnosis. Look for AF, conduction system defects, evidence of previous MI.
- *CXR:* see Figure 6.3. A normal CXR and ECG makes the diagnosis of heart failure very unlikely.
- *ECHO:* This is the key investigation in patients with CHF as it is able to document evidence of cardiac dysfunction at rest and identify any additional valvular problems. Abnormal cardiac function is best described in terms of mild/moderate/severe impairment. Absolute values for ejection fraction are unreliable and do not necessarily reflect the severity of heart failure.
- *Blood tests:* FBC (?anaemia), U&Es, glucose, LFTs, TFTs (hypo- or hyperthyroidism), uric acid.

Investigations to consider for selected patients with heart failure

- Ferritin.
- Immunoglobulins and protein electrophoresis.
- Viral titres.
- BNP: natriuretic peptides are raised in patients with impaired LV function. They appear to have a useful role in 'ruling out' patients to identify those with high levels who go on to have more extensive investigations.
- Coronary angiography (± myocardial biopsy).
- Holter monitoring (± QT dispersion, heart rate variability).
- Cardiopulmonary exercise testing or 6 minute walk test.
- Pulmonary function tests.
- Radionuclide ventriculography.
- Stress imaging (for the assessment of viable/hibernating myocardium).
- Cardiac magnetic resonance.

(a)

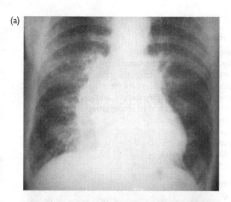

(b)

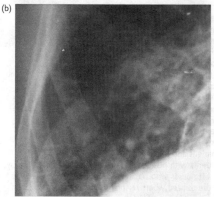

Fig. 6.3 CXR findings in heart failure. **Panel a:** There is cardiomegaly with prominent upper lobe vessels and alveolar oedema ('Bat's wing shadowing'). **Panel b** is a magnification of the right costophrenic angle showing septal lines (Kerley B lines) due to interstitial oedema.

Management

Management outline

- Establish that the patient has heart failure.
- Ascertain severity of symptoms and presenting features: pulmonary oedema, exertional breathlessness, fatigue, peripheral oedema.
- Try to determine the aetiology of heart failure.
- Identify precipitating and exacerbating factors, and any concomitant diseases relevant to heart failure and its management.
- Estimate prognosis.
- Anticipate complications.
- Counsel patient and relatives.
- Choose appropriate management.
- Monitor progress and manage accordingly.

Aims of treatment

1. Prevention of HF
- Prevention and/or controlling of diseases leading to cardiac dysfunction and heart failure.
- Prevention of progression to heart failure once cardiac dysfunction is established.

2. Maintenance or improvement in quality of life

3. Increased duration of life
- It is always better to try and prevent heart failure (HF), than to treat it once it has developed. This includes management of risk factors for ischaemic heart disease, treatment of ischaemia and revascularization where appropriate, early reperfusion therapy for acute MI, aggressive management of hypertension, management of diabetes and valvular heart disease. Stop exacerbating drugs if possible (NSAIDs, steroids, negative inotropes).
- Education of the patient and relatives is an important aspect of the management of patients with heart failure. Many hospitals now employ heart failure specialist nurses who are able to provide an excellent service and should be utilized wherever possible, and formal cardiac rehabilitation classes may be beneficial. It is important to explain the diagnosis, the symptoms, and how the treatment will help, the role of self-weighing, and the importance of exercise. Mild to moderate aerobic exercise can increase functional capacity in these patients.
- General measures include restriction of dietary salt and water intake, smoking cessation, reducing alcohol intake (stopping completely if alcohol is implicated in the aetiology of HF), addressing obesity with a weight reducing program, vaccinations (Pneumovax once and influenza yearly). Patients should also receive counselling on sexual activity.
- Patients should also be counselled about their drug therapy. The desired effects and potential side-effects need to be explained, and that there is a duration of therapy before effects become apparent. Self-management of diuretics may be appropriate for some. The patients need to be aware of drug interactions (e.g. with over-the-counter NSAIDs).

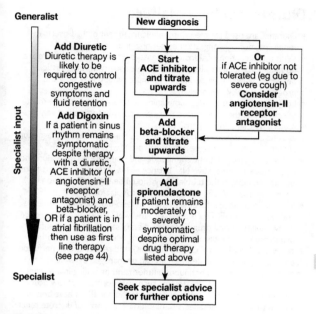

Fig. 6.4 Seeking a specialist opinion for patients with heart failure. Reproduced with permission from NICE guideliness www.nice.org

Diuretics in heart failure

- Diuretics are used for the symptomatic treatment of fluid overload (either pulmonary congestion or peripheral oedema).
- With the exception of aldosterone antagonists (see below), there are no randomized, controlled trials that have shown any prognostic benefit. However they do improve symptoms, and may slow the progression of LV remodelling.
- Loop diuretics (frusemide, bumetanide, and torsemide) are the most effective. Use the lowest dose that controls symptoms effectively.
- If there is insufficient response to diuretic, a combination of a loop diuretic and a thiazide diuretic can be used. Thiazides reduce magnesium absorption and hypomagnesaemia may occur with prolonged use.
- Potassium sparing diuretics (amiloride and triamterene) used alone do not achieve a net negative Na^+ balance as Na^+ retention in heart failure occurs proximal in the tubule. They should be used with caution in conjunction with ACE-inhibitors and spironolactone (result in $\uparrow K^+$)
- 'Diuretic resistance': the effectiveness of loop-diuretics may decrease with worsening HF. This is due to a variety of factors including reduced bioavailability of oral drug, excessive dietary salt intake, compensatory hypertrophy of the distal tubule increasing Na^+ reabsorption, other drugs (e.g. NSAIDs or COX-2 inhibitors), and reduced renal perfusion pressure by volume depletion. This can be managed by switching to IV diuretics (perhaps by continuous infusion) and/or adding in a thiazide. In hospitalized patients treatments such as iv dopamine at low dose and even short term infusion of nesiritide (human BNP) have been shown to enhance the effects of diuretics. Treatment of discrete renal artery stenoses that are amenable to angioplasty may also help diuretic resistance.

Loop diuretics	Initial dose	Maximum dose
Frusemide	20–40 mg od or bd	Titrate to achieve dry weight (up to 400 mg daily)
Bumetanide	0.5–1 mg od or bd	Titrate to achieve dry weight (up to 10 mg daily)
Torsemide	10–20 mg od or bd	Titrate to achieve dry weight (up to 200 mg daily)
Thiazides		
Hydrochlorothiazide	25 mg od	50–75 mg daily
Metolazone	2.5 mg od	10 mg daily
Indapamide	2.5 mg od	2.5 mg daily

Diuretic therapy for heart failure

Initial diuretic treatment

- Loop diuretics or thiazides.
- Always administered in addition to an ACE inhibitor (or ARB).
- If GFR <30 ml/min do not use thiazides, except as therapy prescribed synergistically with a loop diuretics (see below).

Inadequate response

- Increase dose of diuretic.
- Combine loop diuretics and thiazides.
- With persistent fluid retention: administer loop diuretics twice daily and consider changing from frusemide to alternatives that are better absorbed (e.g. bumetanide or torsemide).
- In severe chronic heart failure add a thiazide (e.g. metolazone) with frequent measurement of creatinine and electrolytes.

Potassium-sparing diuretics: triamterene, amiloride, spironolactone

- Use only if hypokalaemia persists after initiation of therapy with ACE inhibitors and diuretics.
- Start 1-week low-dose administration, check serum potassium and creatinine after 5–7 days and titrate accordingly. Recheck every 5–7 days until potassium values are stable.

*Adapted from Remme WJ and Swedberg K (2001) Task Force for the Diagnosis and Treatment of Chronic Heart Failure. *European Heart Journal* 22: 1527–1560.
GFR = glomerular filtration rate; CHF = chronic heart failure; ACE = angiotensin converting enzyme.

ACE inhibitors for heart failure

- ACE inhibitors significantly improve the survival, the symptoms, and reduce hospitalization of patients with moderate and severe HF and LV systolic dysfunction. Thus ACE inhibitors should be used as first-line therapy for patients with a reduced LV systolic function (ejection fraction <40–45%). The absolute benefit is greatest in patients with most severe heart failure (HF).
- In the absence of fluid retention, ACE inhibitors should be given first. In patients with fluid retention diuretics may be added.
- Furthermore, the dosage of ACE inhibitors should be uptitrated to the dosages shown to be effective in the large, controlled trials in heart failure, and not titrated based on symptomatic improvement alone.
- Asymptomatic patients with a documented LV systolic dysfunction benefit from long-term ACE inhibitor therapy. Large trials (SOLVD Prevention Study, SAVE and TRACE) have shown that asymptomatic patients, but with left ventricular dysfunction, will have less development of symptomatic heart failure and hospitalizations for heart failure.
- ACE inhibitors may prevent further deterioration of left ventricular function and attenuate further cardiac dilatation. However, they do not consistently reduce cardiac size.

Starting an ACE-I
- Review diuretic dose and avoid excessive diuresis before treatment.
- Consider giving first dose at night to minimize the hypotensive effect.
- Start with a low dose and build up to target levels.
- Stop treatment if there is a substantial deterioration in renal function.
- Avoid NSAIDS and potassium sparing diuretics.
- Check BP and U/Es 1–2 weeks after each dose increment and at 6 monthly intervals.
- Low BP (systolic <90 mmHg) is acceptable if patient is asymptomatic.

Target doses of various ACE-I

Drug	Initiating dose	Maintenance dose
Captopril	6.25 mg tds	25–50 mg tds
Enalapril	2.5 mg daily	10 mg bd
Lisinopril	2.5 mg daily	5–20 mg daily
Perindopril	2 mg daily	4 mg daily
Ramipril	1.25–2.5 mg daily	2.5–5 mg bd
Quinapril	2–5 mg daily	5–10 mg daily
Trandolapril	1 mg daily	4 mg daily

Which ACE inhibitor and what dose?

Licensed ACE-I	starting dose(mg)	Target dose mg
Captopril	6.25 three times daily	50–100 three times daily
Cilazapril	0.5 once daily	1–2.5 once daily
Enalapril	2.5 twice	10–20 twice daily
Fosinopril	10 once aily	40 once daily
Lisinopril	2.5–5.0 once daily	30–35 once daily
Perindopril	2.0 once daily	4 once daily
Quinapril	2.5–5.0 once daily	10–20 once daily
Ramipril	2.5 once daily	5 twice daily or 10 once daily

*Target dose based on manufacturer's recommendation rather than large outcome study

How to use?

- Start with a low dose (see above).
- Seek specialist advice where the patient is on a high dose (e.g. furosemide 80 mg) of a loop diuretic.
- Double dose at not less than two weekly intervals.
- Aim for target dose (see above) or, failing that, the highest tolerated dose.
- Remember some ACE inhibitor is better than no ACE inhibitor.
- Monitor blood electrolytes (in particular potassium), urea, creatinine and blood pressure.
- When to stop up-titration/down-titration; see 'Problem solving', below.

Advice to patient?

- Explain expected benefits
- Treatment is given to improve symptoms, to prevent worsening of heart failure and to increase survival.
- Symptoms improve within a few weeks to a few months.
- Advise patients to report principal adverse effects, i.e. dizziness/symptomatic hypotension, cough.

Problem solving

- Asymptomatic low blood pressure does not usually require any change in therapy.

Symptomatic hypotension
- If dizziness, light-headedness and/or confusion and a low blood pressure consider discontinuing nitrates, calcium channel blockers[†] and other vasodilators.
- If no signs/symptoms of congestion consider reducing diuretic dose.
- If these measures do not solve problem seek specialist advice.

Cough
- Cough is common in patients with chronic heart failure, many of whom have smoking-related lung disease.
- Cough is also a symptom of pulmonary oedema which should be excluded when a new or worsening cough develops.
- ACE inhibitor induced cough rarely requires treatment dicontinuation.
- If the patient develops a troublesome dry cough which interferes with sleep and is likely to be caused by an ACE inhibitor, consider substituting an angiotensin-II receptor antagonist for the ACE inhibitor.

Worsening renal function
- Some rise in urea, creatinine and K^+ is to be expected after initiation of an ACE inhibitor if the increase is small and asymptomatic no action is necessary.
- An increase in Greatinine of up to 50% above baseline, or to 200 μmol, whichever is the smaller, is acceptable.
- An increase in K^+ to ≤ 5.9 mmol/l is acceptable.
- If urea, creatinine or K^+ do rise excessively consider stopping concomitant nephrotoxic drugs (e.g. NSAIDs), non-essential vasodilators (e.g. calcium antagonists, nitrates), K^+ supplements/retaining agents (triamterene, amiloride) and, if no signs of congestion, reducing the dose of diuretic.
- If greater rises in creatinine of K^+ than those oulined above presist despite adjustment of concomitant medications the dose of the ACE inhibitor should be halved and blood chemistry rechecked, if there is still an unsatisfactory response specialist advice should be sought.
- If K^+ rises to ≥ 6.0 mmol/l or Creatinine increases by >100% or to above 350μmol/l the dose of ACE inhibitor should be stopped and specialist advice sought.
- Blood electrolytes should be monitored closely until K^+ and creatinine concentrations are stable.

Note: it is very rarely necessary to stop an ACE inhibitor and clinical deterioration is likely if treatment is withdrawn; ideally, specialist advice should be sought before treatment discontinuation.

* Adapted from Mc Murray *et al.* Practical recommendations for the use of ACE Inhibitors, beta-blockers and spironolactone in heart failure; putting guidelines into practice. *European journal of Heart Failure* 2001; 3: 495–502.
† Calcium channel blockers should be discontinued unless absolutely essential, e.g. for angina or hypertension.

β-blockers for heart failure

- β-blockers were once contra-indicated in patients with heart failure (HF). However, several studies (Carvedilol studies, Merit-HF, COPERNICUS, see Chapter 15) have shown that they are effective in reducing the risk of sudden cardiac death (of the order of 30%).
- β-blockers are recommended for all patients with HF, whether due to ischaemic heart disease or not and irrespective of the severity of LV dysfunction (NYHA classes II to IV).
- The effect does not appear to be a class effect, and only metoprolol, carvedilol and bisoprolol can be recommended in HF.
- β-blockers should be initiated under careful control as there may be an initial deterioration in heart failure symptoms. The drugs are started at a low dose at up-titrated to target over a period of weeks or months.

Starting a β-blocker

- Patients should be on an ACE-inhibitor if possible.
- Heart failure symptoms should be relatively stable before initiation.
- Start with a low dose and titrate up to target every 1–2 weeks if the preceding dose was tolerated.
- Monitor the patient for symptoms and signs of HF, bradycardia and hypotension.
- If symptoms worsen, increase dose of diuretics or ACE-I initially. β-blocker dose may need to be decreased transiently.
- If hypotensive, reduce dose of vasodilators and reduce dose of β-blockers if necessary.

Titration scheme for β-blockers

Drug	First dose	Increments	Target dose
Carvedilol	3.125 mg bd	6.25, 12.5, 25, 50	50 mg daily
Bisoprolol	1.25 mg od	2.5, 3.75, 5, 7.5, 10	10 mg daily
Metoprolol succinate	12.5 mg daily	25, 50, 100, 200	200 mg daily

NB: Carvedilol max dosage 25 mg bd if severe heart failure. For patients with mild–moderate heart failure max dosage 50 mg bd if weight above 85 kg—otherwise maximum dosage 25 mg bd.

Which beta-blocker and what dose?

Only two beta-blockers are licensed for the treatment of heart failure in the UK at the time of issue of this guideline:

- Bisoprolol (starting dose 1.25 mg once daily; target dose 10 mg once daily)
- Carvedilol (starting dose 3.125 mg twice daily; target dose 25–50mg twice daily)

NB Carvedilol: maximum dose 25 mg twice daily if severe heart failure. For patients with mild to moderate heart failure maximum dose 50 mg twice daily if weight more than 85 kg—otherwise maximum dose 25 mg twice daily.

How to use?

- Start with a low dose (see above).
- Double dose at not less than two weekly intervals.
- Aim for target dose (see above) or, failing that, the highest tolerated dose.
- Remember some beta-blocker is better than no beta-blocker.
- Monitor heart rate, blood pressure, clinical status (symptoms, signs, especially signs of congestion, body weight).
- Check blood eletrolytes, urea and creatinine one to two weeks after initiation and one to two weeks after final dose titration.
- When to down-titrate/stop up-titration, see 'Problem solving', below.

Advice to patient

- Explain expected benefits.
- Emphasize that treatment given as much to prevent worsening of heart failure as to improve symptoms, beta-blockers also increase survival.
- If symptomatic improvement occurs, this may develop slowly—over three to six months or longer.
- Temporary symtomatic deterioration may occur (estimated 20–30% of cases) during initiation/up-titration phase.
- Advise patient to report deterioration (see 'Problem solving', below) and that deterioration (tiredness, fatigue, breathlessness) can usually be easily managed by adjustment of ther medication; patients should be advised not to stop beta-blocker therapy without consulting their physician.
- Patients should be encouraged to weigh themselves daily (after walking, before dressing, after voiding, before eating) and to consult their doctor if they have persistent weight gain.

Problem solving with β-blockers

Worsening symptoms/signs (e.g. increasing dyspnoea, fatigue, oedema, weight gain)
- If marked fatigue (and/or bradycardia, see below) halve dose of β-blocker (if increasing diuretic does not work).
- If increasing congestion double dose of diuretic and/or halve dose of β-blocker (if increasing diuretic does not work).
- Adapted from McMurry *et al.* Practial recommendations for the use of ACE Inhibitors, β-blockers and spironolactone in heart failure: Putting guidelines in to practice. *European Journal of Heart Failure* 2001; **3**: 495–502.
- Review patient in one to two weeks; if not improved seek specialist advice.
- If serious deterioration halve dose of beta-blocker or stop this treatment (rarely necessary); seek specialist advice.

Low heart rate
- If <50 beats/min and worsening symptoms–halve dose beta-blocker or, if severe deterioration, stop beta-blocker (rarely necessary).
- Consider need to continue treatment with other drugs that slow the heart (e.g. digoxin, amiodarone, diltiazem) and discontinue if possible.
- Arrange ECG to exclude heart block.
- Seek specialist advice.

Asymptomatic two blood pressure
- Does not usually require any change in therapy.

Symptomatic hypotension
- If low blood pressure causes dizziness, light-headedness or confusion, consider discontinuing drugs such as nitrates, calcium channel blockers and other vasodialtors.
- If no signs/symptoms of congestion consider reducing diuretic dose.
- If these measures do not solve problem seek specialist advice.

Note: β-blockers should not be stopped suddenly unless absolutely necessary (there is a risk of a 'rebound' increase in myocardial ischaemia/infarction and arrhythmias); ideally specialist advice should be sought before treatment discontinuation.

Angiotensin II receptor antagonists for heart failure

- Angiotensin II receptor blockers (ARBs) are often used in those patients who do not tolerate an ACE-I (because of cough).
- In patients with heart failure (HF), ARBs are as effective as ACE-Is in reducing mortality and morbidity.
- One study (ValHeft II, p588) showed that the combination of an ACE-I and valsartan was better than either drug alone. However, this benefit was reversed in patients also taking a β-blocker. This adverse effect was not seen in the CHARM-Added Trial (p555) which used the ARB candesartan.
- When combined with ACE-inhibitors, ARBs reduce HF hospitalizations.
- In patients with heart failure and preserved LV systolic function (i.e. patients with diastolic dysfunction) the ARB candesartan reduces hospitalization for HF.

Aldosterone receptor antagonists in heart failure

- Aldosterone levels are not reduced by ACE-I, and these raised levels produce myocardial fibrosis and predispose to arrhythmias.
- In the RALES study (p578), spironolactone (an aldosterone receptor antagonist) produced a 30% reduction in total mortality of patients with severe CHF (NYHA classes III and IV) when compared to placebo. The benefit was in sudden as well as cardiac death.
- Long term usage of spironolactone is associated with gynaecomastia, impotence and menstrual irregularities; newer agents have less of this antiandrogenic and progesterone-like effects.
- Eplerenone was evaluated in EPHESUS (Eplerenone Post Acute Myocardial Infarction Heart Failure Efficacy and survival Study). Patients with LV EF <40% were randomized to eplerenone or placebo 3–14 days after acute MI. Eplerenone produced a significant (15%) reduction in mortality. Gynaecomastia, breast tenderness and impotence were no different in the two groups.

Starting spironolactone

- Consider whether a patient is in severe heart failure (NYHA III–IV) despite ACE inhibition and diuretics.
- Check serum K^+ (<5·0 mmol/l) and creatinine (<250 µmol/l).
- Start 25 mg spironolactone daily.
- Check serum K^+ and creatinine after 4–6 days.
- If at any time serum K^+ >5–5·5< mmol/l, reduce dose by 50%. Stop if serum K^+ >5·5 mmol/l.
- If after 1 month symptoms persist and K^+<5.5 mmol/l, increase to 50 mg daily. Check serum potassium/creatinine after 1 week.
- If endocrine related side-effects of spironolactone observed, change to eplerenone.

Which dose of spironolactone?

- 12.5–25 mg daily, although 50 mg be advised by a specialist if heart failure deteriorates and no problem with hyperkalaemia.

How to use?

- Start at 25 mg once daily.
- Check blood chemsitry at 1, 4, 8 and 12 weeks; 6, 9 and 12 months, 6 monthly thereafter.
- If K^+ rises to between 5.5. and 5.9 mmol/l or creatinine rises to 200 μmol/l reduce dose to 25 mg on alternate days and monitor blood chemistry closely.
- If K^+ rises to ≥6.0 mmol/l or creatinine to >200 μmmol/l stop spironolactone and seek specialist advice.

Advice to patient?

- Explain expected benefits
- Treatment is given to improve symptoms, prevent worsening of heart failure and to increase survival.
- Symptom improvement occurs within a few weeks to a few months of starting treatment.
- Aviod NSAIDs not prescribed by a physician (self-purchased 'over the counter' treatment, e.g. ibuprofen).
- Temporarily stop sprionolactone if diarrhoea and/or vomiting and contact physician.

Problem solving—worsening renal function\hyperkalaemia

- See 'How to use'? section, above.
- Major concern is hyperkalaemia (≥ 6.0 mmol/l) though this was uncommon in the RALES clinical trial; a potassium level at the higher end of the normal range may be desirable in patients with heart failure, particularly if taking digoxin.
- Some 'low salt' substitutes have a high K^+ content.
- Male patients may develop breast discomfort and/or gynaecomastia.

---

* Adapted from McMurray et al. Practical recommendations for the use of ACE Inhibitors, beta-blockers and spironolactone in heart failure; putting guidelines into practice. *European Journal of Heart Failure* 2003; **3**: 495–502.

Cardiac glycosides in heart failure

- Digoxin is very useful to aid rate control in supraventricular arrhythmias including AF in the management of patients with chronic HF. Its role in patients with sinus rhythm, however, is less clear.
- Two large digoxin withdrawal trials (RADIANCE and PROVED) demonstrated that patients from whom digoxin was withdrawn were more likely to be admitted with worsening HF.
- The DIG trial enrolled 6800 patients with classes I to III HF with a mean EF of 28%. This showed that there was no increase in mortality in the group given digoxin. There was a trend to a decrease in mortality due to pump-failure, balanced by a slight increase in non-pump failure related cardiac deaths. Digoxin reduced the number of hospitalizations for HF significantly.
- Overall the clinical trials support the use of digoxin in patients in sinus rhythm with mild to moderate HF. Trough levels should be maintained between 0.5–1.0 ng/ml.
- Contraindications: significant bradycardia; heart block, WPW.

Vasodilators in heart failure

- Vasodilators are not a particularly effective method to improve the natural history of chronic HF, but are useful for dealing with acute decompensation. They are also useful in patients intolerant of both ACE-I and ARBs.
- Nitrates are primarily venodilators, but are potent coronary vasodilators making them useful in ischaemic HF.
- Isosorbide dinitrate is the only nitrate formulation that has been shown to increase exercise tolerance, and in combination with hydralazine, prolongs survival in patients with HF.
- The addition of hydralazine appears to attenuate nitrate tolerance by acting as a reducing agent.
- In V-HeFT-II, enalapril was shown to be superior to hydralazine and isosorbide dinitrate except in American Blacks, where the opposite was found: this is still under investigation.
- Nesiritide (human brain natriuretic peptide, hBNP) infusion has been shown to improve haemodynamics and clinical status in patients with decompensated HF, and is less arrhythmogenic than dobutamine. It is in trial as a subcutaneous injection for chronic HF.
- Neutral endopeptidase inhibitors with or without intrinsic ACE-inhibitor activity are being explored for the treatment of chronic HF as they prevent the inactivation of ANP and BNP; promising small trials have been followed by disappointing results in larger scale studies.
- Although all three classes of calcium antagonists are effective arteriolar vasodilators, none produces a sustained improvement in HF. All except amlodipine appear to worsen symptoms.

Phosphodiesterase inhibitors in heart failure

- In large scale placebo controlled trials, selective type III phosphodiesterase inhibitors (PDEI) are associated with an increase in mortality.
- Individual agents like milrinone and enoximone produce sustained inotropic and vasodilator effects when administered intravenously and are useful in the short term in decompensated HF.
- There is no oral PDEI licenced on Europe, but trials are ongoing.

Positive inotropic support

Inotropes (e.g. dobutamine) can be used to limit very severe episodes of heart failure or as a bridge to transplantation in end-stage heart failure. Whist longer term inotropic therapy may improve a patient's quality of life, they also increase mortality and are therefore not recommended.

Antiplatelet agents and anticoagulants

- There has been much controversy regarding the use of aspirin in patients with CHF. As a general rule NSAIDS are avoided due to their fluid retaining and reno-toxic properties. It is also thought that the beneficial effect of ACE-I is reduced by these drugs.
- Generally, patients with ischaemic heart disease as their underlying aetiology should be treated with aspirin, whilst the remainder should not.
- Formal anticoagulation with warfarin is indicated for patients with heart failure and atrial fibrillation (paroxysmal or persistent). It is also often used in those with demonstrated LV thrombus or patients with very large LV cavities where it is thought that the risk of LV thrombus formation is high. There is, however, no randomized data to support this use.

Miscellaneous drugs for heart failure

Patients with CHF may require drug treatment for systems other than the heart:
- Gout is a common problem. Acute flare-ups should be treated with colchicine followed by allopurinol once the acute event has settled.
- Whilst most calcium channel antagonists are avoided in patients with CHF, amlodipine has a neutral effect on prognosis and can be used for the treatment of hypertension or angina.
- Anaemia is frequently seen in CHF patients. Correction of this with iv iron and erythropoietin has been shown to improve symptoms.
- Patients with any severe chronic disease are more likely to become depressed and heart failure is no exception. Tricyclic antidepressants should be avoided because of their pro-arrhythmic potential.

Device therapy for heart failure

Clearly, patients fulfilling the standard indications for permanent pacemaker implantation should undergo this. Wherever possible, dual chamber systems should be implanted to maintain atrioventricular synchrony.

Implantable cardiac defibrillators (ICD) (see p446)

- ICDs are devices that are able to recognize ventricular arrhythmias (VT or VF) and deliver a DC shock to terminate them. They are implanted in the same way as pacemakers.
- Several studies have shown that patients with impaired LV function benefit prognostically from their implantation.
- The MADIT II trial showed an 30% improvement in survival in patients with ischaemic heart disease and an ejection fraction of less than 35%.

Cardiac resynchronization (CRT) (see p406)

- Many patients with CHF have bundle branch block patterns on their ECG, in particular LBBB. A wide QRS duration is associated with a worse outcome in patients with CHF. LBBB results in delayed depolarization and contraction of the lateral LV free wall which is thought to contribute to disease progression.
- Biventricular pacemakers are able to reduce this ventricular dys-synchrony by pacing the LV via a cardiac vein.
- Current indications for implantation include severe symptoms (NYHA III or IV), a broad QRS complex (>130 ms) and impaired LV function (LVEF <35%). These indications alone, however, do not necessarily predict patients who will benefit from resynchronization. Current research is assessing the value of using non-invasive imaging techniques (tissue doppler and MRI) to identify true inter- and intraventricular dys-synchrony.
- Studies in patients with HF undergoing cardiac resynchronization (CRT) have shown an improvement in quality of life, improved exercise capacity (6 minute walk test) and in 1 case, improved survival.
- Biventricular devices can now be combined with ICDs to further improve the outlook of these patients.
- The devices can be difficult to implant, they require close and careful follow-up and are expensive which has reduced their widespread up take.

Surgery for heart failure

Valve surgery

Patients with valve disease as the source of their heart failure should be considered for valve replacement surgery. This is discussed more fully in the chapter on valve disease.

CABG

As shown above, ischaemic heart disease is the commonest cause of heart failure. In some cases, these patients will have evidence of either stress-induced ischaemia or hibernation (muscle that has reduced function due to reduced blood supply). Revascularizing these patients can lead to an improvement in cardiac function.

Transplantation

Cardiac transplantation is reserved for those patients with end-stage heart failure. It is a major undertaking for the patient who must be willing to undergo intensive treatment and is emotionally capable of withstanding the uncertainties that occur both before and after transplantation. There are a number of contraindications, some of which are shown below.

Contraindications for heart transplantation
- Persistent alcohol/drug abuse.
- Treated cancer with remission and <5 years follow-up.
- Systemic disease with multi-organ involvement.
- Infection.
- Fixed high pulmonary vascular resistance.

Despite problems with rejection and complications of immunosuppressive therapy (infection, hypertension, renal failure, malignancy) the 5-year survival is of the order of 70–80% with many patients returning to work.

Assist devices

Because of the lack of organ donors for cardiac transplantation much interest has been shown in the development of LV assist devices (LVAD) and mechanical hearts. LVADs are automatic pumps that take over the work of the heart. They have been used as a bridge to transplantation and also as a bridge to recovery in those with potentially reversible causes for their heart failure (e.g. post-viral).

The next stage up from these large devices is the implantation of a permanent artificial heart. An example is the Jarvik 2000 which has been successfully been implanted in a relatively small number of patients.

Heart transplantation guidelines adapted from ESC/AHA guidelines

Indications	Contraindications and cautions
• Patients must be willing and able to withstand the physical and emotional demands of the procedure and its post-operative sequelae. • Objective evidence of limitation, e.g. peak oxygen consumption less than 10 ml/min/kg on cardiopulmonary exercise test with evidence for anaerobic metabolism. * • Patients dependent on intravenous inotropes and mechanical circulatory support.	• Present alcohol and/or drug abuse. • Chronic mental illness, which can not be adequately controlled • Treated cancer with remission and <5 years follow-up. • Systemic disease with multiorgan involvement. • Uncontrolled infection. • Severe renal failure (creatinine clearance <50 ml/min) or creatinine >200 µmol/l, although some centres accept patients on haemodialysis. • Fixed high pulmonary vascular resistance (6–8 Wood units and mean transpulmonary gradient >15 mmHg and pulmonary artery systolic pressure >60 mmHg). • Recent thromboembolic complication. • Unhealed peptic ulcer. • Evidence of significant liver impairment. • Other disease with a poor prognosis.

* Patients with significant exercise limitation that have a peak oxygen consumption less than 55% predicted or between 11 and 15 ml/min/kg also warrant consideration for cardiac transplantation if they have recurrent unstable myocardial ischaemia untreatable by other means, or recurrent episodes of congestive heart failure in spite of adherence to optimum medical therapy.

Palliative care for heart failure

The demographic spread of most patients with heart failure means that the hi-tech and expensive therapies outlined earlier are not available and consideration must be made about end-of-life issues. Increased input from specialist palliative care teams will help to allow patients and their relatives live with a chronic and terminal disease and die with dignity.

Worsening heart failure

When a patient is seen with worsening heart failure, it is important to try and ascertain the cause. The most frequent reasons for symptom deterioration are shown below.

Causes of worsening heart failure

Non-cardiac
- Non-compliance (lifestyle changes, medication).
- Newly prescribed drugs.
- Renal dysfunction.
- Infection.
- Pulmonary embolus.
- Anaemia.

Cardiac
- Atrial fibrillation.
- Other tachyarryhthmias.
- Bradycardia/heart block.
- Worsening valve disease.
- Myocardial ischaemia (including infarction).

Side effects of drugs for heart failure

Drugs	Complications
Diuretics	**Common:** postural hypotension, gout, urinary urgency.
	Serious: electrolyte imbalance (hypokalaemia, hypomagnesia, hyponatraernia), arrhythmia.
ACE inhibitors	**Common:** cough, hypotension including postural
	Serious : worsening renal function, renal infarction in renal artery stenosis, angio-oedema
β-blockers	**Common:** tiredness, bradycardia, coldness
	Serious: asthmatic attack, exacerbation of heart failure, hear block.
Spironolactone	**Common:** gynaecomastia, tiredness, rashes
	Serious: hyperkalaemia, hypotraemia.
Digoxin	**Comon:** nausea
	Serious: life-threatening arrhythmias
Angiotensin-II receptor antagonists	**Common:** hypotension including postural
	Serious: worsening renal function, renal infarction in renal artery stenosis.
Amiodarone	**Common:** photosensitivity, nausea, thyroid dysfunction, sleep disturbance, corneal microdeposits.
	Serious: thyrotoxic storm, pro-arrhythmia, pulmonary/hepatic fibrosis.
Intropes	**Common:** nausea, palpitation
	Serious: arrhythmia, cardiotoxicity

Diastolic heart failure

Approximately one third of patients with heart failure (HF) have diastolic heart failure. This is defined as symptoms and signs of heart failure but with preserved (normal) LV systolic function.

A number of clinical settings are associated with diastolic dysfunction. Most causes of diastolic dysfunction relate to impaired left ventricular diastolic relaxation. The commonest underlying diseases are hypertension and ischaemia as a result of coronary artery disease. Other causes include aortic stenosis, hypertrophic cardiomyopathy, infiltrative (such as in cardiac amyloidosis) and restrictive cardiomyopathies.

Pericardial restraint such as in constrictive pericarditis and cardiac tamponade impair ventricular filling. In addition mitral valve stenosis causing left ventricular outflow obstruction leads to elevated left atrial pressure and in severe cases, to cardiac failure that is solely due to impaired filling.

Pathophysiology

- Ventricular relaxation may be impaired. This is an energy dependent process and is sensitive to hypoxia. Myocardial ischaemia can induce diastolic dysfunction via this mechanism. Ischaemia may be caused, not only by epicardial coronary artery disease, but possibly also by changes in the microvascular coronary supply.
- Increased compliance of the left ventricle leads to a stiff chamber and impaired filling. There is evidence that this altered compliance is mediated by an increase in myocardial collagen. Most conditions causing left ventricular hypertrophy are associated with impairment of diastolic function; however in conditions where myocardial hypertrophy is not associated with fibrosis such as chronic anaemia, hyperthyroidism and exercise training, diastolic stiffness is normal.

Clinical assessment

Clinical features of HF may be similar whether the LV systolic function is impaired or preserved. The clinical presentation should be considered along with an assessment of systolic and diastolic function.

Diagnostic criteria for diastolic HF	Signs and symptoms of HF plus
Possible diastolic HF	LVEF >50% but not at the time of HF
Probable diastolic HF	LVEF >50% within 72h of HF event
Definite diastolic HF	LVEF >50% within 72h of HF event, and Abnormal LV relaxation, filling and/or distensibility at cardiac catheterization

Adapted from Vasab RS, Levy D.(2000) Defining diastolic heart failure: A call for standardized diagnostic criteria. *Circulation* **101**: 2118.

Diagnosis

A definitive diagnosis of diastolic heart failure can be made when the rate of relaxation of the LV in diastole is slowed. This physiological abnormality is characteristically associated with the finding of an elevated left ventricular filling pressure in a patient with normal left ventricular volumes and contractility.

Noninvasive methods (e.g. Doppler echocardiography) have been developed to assist in the diagnosis of diastolic dysfunction (see Fig. 6.3), but these tests have significant limitations, because cardiac filling patterns are readily altered by nonspecific and transient changes in loading conditions in the heart as well as by aging, changes in heart rate, or the presence of mitral regurgitation.

Every effort should be made to exclude other possible explanations or disorders that may present in a similar manner.

Differential diagnoses with HF and preserved LVEF

- Incorrect diagnosis of HF.
- Inaccurate measurement of LVEF.
- Primary valvular disease.
- Restrictive (infiltrative) cardiomyopathy (e.g. amyloidosis, sarcoidosis, haemochromatosis).
- Pericardial constriction.
- Severe hypertension, ischaemia.
- High-output cardiac failure (anaemia, thyrotoxicosis, AV fistulae).
- Chronic pulmonary disease with right HF.
- Pulmonary hypertension.
- Atrial myxoma.

Adapted with permission from ACC/AHA Guidelines: Hunt *et al.*, Evaluation and Management Of Heart Failure http://www.acc.org/clinical/guidelines/failure/hf_index.htm

Principles of treatment

Unlike LV systolic dysfunction, there is little evidence-based data on how to treat patients with presumed diastolic dysfunction. Causes of diastolic heart failure include ischaemia, hypertension and hypertrophy, which should be identified and treated accordingly. Current recommendations suggest the use of β-blockers, rate slowing calcium channel antagonists (verapamil or diltiazem), ACEI and diuretics. Management of this group is difficult and should probably be tailored to the individual.

- Control of systolic and diastolic hypertension.
- Control of ventricular rate in patients with atrial fibrillation.
- Diuretics to control pulmonary congestion and peripheral oedema.
- Coronary revascularization in patients with coronary artery disease in whom symptomatic or demonstrable myocardial ischemia is judged to be having an adverse effect on diastolic function.
- Restoration of sinus rhythm in patients with atrial fibrillation.

(a) 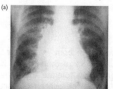 (b)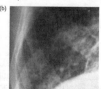

Fig. 6.3 CXR findings in heart failure. Panel a: There is cardiomegaly with prominent upper lobe vessels and alveolar oedema ('Bat's wing shadowing'). Panel b is a magnification of the right costophrenic angle showing septal lines (Kerley B lines) due to interstitial oedema.

High-output heart failure

In high-output states, the only way that the oxygen demands of the peripheral tissues can be met is by an increase in cardiac output. If there is underlying heart disease, it is unable to augment the cardiac output on a long term, and HF results.

Causes of high-output states

- Anaemia
- Acquired arteriovenous fistula
- Haemangioma
- Hereditary haemorrhagic telangiectasia
- Hepatic haemangioendothelioma
- Pregnancy
- Acromegaly
- Thyrotoxicosis
- Beriberi heart disease
- Paget's disease of the bone
- Fibrous dysplasia
- Polycythaemia rubra vera
- Carcinoid syndrome
- Multiple myeloma.

Anaemia
When the Hb levels fall below 8 gm/dl, the anaemia produces a high cardiac output. However, even when severe, anaemia rarely causes heart failure or angina in patients with normal hearts. Look for an underlying cardiac problem or valve disease. Try to determine the aetiology for the anaemia. Patient should be on bed-rest and transfused with packed red blood cells accompanied with iv diuretics.

Systemic arteriovenous fistulas
The increase in cardiac output depends on the size of the fistula. The Branham sign consists of slowing of the heart rate after manual compression of the fistula. It also raises arterial blood pressure. Surgical repair or excision is the ideal treatment.

Pregnancy (see p523)

Thyrotoxicosis
Raised levels of thyroxine produce increased heart rate and cardiac contractility, reduction in systemic vascular resistance and enhances sympathetic activation. Thyrotoxicosis does not usually precipitate heart failure unless there is reduced cardiac reserve. Atrial fibrillation occurs in about 10% of patients exacerbating the HF. Respiratory muscle weakness may contribute to the dyspnoea.

Beriberi (see p512)

Paget's disease
There is a linear relationship between the extent of bone involvement and rise in cardiac output. Involvement of about 15% of the skeleton is required before the rise is seen, and patients may tolerate the early stages well for years. Concomitant valvular disease or iachaemic heart disease results in decompensation. Successful treatment of Paget's with bisphosphonates may reverse the rise in cardiac output over several months.

Chapter 7

Heart muscle diseases

Classification

Heart muscle diseases include a diverse range of cardiomyopathies (literally heart muscle diseases) and myocarditides. Cardiomyopathies have been previously classified as diseases of unknown cause and were therefore distinct from more specific causes of heart muscle disease. However, a better understanding of their aetiology and pathophysiology has lead to this distinction becoming obsolete. As such, they are now reclassified according to the predominant pathophysiological process. Arrhythmogenic right ventricular cardiomyopathy (dysplasia) has been included in its own right and a few conditions remain unclassified as they do not easily fit into any of these categories (systolic dysfunction with minimal dilatation, fibroelastosis, ventricular non-compaction, and mitochondrial disease).

WHO/ISFC classification of cardiomyopathies

- Dilated cardiomyopathy
- Hypertrophic cardiomyopathy
- Restrictive cardiomyopathy
- Arrhythmogenic right ventricular cardiomyopathy (dysplasia)

WHO, World Health Organization; ISFC, International Society and Federation Cardiology

Specific cardiomyopathies are heart muscle diseases associated with specific cardiac or systemic disorders and include conditions previously excluded from this classification.

Specific cardiomyopathies

- Ischaemic
- Valvular
- Hypertensive
- Alcohol
- Metabolic
- Nutritional
- General system disease
- Muscular dystrophies
- Neuromuscular disorders
- Sensitivity and toxic reactions
- Peripartal.

Myocarditis is an inflammatory process involving mycoytes, interstitium, and vascular components ± pericardium and can be caused by a large number of infectious agents.

Dilated cardiomyopathy

Dilated cardiomyopathy (DCM) is characterised by cardiac chamber enlargement and impaired systolic dysfunction, although diastolic dysfunction is almost always also present. Congestive cardiac failure (CCF) often ensues. The prevalence is 5–8 per 100,000 and it is 3 times more frequent in Blacks and males than Whites and females.

Symptoms

Clinical presentation can be abrupt with acute pulmonary oedema, systemic or pulmonary emboli or even sudden death but more often patients present with symptoms of CCF such as breathlessness, in particular exertional dyspnoea, orthopnoea, paroxysmal nocturnal dyspnoea, and fatigue. Arrhythmia (e.g. AF—particularly with high alcohol intake) in are also common and patients are at risk of VT and sudden cardiac death (SCD).

Diagnosis

Diagnosis is established by physical examination, electrocardiography, chest x-ray, and echocardiography.

- **ECG** may show evidence of LVH, previous myocardial infarction, or arrhythmias. A sinus tachycardia is common with non-specific T wave changes and poor R-wave in anterior chest leads.
- **Chest x-ray** may show an enlarged cardiac size and pulmonary oedema (upper lobe venous diversion, interstitial oedema, pleural effusions and Kerley B lines).
- **Echocardiography** allows accurate assessment of cardiac chamber sizes as well as function and importantly valvular function. There is usually biventricular dilatation with poor septal motion (LBBB). There may be mural thrombus in either/both ventricles. There is often a small pericardial collection. Ejection fraction and fractional shortening are low. Dilatation of the ventricles results in motral and tricuspid regurgitation.
- **Exercise testing** with or without measurement of maximum ventilatory oxygen consumption is useful to assess functional capacity.
- **Ambulatory ECG monitoring** is essential to assess for the presence of prognostically significant ventricular arrhythmias.
- **Cardiac catheterization** needs to be undertaken with caution in patients with poor LV function as it may precipitate acute pulmonary oedema, or embolization of mural thrombus.It is useful for:
  - Excluding significant coronary disease.
  - Assessment of severity of mitral regurgitation and pulmonary artery pressures.
  - Ventricular biopsy: not routinely performed now, but may show histological findings of acute myocarditis (lymphocyte infiltration). In situ hybridisation to look for viral genome has not proved to be as revealing as initial studies suggested.

Aetiology of dilated cardiomyopathy

Although originally considered to be idiopathic, experimental and clinical data now suggest that genetic, viral and autoimmune factors play a role in its pathophysiology. Several genetic mutations have been identified as the causative problem in familial DCM while certain viruses have been shown to cause sporadic cases of DCM. The following list is not exhaustive and there is some overlap with specific cardiomyopathies.

- Inherited (may account for >25% of cases).
- Myocarditis (infective, autoimmune, toxic).
- Metabolic (haemochromatosis, thyrotoxicosis).
- Nutritional (vitamin deficiencies—thiamine[Beriberi]).
- Persistent tachycardia (tachymyopathy).

DCM is essentially a diagnosis of exclusion and potentially reversible causes including coronary artery disease, valvular heart disease and adult congenital heart disease should be sought. Careful attention should also be paid to dietary history and alcohol consumption as some reversibility is possible with modification of these factors.

Additional investigations for DCM

- Renal function.
- Liver function tests.
- Serum ferritin, iron, transferrin.
- Thyroid function.
- Viral serology.
- Infective screen (HIV, hepatitis C, enteroviruses).
- Autoantibodies.

Treatment

Management of DCM focuses on relieving symptoms and improving prognosis and is as for CCF. Therapies are designed to correct the maladaptive neurohormonal abnormalities involving the sympathetic system and rein–angiotensin–aldosterone axis. The acute management of heart failure is discussed on pp620–630.

Diuretics

Diuretics, in particular loop diuretics, are useful in relieving symptoms caused by pulmonary and peripheral congestion. Careful monitoring of electrolytes is important as intravascular depletion may cause urea to rise and hypokalaemia is common. Hypokalaemia may be counteracted by the co-administration of a potassium sparing diuretic such as amiloride or spironolactone. Spironolactone is a direct antagonist of aldosterone and blocks its salt and water retaining effects. The recent RALES trial (p608) demonstrated that the use of low dose spironolactone can reduce mortality in patients with severe CCF.

Vasodilators

Angiotensin converting enzyme (ACE) inhibitors have been shown in numerous studies to not only improve symptoms but also prognosis in patients with heart failure, including patients who are asymptomatic. First dose hypotension used to be a concern prompting initiation of therapy to be done preferably in hospital but this is rarely seen with newer ACE inhibitors and usually only in patients who are relatively intravascularly depleted due to the concomitant use of high dose diuretics. Side effects include a dry cough, possibly due to increased levels of bradykinin, angioedema (rare) and should be used with caution in patients with renovascular disease.

Angiotensin receptor$_1$ antagonists (ARBs) can be used as an alternative in patients who are intolerant of ACE inhibitors but have the same problems in patients with renovascular disease. The CHARM-Alternative trial (p555) demonstrated that the ARB, candesartan, was effective in reducing mortality in patients intolerant of ACE-inhibitors.

β-blockers

β-blockers although negatively inotropic have symptomatic and prognostic benefit largely due to improved diastolic filling and possibly by reducing the incidence of arrhythmias. However they should be started in small doses and titrated up. They should not be started in patients with overt heart failure and can be withdrawn if patients decompensate.

Antiarrhythmics

Unfortunately antiarrhythmics have not been shown to reduce the incidence of SCD in patients with DCM. Atrial fibrillation is very common in DCM and should be controlled with appropriate rate limiting medications however, as maintenance of sinus rhythm is unlikely to be sustained in the long-term, the over-use of antiarrhythmics should be avoided.

Anticoagulation

Patients with DCM are prone to thromboembolic complications and should be anticoagulated with warfarin regardless of underlying rhythm.

Non-pharmacological treatments

• Reversible causes of DCM including ischaemic and valvular heart disease should be corrected. Revascularization can improve prognosis in patients with significant coronary artery disease (CAD) and DCM.

• Orthotopic cardiac transplantation using an allograft can be considered in severely symptomatic patients despite maximal medical therapy. The limited availability of donor organs still restricts its role and numerous people die every year on cardiac transplant lists. As a result there is considerable interest in using organs from other species (xenografts). However, technical hurdles still remain before this can be considered a viable option. The artificial heart is another area that has received much interest and publicity and clinical trials are soon to be conducted.

• Cardiac resynchronization therapy (CRT) uses specially designed biventricular pacemakers which pace the right and left ventricle (usually via the coronary sinus) simultaneously, thereby improving cardiac haemodynamics. CRT has been shown in large clinical trials to result in significant improvements in functional capacity and even a small mortality benefit (see p288).

- Although antiarrhythmics have not been shown to reduce mortality in patients with DCM, implantable cardioverter defibrillators (ICD) have demonstrated in large clinical trials considerable efficacy and should be considered in any patient with an ejection fraction <35% especially in conjunction with evidence of non-sustained VT on ambulatory ECG monitoring. Newer devices can combine the benefit of CRT with and ICD (see p288).

Hypertrophic cardiomyopathy

Hypertrophic cardiomyopathy (HCM) is characterized by maladaptive left ventricular hypertrophy (LVH) inappropriate for the degree of afterload. Prevalence is thought to be 1–2 per 1000. The hypertrophy classically is localized to the proximal interventricular septum resulting in a dynamic outflow tract obstruction in association with systolic anterior motion (SAM) of the mitral valve leaflets (present in ~35% of patients).

However there is considerable phenotypic variability and the hypertrophy can be concentric, apical, or mid-cavitary resulting in an intra-cavitary gradient (often in association with an apical aneurysm). In addition genetic studies have demonstrated that affected family members may have little or no cardiac hypertrophy despite the presence of a disease causing mutation (variable penetrance). The reason for this marked phenotypic variability is poorly understood but is almost certainly multi-factorial.

HCM has also been associated with accessory atrio-ventricular pathways and conduction abnormalities in certain families.

Aetiology

HCM is an autosomal dominant inherited cardiac condition. However there is marked allelic and non-allelic heterogeneity with multiple mutations in at least 10 genes now identified as causing the disease. Most of these mutations are in genes encoding proteins of the sarcomere (e.g. β-myosin heavy chain, α-tropomyosin, troponins).

In contrast to mutations causing DCM, mutations frequently affect sarcomeric proteins involved in force generation as opposed to force transmission. This is, however, not consistent and some genes have different mutations causing both HCM *and* DCM (i.e. α-cardiac actin). Other mutations have been found in genes encoding non-sarcomeric proteins.

Histologically there is myofibrillar disarray and extensive fibrosis. Small intramural arterioles are also hypertrophied. The findings may be patchy, but are concentrated in the septum. Sub-valvular obstruction occurs between the anterior leaflet of the mitral valve and the hypertrophied septum. The mitral valve apparatus moves anteriorly in systole (a combination of malaligned papillary muscles and venture effect of a high velocity jet in the outflow tract). The valve becomes thickened and mitral regurgitation occurs.

Obstruction of the LV outflow tract is not always present. It is possible to have asymmetric septal hypertrophy (ASH) alone. Occasionally there is obstruction more evident towards the apex rather than at the outflow tract.

Symptoms

Patients often are asymptomatic and are increasingly picked up incidentally due to the wider use and availability of echocardiography or as part of family screening after identification of an affected family member. Symptoms, when they do occur, may include:
- Fatigue and breathlessness due to impaired diastolic filling and decreased cardiac output. Atrial transport is very important for maintaining cardiac output: symptoms typically get much worse with AF.

- Chest pain (angina) can result from increased cardiac work secondary to the LVH, a relative blood supply–demand mismatch and plugging of intramural arterioles. High diastolic pressures increase the diastolic wall stress and impair diastolic coronary blood flow.
- Atrial and ventricular arrhythmias are common and can result in palpitations, pre-syncope and syncope, or even sudden death.
- Pre-syncope and syncope can also occur due to increased outflow tract obstruction during exercise, at times of relative intravascular dehydration or from certain manoeuvres (i.e. Valsalva).
- Approximately 10–15% of patients may eventually develop left ventricular dilatation and failure.

Sudden cardiac death

The risk of SCD in these patients is extremely difficult to determine due to the marked phenotypic variability and most risk factors have low sensitivity and specificity.

Markers of risk for SCD in HCM

- Early age at diagnosis.
- Family history of SCD.
- Non-sustained VT on ambulatory ECG monitoring.
- Abnormal blood pressure response to exercise.
- Certain genetic mutations.

Diagnosis

The diagnosis is established by physical examination, electrocardiography, and echocardiography. Close attention must be paid to family history and family members should be offered screening. A genetic diagnosis can now be made in select individuals who have a definite family history of HCM. Despite the marked genetic heterogeneity a genetic diagnosis may be established in ~70% of patients with inherited HCM allowing accurate screening of other family members.

Physical examination (See Fig. 7.1)

Evidence of LVH may present with a forceful apical impulse and an S_4 heart sound. Outflow tract obstruction is evident by a double apical impulse and ejection systolic murmur beginning in mid-systole which may be augmented by provocation by manoeuvres such as Valsalva or squatting. A pansystolic murmur due to mitral regurgitation resulting from the systolic anterior movement (SAM) of the mitral valve may also be present.

Investigations

- **ECG** is rarely normal but usually shows voltage criteria for LVH with associated repolarization abnormalities. Features include:
  - LVH with ST and T wave change.
  - Deep Q waves in inferior and lateral leads (septal hypertrophy).
  - Pre-excitation and WPW syndrome.
  - Ventricular ectopics.

- **Echocardiography** is essential for diagnosis allowing accurate measurement of chamber sizes and wall thicknesses. It also facilitates demonstration of outflow tract or intra-cavitary gradients. Features include:
  - ASH: grossly thickened septum compared with posterior LV wall, with reduced septal motion.
  - Small LV cavity with hypercontractile posterior wall.
  - Mid systolic aortic valve closure or fluttering of the aortic valve leaflet tips.
  - SAM: systolic anterior movement of the mitral valve apparatus. There may be contact between the anterior mitral leaflet and septum in systole.
  - Reduced diastolic closure rate of the anterior mitral valve leaflet.
- **Cardiac MRI** may be helpful in borderline cases.
- Other investigations may help in risk stratification although no one investigation accurately predicts those at risk of SCD and negative tests do not exclude the risk of SCD:
  - **Ambulatory ECG monitoring**—atrial and ventricular arrhythmias.
  - **Exercise testing**—functional capacity and blood pressure response to exercise.
  - **Cardiac catheterization**—coronary anatomy and intra-cavitary and outflow tract gradients.
  - **Electrophysiology testing**—VT studies have no proven role in risk assessment but EP studies may be useful to assess suspected accessory AV pathways.
  - **Genetic testing**—only useful for screening family members if causative gene in proband can be identified.

Treatment
Approximately half of sudden deaths in HCM occur during or shortly after strenuous exercise and therefore patients should be advised against competitive sports. Unfortunately this also means that a significant proportion die unexpectedly without any obvious precipitant. Treatment of symptoms usually consists of the following

β-blockers: β-blockers reduce myocardial oxygen demand and improve diastolic filling reducing chest pain and improving breathlessness. They are the mainstay of therapy for angina, dyspnoea, giddiness, and syncope. Large doses may be required.

Calcium channel antagonists: calcium channel antagonists (verapamil and diltiazem) are useful as they are negatively inotropic (reducing outflow tract obstruction) and reduce heart rate during exercise. Use diltiazem cautiously with β-blockers. Avoid verapamil in patients on β-blockers.

Disopyramide: disopyramide is a negatively inotropic antiarrhythmic agent that has been shown to reduce outflow tract gradients. Unfortunately its use is limited by anti-cholinergic side effects.

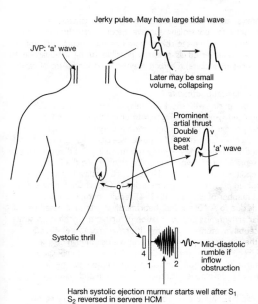

Fig. 7.1 Clinical signs of hypertrophic cardiomyopathy. Reproduced with permission from swanton RH (2003). *Cardiology Pocket Consultant* 5th ed. Blackwell Science: Oxford.

Dynamic manoeuvres to assess LVOT obstruction	
Decreased LVOT obstruction (Murmur softer and shorter)	**Increased LVOT obstruction** (Murmur louder and longer)
↑ *LV volume*	↓ *LV volume*
Squatting	Sudden standing
Handgrip	Valsalva (during)
Passive leg elevation	Sublingual GTN
Valsalva (after release)	Hypovolaemia
Mueller manoeuvre (deep inspiration against a closed glottis)	Dehydration
↓ *Contractility*	↑ *Contractility*
β-blockers (acute i.v.)	β-agonists (e.g. isoprenaline)
↑ *Afterload*	↓ *Contractility*
Phenylephrine	α-blockade
Handgrip	

Antiarrhythmics: other antiarrhythmic drugs such as amiodarone and sotalol are useful for controlling supraventricular arrhythmias but have not been shown to reduce the risk of SCD from ventricular arrhythmias. AF should be cardioverted as soon as possible (using amiodarone to improve chances of success). Digoxin may be used for failure of cardioversion.

Non-pharmacological treatments
- Dual-chamber pacing with short AV delay is used in patients with obstruction and symptoms refractory to drug-therapy. By ensuring ventricular pre-excitation, LV contraction is desynchronized, reducing LVOT gradients. Maintaining RV capture especially during exercise is difficult and shortening the AV delay too much impairs diastolic filling.
- Alcohol septal ablation involves injecting alcohol into the first or second septal perforator artery. This causes a localized infarct of the hypertrophied proximal septum, reducing LVOT gradient. However a significant number of patients (10–15%) require permanent pacing afterwards due to AV block and theoretically there is increased risk of ventricular arrhythmias due to creation of further arrhythmic substrate.
- Surgical septal myotomy–myectomy (Morrow procedure) directly debulks the proximal septum. There is also a risk of high degree AV block requiring permanent pacing and long-term complications include aortic regurgitation. Cardiac transplantation may be necessary in patients who develop left ventricular dilatation and systolic heart failure.
- ICDs should be considered in patients who have survived a cardiac arrest or who have presented with haemodynamically unstable VT. However their role in other patients who may be considered high risk for SCD has not been established.

Restrictive cardiomyopathy

Restrictive cardiomyopathy

Restrictive cardiomyopathy is rare condition characterized by impaired diastolic function due to reduced ventricular compliance. It is very important to distinguish restrictive cardiomyopathy from constrictive pericarditis as the latter can be treated surgically by stripping the pericardium from the myocardium.

Aetiology

The aetiology of truly idiopathic cases remains obscure. A few cases are familial and tend to be associated with skeletal muscle disease. Other cases are associated with systemic diseases, infiltration or endomyocardial fibrosis.

Symptoms

Patients often have severely limited exercise tolerance due to an inability to increase cardiac output as there stroke volume is relatively fixed. There also are limited by breathlessness and have evidence of right heart failure (peripheral oedema).

Diagnosis

Physical examination

In addition to signs of CCF, a loud S_3, S_4 or both may be present. There also may be prominent x and y descents of the JVP and venous pressure may increase on inspiration (Kussmaul sign). The apex beat will be palpable in contrast to constrictive pericarditis.

Investigations

* **ECG** may show P-mitrale or -pulmonale, reduced precordial QRS voltages, and atrial arrhythmias.
* **Echocardiography** may be normal or at least demonstrate normal systolic function. Alternatively systolic function may be reduced in advanced cases. Infiltration may be evident by hypertrophied ventricles, thickened intra-atrial septum and the myocardium may appear speckled. Biatrial enlargement may also be present. A restrictive mitral inflow pattern is seen on Doppler tracing.
* **Laboratory test** are aimed at determining causes of infiltration. Left and right heart catheterization may be necessary to help to exclude constrictive pericarditis (difference in LVEDP and RVEDP >7 mmHg at end-expiration makes constriction unlikely).
* **CT and MRI scanning** are useful to look at pericardial disease.

Treatment

Treatment is aimed at the symptoms of CCF and the underlying condition. Rate control in atrial fibrillation is important as reducing ventricular filling times will have significant impact.

❶ Patients with amyloid are very sensitive to digoxin.

Causes of restrictive cardiomyopathy

Myocardial

- Non-infiltrative.
  - Idiopathic.
  - Scleroderma.
- Infiltrative.
  - Amyloid.
  - Sarcoid.
- Storage Diseases.
  - Lysosomal storage diseases (Gaucher's, Hurler's, Fabry).
  - Glycogen storage disease.
  - Haemochromatosis.

Endomyocardial

- Endomyocardial fibrosis.
- Hypereosinophilic syndrome.
- Metastatic malignancies.
- Carcinoid.
- Iatrogenic (radiation, anthracyclines).

Arrhythmogenic right ventricular cardiomyopathy

Arrhythmogenic right ventricular cardiomyopathy (ARVC) is a disease in which the normal right ventricular myocardium is replaced by a fibro-fatty infiltrate. It was originally termed a dysplasia reflecting the idea that it was somehow a developmental defect but further understanding has lead to the appreciation that it is a continuing process and has subsequently been reclassified as a cardiomyopathy. It can progress to right ventricular dilatation and failure and in some cases there may also be left ventricular involvement.

Aetiology

Fifty per cent of cases are familial with an autosomal dominant pattern of inheritance. Disease causing genes have not been found but several loci have been mapped to chromosomes 1, 2, 3, 10, and 14 and an autosomal recessive variant, which is characterized by ARVC, palmoplantar keratosis, and wooly hair (Naxos disease) has been mapped to chromosome 17.

Symptoms

Patients are usually asymptomatic and presentation is usually in the form of ventricular arrhythmias with typical LBBB pattern indicating probable origin from the right ventricle. Therefore otherwise healthy young individuals can present with cardiac arrest or SCD. Other patients present in later life with symptoms of CCF with or without ventricular arrhythmias and are misdiagnosed as having DCM.

Diagnosis

Diagnosis of affected individuals can be very difficult especially during family screening as standard non-invasive investigations have poor sensitivity. Only a minority may have classic findings of typical right ventricular arrhythmias with LBBB pattern, abnormal depolarization/repolarization abnormalities, particularly on right precordial ECG leads, and evidence of structural abnormalities of the right ventricle. Right ventricular free wall abnormalities are best characterized by MRI but this too has limitations and therefore patients with suspected ARVC but negative investigations may need repeated studies.

There are no established or proven specific risk factors for SCD but markers of increased risk include young age at diagnosis, malignant family history, syncope, right ventricular dysfunction and left ventricular involvement, and presence of VT on ambulatory monitoring.

Therefore baseline investigations in addition to a carefully taken history should include:
- 12 lead and signal averaged ECG.
- 24 hour ambulatory ECG monitoring.
- Exercise testing.
- Echocardiogram (±MRI scan).

Treatment

There are no established best treatment options for patients with ARVC, and, as the disease is progressive, antiarrhythmic options are used for symptomatic benefit in patients with haemodynamically well tolerated ventricular arrhythmias. Patients who have developed RV ± LV dysfunction can be managed with standard treatments for CCF and in severe case transplantation may be an option.

Antiarrhythmics

β-blockers alone or in combination with class I and III antiarrhythmics are the most effective in reducing symptomatic but well tolerated ventricular arrhythmias. Sotalol and amiodarone have been shown to be most effective.

Patients with more sustained ventricular arrhythmias may have their drug therapy guided by their response during programmed electrical stimulation but this has no proven benefit in reducing the risk of SCD.

Radiofrequency ablation

In a small subset of patients with drug refractory arrhythmias who are felt to have fairly localized disease may be amenable to electrophysiologic mapping and radiofrequency ablation. However it must be remembered that ARVC is progressive disease and this can only be viewed as a palliative procedure.

Implantable cardioverter defibrillators

In patients with life threatening or drug refractory ventricular arrhythmias and widespread disease, ICDs probably offer the best protective measure against SCD.

Ischaemic cardiomyopathy

This is a condition in which coronary artery disease (CAD) causes a picture which is often indistinguishable from DCM with or without a preceding history of angina or myocardial infarction. Often the degree of dysfunction is inconsistent with the extent of CAD. It is important to recognize patients with hibernating myocardium as they will benefit from revascularization.

Valvular cardiomyopathy

Patients with valvular heart disease will develop a cardiomyopathy dependent on the predominant valvular lesion. Often significant improvement in cardiac function can be seen after correction of the valve disease.

Hypertensive cardiomyopathy

Hypertension causes LVH in response to increased afterload which is compensatory and protective to a point. However there are ultimately detrimental effects on systolic and diastolic ventricular function. Hypertension also leads to accelerated atherosclerosis and ischaemic heart disease. Hypertensive cardiomyopathy is the commonest form of CCF outside the Western world.

Alcoholic cardiomyopathy

Chronic alcohol excess is the commonest 2° cause of DCM in the Western world. Proposed mechanisms include (1) direct toxic effect, (2) concomitant nutritional deficiencies (esp. thiamine), and (3) rarely toxic effects of additives (cobalt). Unlike other forms of DCM, abstinence from alcohol early in the disease process may stop progression or even result in significant improvement in cardiac function.

Metabolic cardiomyopathy

Various abnormalities in metabolism can result in cardiomyopathy. As already mentioned, lysosomal and glycogen storage diseases can cause a form of restrictive cardiomyopathy. Haemochromatosis also causes restrictive cardiomyopathy by unknown mechanisms. Acquired errors of metabolism such as acromegaly result in biventricular hypertrophy. Diabetes mellitus can cause cardiomyopathy with systolic and/or diastolic dysfunction even in the absence of significant epicardial CAD.

General system disease

Systemic lupus erythematosis can cause heart disease in many ways. Approximately 10% of patients with SLE have evidence of myocarditis. Patients with associated antiphospholipid antibody syndrome have increased risk of valvular abnormalities and DCM due to thrombotic occlusions of the microcirculation without vasculitis. They also have increased atherogenesis.

Pulmonary hypertension due to pulmonary vasculitis is an uncommon cause of cardiomyopathy in patients with rheumatoid arthritis.

Nutritional cardiomyopathy

Thiamine is an important co-enzyme in the hexose monophophate shunt. Infants breast fed in areas with diets deficient in thiamine develop mainly right ventricular failure between 1 and 4 months of age. Prompt correction of the vitamin deficiency results in rapid improvement in the cardiac abnormalities without long-term consequence.

Protein–calorie malnutrition (Marasmus, Kwashiorkor) results in thinning and atrophy of muscle fibers and ultimately DCM. Careful treatment may result in marked improvement over several months provided the patient survives the initial period.

Muscular dystrophies

The large number of muscular dystrophies can be associated with either DCM or HCM and this can be the commonest cause of death in these patients. Myotonic dystrophy is associated with AV conduction abnormalities and arrhythmias rather than cardiomyopathy. All patients need careful long-term follow-up.

Neuromuscular disorders

Cardiac involvement in Friedreich's ataxia is relatively common although usually asymptomatic. It is most commonly associated with HCM which is distinct from the genetic variety by lack of myofibrillar disarray and malignant ventricular arrhythmias. Rarely, it is associated with DCM.

Sensitivity or toxic reactions

A large number of non-infectious agents can damage the myocardium. The damage can be acute with evidence of an inflammatory reaction, or there may be no inflammation and necrosis as in hypersensitivity reactions. Other agents lead to chronic changes with progressive fibrosis and an ultimate picture similar to DCM. Numerous chemical and industrial agents can cause myocardial damage as well as radiation and excessive heat.

Peripartum

Peripartum cardiomyopathy is a form of DCM. Symptoms occur in the third trimester and the diagnosis is made in the peripartal period. Approximately half will show complete or near complete resolution over the first six months post-partum. Of the remainder, some will continue to deteriorate and result in death or transplantation while others continue to experience chronic CCF. Its diagnosis is established by excluding other causes of DCM and the cause is unknown. (Also see Chapter 14.)

Myocarditis

Myocarditis is the process whereby the myocardium becomes inflamed by one of a large range of infectious agents. Unfortunately the infectious agent is rarely identified. Numerous bacteria, viruses, spirochetes, fungi, parasites and rickettsia can cause myocarditis.

Aetiology

Damage can result from a number of mechanisms including direct toxic effect on the myocyte, production of a toxin (e.g. diphtheria), and immunologically mediated cell damage. Histological findings depend on a number of factors including the infectious agent, stage of disease and the mechanism of damage. Damage can be focal or diffuse and is randomly distributed throughout the myocardium.

Symptoms

The clinical consequences of the damage can range from asymptomatic subclinical infection to rapidly progressive and ultimately fatal CCF.

Long-term consequences are also variable. Patients who were initially asymptomatic can present after a prolonged latency period with DCM or have complete recovery. Patients who present early, even with fulminant CCF, can also have complete recovery. Patients with non-fulminant presentations can gradually deteriorate are recover gradually.

Diagnosis

The diagnosis is often established by identifying the associated systemic illness. Isolation of the infectious agent is rarely achieved although clearly supportive of the diagnosis if positive. Endomyocardial biopsy can be useful in confirming the diagnosis but is frequently negative.

Treatment

Management of patients with myocarditis is largely supportive. Physical activity should be restricted as in animal models exercise was found to be detrimental to cardiac function. Standard management of CCF and eradication of the infectious agent are the main stay of treatment. Symptomatic arrhythmias should be controlled and β-blockers may be cardioprotective.

Trials of immunosuppressive therapy in patients with myocarditis have been largely disappointing. The use of steroids in acutely ill patients could be considered but any benefit is unproven.

Viral myocarditis

- In Western countries the **enterovirus** (especially **Coxsackie B**) is the commonest cause of myocarditis. This is usually mild and self-limiting, although can be particularly virulent in neonates and young children. Clinical manifestations in adults include myalgia, pleuritic chest pains, upper respiratory tract symptoms, arthralgia, palpitations, and fever. The ECG is usually abnormal with ST and T wave changes, VEs and AV conduction abnormalities. Cardiac enzymes may be elevated or normal reflecting the degree of myocardial necrosis. ECHO may show diffuse or regional LV dysfunction. Most make an uneventful recovery within weeks. Treatment is symptomatic.
- Other viruses such as CMV, Dengue, hepatitis, EBV, influenza and varicella are rarely associated with cardiac involvement. ECG changes and cardiac enzyme release makes the diagnosis. With mumps, myocarditis is rarely recognised, but pathologically is common. Myocarditis generally occurs in the first week of illness and is transient. Rubella infection in 1st trimester of pregnancy results in congenital lesions such as patent ductus or pulmonary artery maldevelopment; myocarditis is rare but causes fetal/neonatal heart failure.
- Cardiac involvement is common in patients with **HIV** (up to 50%) but only clinical evident in ~10%. The usual presentation is with CCF and DCM, due to a direct effect of HIV on the myocardium, although opportunistic infection in AIDS patients is another important cause of myocarditis.

Rickettsial myocarditis

- Q fever (*R. burnetti*) typically causes endocarditis; pericarditis (chest pain and dyspnoea) is also common. Myocarditis is uncommon and produces ECG changes such as transient ST and T wave changes).
- Rocky Mountain spotted fever (*R. rickettsii*) produces a widespread vasculitis that involves the myocardium. ECHO shows unexpected LV dysfunction which may persist even after the infection is cleared.
- Scrub typhus (*T. rsutsugamushi*) produces a panvasculitis that may involve the myocardium producing haemorrhage into the myocardium and subepicardial petichiae. Long-term damage appears to be infrequent.

Bacterial myocarditis

- **Diptheria:** myocarditis occurs in up to 20% and is due to the production of a toxin that inhibits protein synthesis. Clinical signs appear towards the end of the first week of infection with CCF, and cardiomegaly. ECG changes are seen and may persist after recovery. Treatment with antitoxin should be given early in the course of the disease. Corticosteroids do not appear to be helpful. However treatment with carnitine seems to reduce the incidence of heart failure, need for pacemaker and lowers mortality.
- **Meningococcus:** myocarditis is associated with increased mortality, and results in haemorrhagic lesions and intracellular organisms. Clinical features include CCF, an pericardial effusion with tamponade. Patients with septicaemia should be monitored especially if there are ECG abnormalities.
- **Mycoplasma:** ECG changes are not uncommon in patients with *Mycoplasma* pneumonia. Other manifestations include pericarditis and CCF. No specific treatment for the carditis is usually indicated.
- **Whipple's disease** (*Tropheryma whippelli*) may involve the myocardium with infiltration with PAS-positice macrophages. Coronary artery lesions may be seen. Pulmonary arterial hypertension can occur. Valve fibrosis produces aortic and mitral regurgitation. Antibiotic therapy appears to be effective, but relapses are not uncommon.
- Other bacterial infections occasionally associated with cardiac involvement include Legionella, Salmonella, Psittacosis and Streptococcus (acute rheumatic fever—p60). Tuberculous myocarditis is rare unless there is pericarditis (p342).

Spirochetal myocarditis

- About 10% of patients with **Lyme disease** (caused by the tickborne spirochete *Borrelia burgdorferi*) have evidence of cardiac involvement; a combination of direct muscle invasion by the spirochete together with immune-mediated damage. Although this normally takes the form of AV conduction abnormalities, LV dysfunction can be present. Syncope due to complete heart block is frequent and there is often associated ventricular escape rhythms. VT is uncommon. A positive gallium or indium antimyosin antibody scan may point toward suspected cardiac involvement. Patients with 2nd or 3rd degree heart block require hospital admission and monitoring. Treatment with iv penicillin, temporary pacing (if required). The role of steroids and aspirin is unclear.
- **Leptospirosis** (Weil disease): cardiac involvement is seen in the more severe presentations. Interstitial myocarditis with involvement of the papillary muscles is seen; conduction defects, aortitis, and coronary arteritis have been described.
- **Syphillis** most commonly produces an aortitis, and direct involvement of the myocardium with gummae is rare (see p508).

Protozoal myocarditis

- In South America the parasite *Trypanosoma cruzi* causes the myocarditis **Chagas' disease** which is a significant public health problem (see p506). In the acute phase it can cause severe myocarditis resulting in CCF and death. Histologically, parasites can be seen lying alongside the myofibers. Immune lysis by antbody and cell-mediated immunity directed against *T. cruzi* antigens adsorbed onto the myocardium appears to be the mechanism of damage. Young children more commonly develop the acute disease and are more severely affected than adults.
- After an average of 20 years, approx. 30% of patients develop findings of chronic Chagas' disease. Clinical manifestations vary from asymptomatic seropositivity to progressive cardiac chamber dilatation with resultant severe CCF. AV conduction defects also occur. Histologically there is extensive fibrosis but no parasites are seen. Fatigue, peripheral oedema, ascites, and hepatomegaly are seen. Ventricular arrhythmias are common: multifocal VEs and bouts of VT occur, culminating in syncope and sudden cardiac death. ECHO shows features of dilated cardiomyopathy; in advanced cases the appearances are distinctive with posterior hypokinesis with relativly preserved septal motion.
- Diagnosis is with the complement fixation test (Machado-Guerreiro), indirect immunofluorescence, or ELISA. Treatment is supportive; amiodarone is useful for ventricular arrhythmias; anticoagulation prevents thrombolism. Anti-parasitic agents reduce parisitaemia, but there is no evidence that they cure the disease.
- Myocardial involvement with other protozoa (e.g. trypanosomes, Toxoplasma or malaria) is rare and usually asymptomatic. Severe fatal disease is occasionally seen.

Fungal myocarditis

- Fungal infection is rare and seen in patients with concomitant malignant disease or those receiving chemotherapy, steroids or other immunosuppressive therapy. Other predisposing factors include cardiac surgery, HIV infection, and IV drug use.
- Organisms implicated include *Actinomyces*, *Aspergillus*, *Candida*, *Cryptococcus* and *Histoplasma*. Generalized coccidioidomycosis generally causes epicardial lesions with pericarditis, progressing on to constrictive pericarditis (see p334). Myocardial involvement has been described.

Toxic and metabolic myocarditis

A variety of drugs, chemical agents, physical agents (e.g. radiation, heat) may result in myocardial damage. Cardiac involvement in systemic disease is discussed in Chapter 14.

Anthracylines (daunorubicin and adriamycin): these drugs inhibit nucleic acid synthesis and can produce acute and late toxicity. Acute cardiotoxicity includes arrhythmias, acute LV dysfunction, a pericarditis-myocarditis syndrome, myocardial infarction, and sudden cardiac death. Late cardiotoxicity is due to a dose-dependent degenerative cardiomyopathy that manifests anywhere from weeks to months after the last dose. Symptoms can be difficult to control with conventional therapy and cardiac transplantation has been used in cases where 'cancer cure' has been achieved.

Cocaine: this produces chest pain, sweating, and palpitations. In a minority there is myocardial ischaemia due to coronary vasoconstriction or thrombotic occlusion of the coronary. Associated findings include ventricular arrhythmias, and sudden cardiac death. Treatment is supportive and with β-blockers.

Catecholamines: severe reversible dilated cardiomyopathy has been described with phaeochromocytoma, as well as treatment with high doses of catecholamines and excessive doses of β-agonists in decompensated pulmonary disease. Aspirin and dipyridamole may offer some protection suggesting a role for platelets in the pathogenesis.

Carbon monoxide: poisoning usually results in CNS depression, but subendocardial myocardial necrosis is seen. Palpitations, sinus tachycardia, AF and ventricular arrhythmias may be seen. ECG abnormalities are common. Treatment with 100% oxygen, bed rest, and supportive treatment for arrhythmias is usually effective.

Electrolyte abnormalities: chronic hypocalcaemia is associated with CCF that only responds to restoration of serum calcium. Rapid blood transfusion (citrated blood) has been described to result in transient LV dysfunction due to low serum calcium levels. Severe hypophosphataemia can also result in reversible LV impairment, restored by correcting the phosphate levels. Hypomagnesaemia is associated with SVT and VT (esp. in the context of digitalis toxicity) and focal myocardial necrosis is seen.

Deficiency of taurine and carnitine is associated with a DCM, and in the case of carnitine, supplementation can lead to symptomatic and functional improvement. Myocardial carnitine levels are reduced in patients with DCM but the significance of this is still debated. Selenium deficiency accounts for a type of DCM seen in parts of rural China, and is occasionally seen in patients on TPN without selenium supplements.

Hypersensitivity myocarditis (eosinophilia and myocardial infiltraton with eosinophils and giant cells) has been described with a variety of drugs including antibiotics (penicillins, amphotericin, chloramphenicol, tetracycline, sulphonamides), antiepileptics (phenytoin, carbamazepine), antituberculous drugs (isoniazid), NSAIDs (indomethacin, phenylbutazone), diuretics (spironolactone, chlorthalidone, hydrochlorothiazide, acetazolamide), sulphonylureas and amitryptilline. It is rarely recognised clinically. The offending drug should be stopped and steroids may be required in severe cases.

Chapter 8

Pericardial diseases

Aetiology

The pericardium may be involved in the large number of disease pro
cesses listed in the table below. In some patients, pericardial disease is
the primary disease process dominating the clinical picture whereas in
others it is a manifestation of a systemic disease. The most common
causes are idiopathic (or viral), uraemic, neoplastic, tuberculous pericarditis, and acute myocardial infarction. The spectrum of pericardial disease
is determined by the age and social circumstances of the patient. In
an elderly North American and Western European population, the
commonest causes are malignancy, followed by uraemia and myocardial
infarction. In less privileged communities and in developing countries,
tuberculosis is still the predominant cause of pericardial disease.

Aetiology of pericardial diseases	
Infections	*Bacterial:* Mycobacterium tuberculosis, Staphylococcus, Pneomococcus, Meningococcus, Mycoplasma.
	Viral: Coxsackie, CMV, ECHO, EBV, influenza, HIV, mumps, parvo B19, rubella, varicella.
	Fungal: Histoplasmosis, Blastomycosis.
	Parasitic: *Amoebiasis.*
Autoimmune and hypersensitivity diseases	*Collagen vascular diseases:* systemic lupus erythema-tosus, polyarteritis nodosa, scleroderma, dermato-myositis.
	Type 2 auto-immune disorders: rheumatic fever, autoreactive pericarditis, postmyocardial infarction, and postpericardiotomy syndromes.
	Drug-induced: hydralazine, procainamide, penicillin, phenylbutazone.
	Other autoimmune disorders: rheumatoid arthritis, ankylosing spondylitis.
Pericardial involvement by disease in surrounding organs	*Heart:* acute myocardial infarction, myocarditis.
	Lung: pulmonary infarction, pneumonia.
Malignant disease	*Primary:* mesothelioma, sarcoma, fibroma, lipoma.
	Secondary: lung carcinoma, breast carcinoma, mela-noma, lymphoma, leukaemia.
Bleeding into the pericardium	*Trauma:* penetrating and non-penetrating.
	Dissecting aortic aneurysm.
	Haemorrhagic diathesis: leukemia, scurvy.
	Anticoagulants: warfarin.
Metabolic disorders	Uraemia, dialysis-related, myxoedema, gout.
Miscellaneous	Acute idiopathic pericarditis, radiation, sarcoidosis, amyloidosis, familial mediterranean fever.

Syndromes of pericardial disease

Pericardial reaction to the various disease processes is limited, and we are thus able to distinguish the following five clinical and pathological forms of pericarditis:
(1) Acute pericarditis without effusion,
(2) Pericardial effusion with or without tamponade,
(3) Constrictive pericarditis,
(4) Effusive-constrictive pericarditis
(5) Calcific pericarditis without constriction.

Acute pericarditis without effusion

('Dry' pericarditis)

Aetiology: Any of the causes listed in the table on p328 may cause dry pericarditis. The clinical syndrome is commonly seen in acute viral pericarditis or after myocardial infarction.

Pathology: there is a fibrinous exudate with an inflammatory reaction involving the visceral and parietal pericardium. The epicardium is also involved and this accounts for the ECG changes that are seen, and the rise in cardiac enzymes (e.g., troponin I).

Symptoms: sharp, stabbing, central chest pain is common, with radiation to the shoulders and upper arm. It is relieved by sitting up and leaning forward, and aggravated by lying down, and may be accentuated by inspiration, cough, swallowing, or movement of the trunk. Fever, night sweats, and other constitutional symptoms may be present, depending on the underlying cause.

Signs: a pericardial friction rub is frequently heard. This is a superficial, scratchy, grating sound that is best heard in the second to fourth intercostal spaces when pressure is exerted on the diaphragm of the stethoscope. Positioning the patient leaning forward and listening in held inspiration may bring it out. The rub is classically described as being triphasic. Usually you hear at least two components due to atrial systole and ventricular systole. Occasionally a third component attributed to rapid ventricular filling is heard.

ECG: the patient is usually in sinus rhythm but atrial fibrillation may occur. In the early stages there is widespread S-T segment elevation with concavity directed upwards, and PR segment deviation opposite to the polarity of the P wave. After a few days the ST segments followed by PR segments return to normal, and T waves become inverted.

CXR: the cardiac shadow is not enlarged in dry pericarditis.

Differential diagnosis: acute pericarditis must be differentiated from myocardial infarction, spontaneous pneumothorax, and pleurisy.

Diagnosis is of acute pericarditis is based on typical symptoms of chest pain, pericardial rub, and/or characteristic ECG changes.

Management: treat underlying cause. Good pain relief can be achieved by the use of nonsteroidal anti-inflammatory agents (NSAIDs).

Pericardial effusion ± tamponade

Aetiology

Any of the causes listed in the table on p328 may cause pericardial effusion. Large effusions are common with neoplastic, TB, uraemic pericarditis, and myxoedema.

Pathology

In addition to fibrinous inflammation, there is significant fluid exudation. The pericardial fluid may be serous, sero-sanguineous, haemorrhagic or purulent depending on the underlying cause. Haemorrhagic effusion is common in tuberculosis or neoplasia. Brownish fluid with an anchovy sauce appearance of the pus is highly suggestive of amoebic pericarditis.

Clinical features

The clinical presentation varies depending on the rate of accumulation of the fluid, the amount of fluid that accumulates, and the stage at which the patient is first seen.

Symptoms: chest pain may be typically pericardial (as described under dry pericarditis), or it may be dull and heavy due to distension of the pericardium. Dyspnoea is common, and orthopnoea may occur later in the course of the disease. Cough may be present due to compression of surrounding structures. Constitutional symptoms may be present depending on the cause of the disease.

Signs: typically, praecordial dullness extends beyond the apex beat (which may be impalpable), and dullness is present to the right of the sternum. Dullness and bronchial breathing (Ewart's sign) at the left base posteriorly due to compression of the left lower lobe bronchus may be found. Cardiac tamponade should be considered in a patient with hypotension, raised JVP, and quiet heart sounds (Beck's triad). The primary defect in cardiac tamponade is interference with diastolic filling of the heart. The other clinical features of cardiac tamponade are presence of tachycardia, pulsus paradoxus (fall is systolic blood pressure on inspiration of >10 mmHg or inspiratory fall in systolic blood pressure that exceeds half the pulse pressure), elevated JVP with brisk 'x' descents and absent 'y' descents, rise in JVP on inspiration (Kussmaul's sign), dyspnoea or tachypnoea with clear lungs, and hepatomegaly.

ECG

Sinus tachycardia, generalized low voltage QRS complexes with non-specific S-T segment and T-wave changes. Electrical alternans, involving the QRS complex, suggests the presence of a massive pericardial effusion. Total electrical alternans (P-QRS-T), which is uncommon, is pathognomonic of cardiac tamponade.

CXR

This commonly shows a large globular heart usually with clear lung fields.

Echocardiography is diagnostic, showing an echo free zone surrounding the heart. The fluid may not be evenly distributed. Diastolic collapse of the right ventricle and right atrium indicate cardiac tamponade.

The following features are more common in patients with marked inflammatory or malignant causes of pericardial effusion:

- soft tissue density masses,
- thickening of the visceral pericardium, and
- presence of fibrinous strands.

The hallmark of benign, idiopathic effusion is a clear echo-free space, whereas malignancy, bacterial infection, and haemorrhagic effusions are more likely to have solid components or stranding.

Cardiac catheterization can establish the diagnosis and severity of tamponade but is rarely necessary. The important findings are

1. Equilibration of mean right atrial, right ventricular end-diastolic, and mean capillary wedge pressure,
2. Rapid 'x' descent on the right atrial pressure waveform, and
3. Pulsus paradoxus.

Differential diagnosis

Myocardial infarction and pulmonary embolism.

Management

- When an effusion does not cause haemodynamic impairment and the cause is known (e.g., uraemia, myxoedema), then no further investigations are necessary and the treatment consists of treating the underlying cause.
- If the cause is not known, then pericardiocentesis must be considered. Aspiration of the fluid helps to establish the nature of the effusion.
- Cardiac tamponade is a life-threatening condition. Urgent pericardial aspiration necessary (See section on 'Pericardiocentesis' p698). Surgical drainage is indicated for haemopericardium or purulent pericarditis.

Constrictive pericarditis

Aetiology: constrictive pericarditis is usually due to tuberculosis. Other causes are mediastinal irradiation, purulent pericarditis, previous trauma (surgical or non-surgical) with infection of the pericardial space, and, very rarely, viral pericarditis.

Pathology: the pericardium becomes a dense mass of fibrous tissue and this may be calcified. This results in the encasement of the heart within a non-expansile pericardium.

Clinical features

Symptoms: dyspnoea, oedema and abdominal swelling due to ascites and hepatomegaly.

Signs: small volume pulse and pulsus paradoxus. JVP is always elevated, usually very high with prominent 'x' and 'y' descents. A diastolic knock is usually felt at the left sternal border due to the sudden halting of the ventricles during diastolic filling. Apex beat may be impalpable. Heart sounds are usually soft, and an early third sound coincident with the diastolic knock is usually heard. In the pulmonary area there is sudden instantaneous widened splitting of the second sound that occurs following the first heartbeat of inspiration (Vogelpoel–Beck sign). The liver is commonly grossly enlarged, ascites is marked and peripheral oedema is present.

ECG is abnormal in virtually every case, but changes are non-specific. (i.e., generalized low voltage QRS complexes, and widespread flattening and inversion of T waves). Atrial fibrillation is common in the chronic form.

CXR: a normal or near normal cardiac size in the presence of marked venous distension or heart failure is suggestive of constrictive pericarditis or restrictive cardiomyopathy. Pericardial calcification is diagnostic but its incidence varies from 5% to 70% of cases in different series.

Echocardiography: pericardial thickening may be present. A restrictive mitral filling pattern on Doppler, with respiratory variation of > 25% over the atrio-ventricular valves.

CT and MRI scan: these techniques demonstrate pericardial thickening (>5 mm).

Cardiac catheterization: this demonstrates elevation and equalization of filling pressures. In the typical case, the difference in filling pressures between the right ventricle and left ventricle does not exceed 6 mmHg. The right atrial waveform shows rapid 'x' and 'y' descents, and the mean pressure does not decrease normally with inspiration or may show Kussmaul's sign.

Management: constrictive pericarditis is treated by surgical removal of the fibrous constrictive tissue (pericardiectomy).

Effusive–constrictive pericarditis

Aetiology: this is characteristically encountered in active TB pericarditis where there are signs of both pericardial effusion or tamponade and constriction. It may also occur in neoplastic, radiation, and septic pericarditis.

Clinical presentation: symptoms are usually those of constriction. Examination reveals pulsus paradoxus, raised JVP with prominent 'x' and 'y' descents. The CXR shows an enlarged cardiac silhouette like that of pericardial effusion.

Diagnosis: the clue to diagnosis is persistent signs of constriction following adequate pericardial drainage.

Management: treatment of the underlying cause and pericardial drainage if indicated. Pericardiectomy is indicated should haemodynamics not improve.

Calcific pericarditis without constriction

This condition is usually discovered during routine radiological examination, which demonstrates pericardial calcification. There are no symptoms and signs of constriction and the cause is usually unknown.

Viral pericarditis

Clinical presentation: most patients present with a history of upper respiratory tract infection within the preceding three weeks. The viruses most frequently responsible include coxsackie B, echo, mumps, influenza, and varicella. Pericardial pain, fever, and malaise are typical. The physical examination reveals a pericardial friction rub and/or characteristic changes of acute pericarditis on ECG.

Course: in the majority of patients the illness resolves spontaneously in one to two weeks. In some patients, the illness recurs on at least one occasion in the next few weeks or months, and in 20% of patients there are multiple recurrences in the ensuing months or years (benign relapsing pericarditis).

Diagnosis: it is important to search for an underlying disease (see table p328) that may require specific therapy. In most cases of suspected viral pericarditis special studies for aetiologic agents are not necessary because of low diagnostic yield of viral studies and lack of specific therapy for viral disease.

Management

- NSAIDs are effective in most patients with viral pericarditis. There are no data from randomized controlled trials to guide treatment for relapsing patients who do not respond to NSAIDs.
- Corticosteroids (prednisone 1–1.5 mg/kg for at least 1 month) provide symptomatic relief in most patients; symptoms recur in many patients when prednisone dose is reduced.
- Colchicine (2 mg/day for 1–2 days, followed by 1 mg/day) may be effective when NSAIDs and corticosteroids fail to prevent relapses.
- If patients do not respond adequately, azathioprine (75–100 mg/day) or cyclophosphamide may be added.
- Pericardiectomy is indicated only in frequent and highly symptomatic recurrences resistant to medical therapy. However, postpericardiectomy recurrences may occur, possibly due to incomplete resection of the pericardium.

Tuberculous pericarditis

Tuberculous (TB) pericarditis is uncommon in the First World, but is very common in developing countries, and the incidence appears to be increasing in sub-Saharan Africa in parallel with the HIV/AIDS epidemic. The disease presents in three forms: constrictive pericarditis, effusive-constrictive pericarditis, and pericardial effusion.

Tuberculous pericardial constriction

Clinical presentation: most cases have an active inflammatory fibro-caseous tissue surrounding the heart, and involve visceral and parietal pericardium. The clinical presentation is highly variable. Patients range from being asymptomatic to showing severe signs and symptoms of constriction. The diagnosis is often missed on cursory clinical and echo-cardiographic examination. It is uncommon to find concomitant pulmonary tuberculosis, and pericardial calcification is found in <5% of cases.

Treatment: the initial management of patients with non-calcific TB constrictive pericarditis is with anti-TB therapy, and since the process is an active fibro-caseous condition, resolution of constriction occurs in 15–20% of patients with medical management over three to four months. Pericardiectomy is recommended if no improvement has occurred after 6 weeks of anti-TB treatment or unsatisfactory improvement after several months of treatment. By contrast, calcific TB pericarditis is treated by early pericardiectomy and anti-TB chemotherapy.

Effusive–constrictive TB pericarditis

Features: this mixed form is a common presentation of TB pericarditis. There is increased pericardial pressure due to effusion in the presence of visceral constriction. The echocardiogram shows porridge-like exudation with loculation of the fluid.

Treatment of this condition is by standard four-drug therapy. The role of adjuvant steroids is not known. The mortality is about 10% and about 30% of cases will come to pericardiectomy over two years of follow-up.

Tuberculous pericardial effusion

Pathology: pericardial effusion is the commonest mode of presentation with or without tamponade. The effusion is bloodstained in over 95% of cases, and may even resemble venous blood. The absence of parenchymatous lung disease and the presence of hilar lymphadenopathy in many of these patients suggest a direct spread from a TB hilar node to the pericardium.

Clinical presentation: systemic symptoms are variable.   Typical pericardial pain is uncommon and the classic ECG features of pericarditis are not seen.   CXR shows an enlarged globular heart, small pleural effusions on one or both sides, and evidence of pulmonary tuberculosis in only 30% of cases.   The echocardiogram shows features of pericardial effusion, typically associated with soft tissue density masses, thickening of the visceral pericardium, and fibrinous strands.

Diagnosis: a *definite diagnosis* of TB pericarditis is based on the demonstration of tubercle bacilli in the pericardial fluid or on histologic section of the pericardium. Pericardial effusion should be confirmed by pericardiocentesis. Fluid should be sent for microscopy (to identify acid-fast bacilli [AFB]) and culture of tubercle bacilli. The chances of a positive culture are improved by bedside inoculation of the fluid into double-strength Kirschner culture medium. Pericardial biopsy and drainage offer the advantage of a histological diagnosis and early complete drainage of the pericardium. This can be performed via the sub-xiphisternal approach under local anaesthesia.

A *probable diagnosis* is made when there is proof of tuberculosis elsewhere in a patient with unexplained pericarditis. Palpation in the supra-clavicular fossa will frequently reveal enlarged lymph nodes, which should be biopsied. AFB positive sputum will only be found in about 10% of cases.   Tuberculin skin testing is of little value in endemic and non-endemic areas. It is not known whether the enzyme-linked immunospot (ELISPOT) test that detects T-cells specific for *M tuberculosis* antigen will perform better in TB pericarditis than the tuberculin skin test.

Several tests have been developed for the rapid diagnosis of TB in the pericardial fluid. PCR can identify DNA of *M. tuberculosis* rapidly from only 1 µl of pericardial fluid (sensitivity 75%, specificity 100%). An adenosine deaminase (ADA) level >40 U/l has a sensitivity of 83% and a specificity of 78%. A high interferon γ level is also a highly sensitive (92%) and specific (100%) marker of pericardial TB.

Treatment is by means of standard four-drug anti-TB chemotherapy for 6 months. Overall mortality is about 8%. Repeat pericardiocentesis is required in about 15% of patients, and during a two-year follow-up period, about 10% of patients will require surgical pericardiectomy. While some favour the addition of steroids to conventional therapy, their role in improving survival on not clearly established, particularly in HIV infection.

Uraemic pericarditis

Pathology: uraemia produces a fibrinous, often haemorrhagic inflammation that may lead to tamponade, and constriction in some cases.

Management: symptomatic pericarditis that occurs before the initiation of dialysis will respond to repeated peritoneal or haemodialysis. Heparin-free haemodialysis should be used to avoid haemopericardium. Many patients who develop pericardial effusion while on dialysis (dialysis-associated pericarditis) will respond to intensification of the dialysis regime. Those who do not respond will require drainage either by subxyphoid pericardiotomy or pericardial window. Pericardiocentesis is associated with a high risk of intrapericardial haemorrhage.

Neoplastic pericardial disease

Aetiology: usually secondary to malignancy of the bronchus, breast, or kidney. Primary tumours of the pericardium are rare and usually a result of mesothelioma following asbestos exposure.

Diagnosis: metastases may produce a large haemorrhagic effusion or severe constriction when tumour encases the heart. Malignant cells may be found in 85% of cases of aspirated pericardial fluid. Tumour markers such as carcinoembryonic antigen (CEA), alpha-feto protein (AFP), and carbohydrate antigens (e.g., CA 125) have been used in the diagnosis of malignant effusion. The differentiation of TB and neoplastic effusion is virtually absolute with low ADA and high CEA levels.

Management: depends on the type and stage of malignancy, condition of the patient, and presence of cardiac compression Pericardiocentesis is effective in relieving neoplastic cardiac tamponade in the vast majority of cases. Commonly, neoplastic pericardial disease is a pre-terminal event. Palliation for recurrent tamponade can be obtained by subxyphoid surgical pericardiotomy (which can be performed under local anaesthesia) or by percutaneous balloon pericardiotomy to create a pleuro-pericardial window to allow fluid drainage into the pleural space in large malignant pericardial effusions with and a limited life expectancy. Partial pericardiectomy (pericardial window) through a left thoracotomy should be reserved for patients who have a better prognosis and are likely to respond to chemotherapy or radiation.

Intrapericardial instillation of cytostatic/sclerosing agents has also been used to prevent recurrences of large pericardial effusion. Intrapericardial treatment related to the type of tumour indicates that cisplatin may be effective in secondary lung cancer and thiotepa may be effective in metastatic breast cancer. Tetracycline as a sclerosing agent controls malignant pericardial effusion in up to 85% of cases, but side-effects such as fever, chest pain, atrial arrhythmias, and constriction in long-term survivors, are common.

Myxoedematous effusion

Clinical presentation: effusion with high protein content is common in untreated myxoedema. Myxoedema must always be excluded in a patient with chronic, asymptomatic, pericardial effusion, associated with bradycardia, low voltage of the QRS complexes, and a history of radiation induced thyroid dysfunction. Cardiac tamponade does not occur.

Diagnosis: this is based on serum levels of thyroxine and thyroid stimulating hormone.

Treatment with thyroid hormone causes resolution of the pericardial effusion.

Nontuberculous bacterial (purulent) pericarditis

Predisposing conditions: immunosuppression (e.g., immunosuppressive drugs, lymphoma, or HIV/AIDS); pre-existing pericardial effusion; cardiac surgery; and chest trauma. Children—pharyngitis, pneumonia, otitis media, endocarditis, and arthritis.

Precipitating factors: cardiac surgery, pericardial aspiration, extension of aortic root endocarditis into the pericardial sac, or haematogenous spread from a septic focus such as osteomyelitis or pneumonia.

Causative organisms: adults—*Staphylococcus aureus*, gram-negative bacilli, and anaerobes. Children—*Haemophilus*, *Staphylococcus aureus*, and *N. meningitides*.

Clinical presentation: rare in adults. Presents as an acute, fulminating infectious illness and is fatal if not treated. The most important reason for this poor outlook is failure to suspect the condition in debilitated patients with overwhelming systemic infection.

Diagnosis: pericardiocentesis shows purulent fluid, with high white cell count, low glucose, positive Gram stain for organism, and positive pericardial fluid and blood culture.

Treatment: complete pericardial drainage preferable through a subxyphoid pericardiotomy, and systemic antibiotic therapy. The mortality rate is 40% even with appropriate management.

Radiation pericarditis

Clinical features: usually follows treatment for lymphoma and breast cancer. Incidence of pericarditis depends on how much the heart is included in the field of radiation, the dose, the duration of treatment, and age of patient. Radiation is a common cause of effusive–constrictive pericarditis and also may result in myocarditis and premature coronary atherosclerosis.

Clinical evidence of pericarditis may occur during, or shortly after treatment, but is more usually delayed for approximately 1 year. The presentation is one of pericarditis with some effusion. In about 50% of cases there is evidence of tamponade, which requires drainage.

Management: up to 20% of patients will require pericardiectomy because of severe constriction. The operative mortality is high (21%) and the postoperative 5-year survival is very low (1%), mostly due to underlying myocardial fibrosis and severe thickening of the visceral pericardium.

Drugs/toxin-induced pericarditis

Aetiology: pericardial reactions to drugs and toxins are rare. Pericarditis may develop as part of the lupus erythematosus-like syndrome (hydralazine, INH, procainamide, methyldopa, reserpine), hypersensitivity reaction (cromolyn sodium, penicillins, streptomycin), serum sickness or envonomation (scorpion fish sting).

Management: consists of the removal of the causative agent and symptomatic treatment.

Postcardiotomy syndrome

Clinical presentation: the syndrome occurs in approximately 30% of patients undergoing any form of cardiac surgery. It is more common in patients receiving aminocaproic acid during the operation. After a latent period of 2–3 weeks there is fever, pericarditis, pleuritis, and pneumonitis with a marked tendency to relapse. 'Dry' pericarditis or pericarditis with effusion may occur. The illness is self-limited, varies in intensity and duration, but usually lasts only 2–4 weeks.

Treatment: NSAIDs, analgesics such as aspirin or colchicine. Steroids (oral or intrapericardial) induce prompt relief of symptoms, but should be reserved for severely affected patients since relapse may occur when they are discontinued and dependency may result. Anticoagulants should be avoided because of the risk of haemopericardium.

Post-infarction pericarditis

Clinical presentation: two forms of post-infarction pericarditis may be distinguished:

(1) The usual early form of pericarditis occurs within a week in at least 20% of patients with transmural myocardial infarction. It is a result of pericardial irritation by adjacent infracted myocardium.

(2) Less commonly, a delayed autoimmune reaction may produce pericarditis 2 weeks to a few months after the infarct (Dressler syndrome). The delayed form behaves very similarly to the postcardiotomy syndrome.

Treatment: ibuprofen is said to increase coronary flow, and is the NSAID of choice. Aspirin, up to 650 mg every 4 hours for 2–5 days, has also been used successfully. Occasionally steroids may be required for relapse, but should be avoided as they may delay myocardial healing. Anticoagulants should be avoided because of the risk of haemopericardium.

Rheumatic fever

This is an important cause of pericarditis world-wide, almost invariably associated with severe pancarditis and valvular involvement. Rheumatic pericardial effusion is usually clear, straw-coloured, and sterile. Cardiac tamponade is rare and the fluid usually reabsorbs rapidly in response to salicylates or steroid therapy. Chronic constrictive pericarditis is never rheumatic in origin but adherent pericardium with flecks of calcification is not uncommon.

Autoimmune pericarditis

Pericarditis may be the presenting feature of systemic lupus erythematosus, or complicate scleroderma and polyarteritis nodosa. Dry or effusive pericarditis may occur; and it is important to exclude these disorders in patients presenting with idiopathic benign pericarditis. Generally, other signs and symptoms of these collagen vascular diseases will be present.

Granulomatous pericarditis is a complication of rheumatoid arthritis and ankylosing spondylitis, leading to effusion and occasionally constriction. Aortitis and aortic insufficiency may be associated and occasionally there is invasion of the interventricular septum, producing heart block.

Traumatic pericarditis

This produces two forms of pericarditis. One is a direct result of trauma with haemorrhage into the pericardial cavity and formation of haemopericardium. If associated myocardial or valvular injury is absent, complete recovery is the rule, although chronic constriction may develop.

The second type is a form of recurrent pericarditis allied to the postcardiotomy and post myocardial infarction syndromes, which may also result in chronic constriction.

Fungal pericarditis

Clinical presentation: fungal pericarditis occurs as a rare opportunistic infection in immunocompromised patients (e.g., immunosuppressive therapy, HIV/AIDS). It is caused by endemic fungi (*Histoplasma, Coccidioides*), non-endemic opportunistic fungi (candida, *Aspergillus, Blastomyces*) and semi-fungi (*Norcadia, Actinomycosis*).

Diagnosis: fungal pericarditis may resemble TB pericarditis. Fungal staining and culture of aspirated pericardial fluid and pericardial biopsy are necessary to make the distinction.

Treatment: antifungal treatment with fluconazole, ketoconazole, itraconazole, amphotericin B or amphotericin B lipid complex is indicated. NSAIDs are used for symptomatic relief. Sulfonamides are the drug of choice for *Norcadiosis*, and a combination of three antibiotics including penicillin should be given for *Actinomycosis*.

Amoebic pericarditis

Pathology: amoebiasis (caused by *Entamoeba histolytica*) occurs mainly in endemic areas and in travellers from them (in whom the syndrome may appear years later). Pericardial complications are rare but when they occur, they carry a high mortality, especially with delayed or missed diagnosis. The usual cause of amoebic pericarditis is extension from an amoebic liver abscess in the left lobe. Rarely, spread may also occur from the right lobe or disease may reach the pericardium from an amoebic lung abscess.

Clinical presentation: there are two modes of presentation

(1) **Hepatic presentation:** an abscess near the pericardium, which has not yet ruptured, can cause a pericardial friction rub, a non-purulent pericardial effusion, and ECG/CXR signs of pericarditis.
(2) **Cardiac presentation:** perforation of a liver abscess into the pericardium results in a purulent pericarditis. The onset can be acute, with shock and death within a short time, or the onset may be gradual with signs of tamponade as a result of the pericardial fluid.

Diagnosis is difficult but should be suspected if, in a patient with a purulent pericarditis and signs of cardiac failure, tenderness of the liver in the epigastrium is much more marked than the rest of the palpable liver. A high and immobile left hemidiaphragm detected by fluoroscopy or CT scan is also suggestive. Definite diagnosis is by pericardiocentesis (which typically shows brownish fluid; the pus may simulate anchovy sauce) and serological testing for antibodies resulting from invasive amoebiasis (fluorescent antibody test or amoebic enzyme immunoassay or amoebic gel diffusion test).

Treatment: Hepatic presentation—the pericardial disease resolves with successful treatment of the liver abscess. Cardiac presentation—pericardial drainage and metronidazole. Constrictive pericarditis is an occasional complication.

Constrictive pericarditis vs. restrictive myocardial disease

It is difficult to separate congestive pericarditis from restrictive myocardial disease. The distinction is vital because pericardiectomy is one of the most satisfying operations in terms of cure. Points of differentiation are as follows:

1. **Clinical:** murmurs of mitral and tricuspid regurgitation are strong pointers against constrictive pericarditis.
2. **ECG:** left axis deviation favours myocardial damage.
3. **CXR:** pericardial calcification favours constrictive pericarditis.
4. **ECHO:** concentric left ventricular hypertrophy with a 'sparkling granular' appearance in amyloid. Left ventricular hypertrophy may be present in haemochromatosis. Endomyocardial fibrosis is characterized by obliteration of the left ventricular wall. The ejection fraction is normal in constrictive pericarditis, whereas in heart muscle disease left ventricular function is frequently depressed. On tissue Doppler imaging, a peak early velocity of longitudinal expansion (peak E_a) of ≥ 8.0 cm/s differentiates patients with constriction from restriction with 89% sensitivity and 100 % specificity.
5. **CT and MRI scan:** these are diagnostic when they show thickened pericardium ≥ 3 mm.
6. **Cardiac catheterization:** when the right ventricular and left ventricular end-diastolic pressures differ by more than 6 mmHg, restrictive cardiomyopathy is likely present. A pulmonary artery pressure of more than 50 mmHg strongly favours restrictive cardiomyopathy.
7. **Endomyocardial biopsy:** diagnostic of infiltration in amyloid disease and haemochromatosis. Extensive fibrosis is indicative of restrictive cardiomyopathy.

An **exploratory thoracotomy** is justified if all these tests fail to make a distinction between the two entities.

Pericardial fluid analysis

Analyses of pericardial effusion can establish the diagnosis of viral, bacterial, TB, fungal, amoebic, and malignant pericarditis. The appearance of the pericardial fluid should be noted. The tests should be ordered according to the clinical presentation of the patient.

However, the following routine samples are useful:
- Biochemistry sample for protein and LDH estimation to distinguish between and exudate and a transudate.
- Microbiology specimen for microscopy, culture, and sensitivity testing.
- Cytology specimen.

The following tests are requested for the diagnosis of the specific forms of pericarditis:
- Viral pericarditis—PCR for cardiotropic viruses.
- Purulent pericarditis—Gram stain, at least 3 blood cultures of pericardial fluid for aerobes and anaerobes and blood cultures.
- TB pericarditis—staining for acid fast bacilli; bedside inoculation of pericardial fluid into double-strength Kirschner transport medium and culture; ADA level.
- Fungal pericarditis—microscopy and culture.
- Amoebic pericarditis—brownish pericardial fluid with anchovy sauce appearance of pus.
- Malignant effusion—cytology and tumour markers (e.g., CEA).

Pericardiocentesis

See p698.

Further reading

- Chesler E (1992). *Clinical Cardiology*, 5th ed. Springer-Verlag: New York.
- Commerford PJ, Strang JIG (1991). Tuberculous pericarditis. In: Coovadia HM, Benatar SR, eds. *A century of tuberculosis: South African perspectives.* Oxford University Press: Cape Town pp.123–36.
- Maisch B et al (2004) *Eur Heart J* 25:587–610.
- Mayosi BM, Volmink JA, Commerford PJ (2002). Pericardial disease: an evidence based approach to diagnosis and treatment. In: Yusuf S, Cairns JA, Camm AJ, Fallen EL, Gersh BJ, eds. *Evidence Based Cardiology.* 2nd edition. BMJ Books BMA House: London.

Chapter 9

Arrhythmias

The cardiac conduction system

Cardiac action potential

The resting cardiac myocyte is electrically negative with a transmembrane voltage of between −50 mV to −95 mV. This is due to the distribution of K^+, Na^+, Cl^- and Ca^{2+} ions across the cell membrane. The negativity is maintained by the energy consuming Na/K pump which transports three Na^+ ions out of the cell for two K^+ ions inward. During phase 4 of the action potential the voltage slowly increases until a threshold of −60 mV is reached which opens voltage gated Na^+ channels and triggers depolarization. The voltage changes in one cell are spread to adjacent cells via gap junctions between them, such that a wavefront of electrical activation is propagated. At least ten distinct ion channels modulate the voltage changes that occur in the action potential (Fig. 9.1).

Automaticity

This is the ability of all cardiac cells to spontaneously depolarize. It is caused by the inward flow of positive ions during diastole. At potentials more negative than −60 mV ion channels open allowing in a slow influx of cations. In the sinoatrial node (SAN) the slow influx of Ca^{2+} allows it to depolarize more rapidly and therefore suppress other potential pacemaker sites.

Sinoatrial node

The SAN sits high in the lateral right atrium (RA) just below the superior vena cava (SVC). It is 1–2 cm in length, 2–3 mm wide and less than 1 mm from the epicardial surface. It is the dominant site of impulse generation which are conducted out of the sinus node to depolarize the surrounding RA. The SAN is richly innervated with both adrenergic and cholinergic receptors, which alter the rate of depolarization hence controlling heart rate. Activation spreads out from the SAN to the rest of the RA and left atrium (LA) via specialised interatrial connections including Bachmann's bundle.

Atrioventricular node

The atrioventricular node (AVN) is found in the RA anterior to the mouth of the coronary sinus and directly above the insertion of the septal leaflet of the tricuspid valve. It is the only electrical connection to the ventricle, via the bundle of His which. Like the SAN it is also densely innervated with sympathetic and parasympathetic fibres.

His–Purkinje system

The electrical impulse conducts rapidly through the bundle of His into the upper part of the interventricular septum where it splits into two branches. The right bundle branch which continues down the right side of the septum to the apex of the right ventricle and the base of the anterior papillary muscle and the left bundle branch which further splits into two fascicles, anterior and posterior. The terminal Purkinje fibres connect with the ends of the bundle branches forming an interweaving network on the endocardial surface so that a cardiac impulse is transmitted almost simultaneously to the entire right and left ventricles.

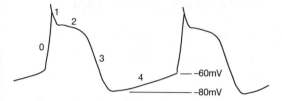

Fig. 9.1 The cardiac action potential.

The action potential has five parts:7

0 rapid influx of Na causing fast depolarization.

1 rapid early repolarisation due to efflux of Na^+.

2 plateau phase where repolarisation is slowed by an influx of Ca^{2+}.

3 repolarisation due to the the efflux of K^+.

4 diastole with a steady state resting transmembrane voltage.

The plateau phase distinguishes the cardiac from neuronal action potential. The release of Ca^{2+} during phase 3 triggers mechanical contraction of the cell.

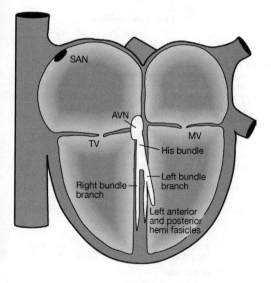

Fig. 9.2 Anatomy of the normal conduction system.

SAN, sinoatrial node; TV, tricuspid valve; AVN, atrio ventricular node; MV, mitral valve.

Bradyarrhythmias: general approach

- Ask specifically about previous cardiac disease, palpitations, blackouts, dizziness, chest pain, symptoms of heart failure, and recent drugs.
- Examine carefully, noting the BP, JVP waveform (?cannon waves), heart sounds and murmurs, and signs of heart failure.

Investigations

• 12 lead ECG & rhythm strip	Look specifically for the relationship between P waves and QRS complex. A long rhythm strip is sometimes necessary to detect complete heart block if atrial and ventricular rates are similar.
• Blood tests	FBC, biochemistry, glucose (urgently). Ca^{2+}, Mg^{2+} (especially if on diuretics). Biochemical markers of cardiac injury.
• Where appropriate	Blood cultures, CRP, ESR. Thyroid function tests. Drug levels. Arterial blood gases.
• Chest x-ray	Heart size. ?signs of pulmonary oedema.

Management

Haemodynamically unstable patients:

- Give **oxygen** via facemask if the patient is hypoxic on air.
- **Keep NBM** until definitive therapy has been started to reduce the risk of aspiration in case of cardiac arrest or when the patient lies supine for temporary wire insertion.
- Secure peripheral venous access.
- Bradyarrhythmias causing **severe haemodynamic compromise** (cardiac arrest, asystole, SBP <90 mmHg, severe pulmonary oedema, evidence of cerebral hypoperfusion) require immediate treatment and temporary pacing (The technique is described on p692).
- Give **atropine 1 mg IV** (Min-I-Jet®) bolus; repeat if necessary up to a maximum 3 mg.
- Give **isoprenaline 0.2 mg IV** (Min-I-Jet®) if there is a delay in pacing and the patient remains unstable. Set up an infusion (1 mg in 100 ml bag N saline starting at 1 ml/min titrating to HR).
- Set up **external pacing system** if available, and arrange for transfer to a screening room for trans-venous pacing.
- Bradycardia in shock is a poor prognostic sign. Look for a source of blood loss and begin aggressive resuscitation with fluids and inotropes.

Haemodynamically stable patients:

- Admit to CCU with continuous ECG monitoring.
- Keep atropine drawn up and ready in case of acute deterioration.
- Does the patient require a temporary wire immediately? (See p690.) It may be of value to have appropriate central venous access (femoral or internal jugular vein) in place in case of the need for emergency temporary wire insertion.

External cardiac pacing

- In emergencies, external cardiac pacing may be used first but this is painful for the patient and is only a temporary measure until a more 'definitive' trans-venous pacing wire can be inserted.
- External cardiac pacing is useful as a standby in patients
- post-myocardial infarction when the risks of prophylactic trans-venous pacing after thrombolysis are high.
- Haemodynamically stable patients with anterior myocardial infarction and bifasicular block may be managed simply by application of the external pacing electrodes and having the pulse generator ready if necessary.
- Familiarize yourself with the machine in your hospital when you have some time—a cardiac arrest is not the time to read the manual for the apparatus!

Sinus bradycardia

The sinoatrial node (SAN) discharges <60/min. P waves are normal but slow. It may be normal (e.g. in sleep, healthy resting hearts).

Causes

- Young athletic individual
- Drugs-(β-blockers, morphine, amiodarone, calcium channel blockers, lithium, propafenone, clonidine)
- Hypothyroidism
- Hypothermia
- Increased vagal tone
  - vasovagal attack
  - nausea or vomiting
  - carotid sinus hypersensitivity
  - acute MI (especially inferior)
- Ischaemia or infarction of the sinus node
- Chronic degeneration of sinus or AV nodes or atria
- Cholestatic jaundice
- Raised intracranial pressure
- Drugs-(β-blockers, morphine, amiodarone, calcium channel blockers, lithium, propafenone, clonidine).

Management

- If hypotensive or pre-syncopal:
  - Atropine 600 µg–3 mg IV bolus repeating as necessary.
  - Isoprenaline 0.5–10 µg/min IV infusion.
  - Temporary pacing.
  - Avoid and take steps to correct precipitants
  - Stop any drugs that may suppress the sinus or AV nodes.
- Long term treatment:
  - If all possible underlying causes removed and if symptomatic bradycardia remains, refer for permanent pacing.
  - Consider Holter monitoring in patients with possible episodic bradycardia. R-R intervals >2.5 seconds may require permanent pacing, especially if associated with symptoms.

Sinus pause

The SAN fails to generate impulses (sinus arrest) or the impulses are not conducted to the atria (SA exit block). A single dropped P wave with a PP interval that is a multiple of the basic PP interval suggests exit block. A period of absent P waves suggests sinus arrest. Causes include, excess vagal tone, acute myocarditis, MI, aging (fibrosis), stroke, digoxin toxicity, and anti-arrhythmic drugs.

Sick sinus syndrome

This syndrome encompasses a number of conduction system problems: persistent sinus bradycardia not caused by drugs, sinus pauses, AV conduction disturbances, and paroxysms of atrial or junctional tachyarrhythmias. It is usually diagnosed by ambulatory cardiac monitoring.

Atrioventricular block

This can occur at the AVN (nodal) or His–Purkinje system (infranodal). Common causes are ischaemic heart disease, conduction system fibrosis (aging), calcific aortic stenosis, congenital, cardiomyopathy, hypothermia, hypothyroidism, trauma, radiotherapy, infection, connective tissue disease, sarcoidosis, and anti-arrhythmic drugs. AV block is further classified:

First degree AV block

Every impulse conducts to the ventricle but conduction time is prolonged. Every P wave is followed by a QRS but with a prolonged PR interval (>200 ms). If the QRS width is normal then the block is at the AV node, If the QRS shows aberration (RBBB or LBBB) then the block may be at the AV node or the His–Purkinje system.

Second degree AV block

Mobitz 1. (Wenckebach). ECG shows the PR interval prolongs until a P wave is not conducted P wave. The PR interval following the dropped P wave must be the shortest. The RR interval is therefore irregular. This block is characteristic of the AVN.

Mobitz 2. ECG shows a fixed P to QRS ratio of 2:1, 3:1 or 4:1. Block is predominantly at the His bundle and there is often an aberrant pattern to the QRS complex.

Third degree AV block (complete heart block)

There is no conduction to the ventricle. The ECG shows dissociation between P and QRS complexes. An escape pacemaker rhythm takes over. A narrow QRS indicates AVN block and the His bundle is the pacemaker, which is faster and more stable than more distal sites. A wide QRS indicates infra nodal block and a distal ventricular pacemaker site. This carries a worse prognosis.

Causes of atrioventricular block

- Associated with acute infarction or ischaemia.
- Drugs (β-blockers, digitalis, Ca^{2+}-blockers).
- Conduction system fibrosis (Lev and Lenegre syndromes).
- Increased vagal tone.
- Trauma or following cardiac surgery.
- Hypothyroidism (rarely thyrotoxicosis).
- Hypothermia.
- Hyperkalaemia.
- Hypoxia.
- Valvular disease (Aortic stenosis, incompetence, endocarditis).
- Myocarditis (diphtheria, rheumatic fever, viral, Chagas' disease).
- Associated with neuromuscular disease i.e. myotonic dystrophy.
- Collagen vascular disease (SLE, RA, scleroderma).
- Cardiomyopathies (haemochromotosis, amyloidosis).
- Granulomatous disease (sarcoid).
- Congenital heart block.
- Congenital heart disease (ASD, Ebstein's, PDA).

Bundle branch block

Due to disease in the His–Purkinje system causing a QRS >120 ms. Common causes are conduction system fibrosis (aging), ischaemic heart disease, hypertension, cardiomyopathies, cardiac surgery, infiltrative diseases.

LBBB: left ventricular depolarization is delayed giving large notched R waves in leads I and V6 and an 'M' pattern in V1. Block confined to the anterior or posterior fascicles of the left bundle gives left axis or right axis deviation respectively on the ECG. BBB leads to asynchronous contraction of the left and right ventricle which worsens function.

RBBB: right ventricular depolarization is delayed giving an RSR pattern in V1 and a prominent S wave in I and V6. This can be a normal variant but more commonly by causes listed above and in addition; ASD, PE, cor pulmonale.

Bifasicular block = RBBB + left anterior hemiblock (left axis deviation on ECG), RBBB + left posterior hemiblock (right axis deviation on ECG) or LBBB. All of these may progress to complete AV block. *Trifasicular block* = bifasicular block + 1st degree AV block.

Management

- Interventricular conduction disturbances on their own do not require temporary pacing. However, when associated with haemodynamic disturbance or progression to higher levels of block (even if intermittent) must consider insertion of a transvenous pacing wire. The need for longer term pacing is dependent on the persistence of symptoms and underlying cause. Consult a cardiologist. See p690 for situations where temporary pacing is indicated.

Common causes of bundle branch block
- Ischaemic heart disease.
- Hypertensive heart disease.
- Valve disease (especially aortic stenosis).
- Conduction system fibrosis (Lev and Lenegre syndromes).
- Myocarditis or endocarditis.
- Cardiomyopathies.
- Cor pulmonale (RBBB) (acute or chronic).
- Trauma or post-cardiac surgery.
- Neuromuscular disorders (myotonic dystrophy).
- Polymyositis.

Tachyarrhythmias: general approach

Tachyarrhythmias may present with significant symptoms and haemo-dynamic compromise. The approach to patients depends upon:
1. The effects of the rhythm on the patient.
2. The diagnosis from the ECG and rhythm.
3 Any underlying cardiac abnormality or identifiable precipitant.

The effect of the rhythm on the patient

1. Patients with signs of severe haemodynamic compromise:
- Impending cardiac arrest.
- Severe pulmonary oedema.
- Shock—systolic BP <90 mmHg.
- Depressed consciousness.

Treat immediately with unsynchronized external defibrillation for tachar-rhythmia and temporary pacing for bradyarrhythmia.

2. Patients with mild-moderate compromise:
- Mild pulmonary oedema.
- Low cardiac output with cool peripheries and oliguria.
- Angina at rest.

Try to record an ECG and long rhythm strip before giving any pharma-cological agents and/or defibrillation. This will be invaluable for long-term management. If they deteriorate, treat as above.

Diagnosing the arrhythmia

The main distinctions to make are:
- Tachy- (>120/min) vs brady- (<60/min) arrhythmia.
- Narrow (≤120 ms or 3 small sq.) vs. broad QRS complex.
- Regular vs irregular rhythm.

Precipitating factors (multiple, common ones listed below)

Underlying cardiac disease
- Ischaemic heart disease
- Acute or recent MI
- Angina
- Mitral valve disease
- LV aneurysm
- Congenital heart disease
- Abnormalities of resting ECG
- Pre excitation (short PR interval)
- Long QT (congenital or acquired).

Drugs
- Anti-arrhythmics
- Sympathomimetics
- (β_2 agonists, cocaine)
- Antidepressants (tricyclic)
- Adenylate cyclase inhibitors (aminophylline, caffeine)
- Alcohol.

Metabolic abnormalities
- ↓ or ↑ K^+
- ↓ or ↑ Ca^{2+}
- ↓ Mg^{2+}
- ↓ P_aO_2
- ↑ P_aCO_2
- Acidosis.

Endocrine abnormalities
- Thyrotoxicosis
- Phaeochromocytoma.

Miscellaneous
- Febrile illness
- Emotional stress
- Smoking
- Fatigue.

Investigations for patients with tachyarrhythmias

12 lead ECG & rhythm strip	• Regular vs. irregular rhythm. • Narrow vs. broad QRS complex.
Blood tests	• FBC, biochemistry, glucose (urgently). • Ca^{2+}, Mg^{2+} (especially if on diuretics). • Biochemical markers of myocardial injury.
Where appropriate	• Blood cultures, CRP, ESR. • Thyroid function tests. • Drug levels. • Arterial blood gases.
Chest x-ray	• Heart size. • Evidence of pulmonary oedema. • Other pathology (e.g. Ca bronchus→AF, pericardial effusion→sinus tachycardia, hypotension ± AF).

- **Narrow complex tachycardias** originate in the atria or AV node (i.e. supraventricular tachycardias SVT).
- **Irregular, narrow complex tachycardia** is most commonly AF or atrial flutter with varying AV block.
- **Broad complex tachyarrhythmias** may originate from either the ventricles (VT) or from the atria or AV node (SVT) with aberrant conduction to the ventricles (RBBB or LBBB configuration).
- If the patient has previous documented arrhythmias, compare the morphology of the current arrhythmia to old ECGs. The diagnosis of VT vs. SVT and therapy may be evident from the last admission.

Tachyarrhythmias: classification

Fast heart rates can be classified in various ways, however, an anatomical approach should be used which can then be subdivided mechanistically. This provides a simple foundation for understanding the ECG appearance and the tachycardia mechanism.

Atrial tachyarrhythmias: contained completely in the atria (or SAN).
- Sinus tachycardia.
- Sinus node reentrant tachycardia (SNRT).
- Atrial fibrillation.
- Atrial tachycardia.
  - Focal atrial tachycardia.
  - Macro-reentrant atrial tachycardia (= atrial flutter).

Atrio-ventricular tachyarrhythmias: dependent on activation between the atrium and ventricle (or AV node).
- Atrio-ventricular reentry tachycardia (AVRT). ~ WPV.
- Atrio-ventricular nodal reentry tachycardia (AVNRT).
- Junctional tachycardia.

Ventricular tachyarrhythmias: contained in the ventricle.
- Ventricular tachycardia (VT).
  - Monomorphic VT.
  - Polymorphic VT (Torsades de Pointes).
- Ventricular fibrillation.

Features of a broad complex tachycardia suggesting ventricular origin:
- AV dissociation (NB VA conduction may be present during VT).
  - Independent p waves.
  - Capture and fusion beats.
- QRS width >140 ms (if RBBB appearance) *or*
            >160 ms (if LBBB appearance).
- QRS axis < −30 or > +90.
- Concordance of QRS complexes in precordial leads (all positive or all negative).

Supraventricular causes of a broad complex tachycardia:
- SVT + aberrancy (bundle branch block).
- SVT + pre excitation (activation of the ventricle over a pathway other than the AV node).
- Antidromic AVRT.
- SVT + class 1c drug (flecainide).

ECG diagnosis of tachyarrhythmias

By following simple rules when interpreting the ECG, any tachycardia can be classified to the categories described earlier, however the ECG should always be considered in the clinical context. A broad complex tachycardia (BCT) must *always* be diagnosed as VT in the acute setting as treating such patients incorrectly may be fatal. View the ECG in both tachycardia and the patients usual rhythm to make a diagnosis (e.g. may see features of WPW). For narrow complex tachycardias (NCTs) use carotid sinus massage or adenosine boluses to see the underlying atrial rhythm. A simple approach follows:

1. Is the tachycardia regular?

Grossly irregular RR intervals regardless of other ECG features indicate AF (or VF, however expect the patient to be unconscious!). A slight irregularity can occur in other tachycardias, particularly at their onset. Alternatively multiple atrial and/or ventricular ectopic beats or atrial tachycardia with variable AV block can give irregularity.

2. Is the QRS complex broad (>120 ms)?

Yes—ventricular in origin, No—supraventricular.

SVT should only be considered for a broad complex tachycardia (BCT) when there is strong clinical suspicion (e.g. young patient, no previous cardiac history, normal RV and LV function, no accompanying cardiovascular compromise) and after discussion with senior colleagues. *NB* Look at the SR ECG (if available) for pre-existing bundle branch block or pre excitation (suggesting an accessory pathway).

3. Identify p waves, their morphology and p:r ratio

- *1:1 P:R, normal P wave morphology:* sinus tachycardia, focal atrial tachycardia originating from close to the SA node (high crista terminalis or right superior pulmonary vein) or rarely SNRT.
- *1:1 P:R, abnormal P wave morphology:* focal atrial tachycardia. AVRT or AVNRT (if slow activation from ventricle to atrium = long RP tachycardia).
- *P waves not visible:* AVRT or AVNRT (with fast activation from ventricle to atrium). Compare QRS morphology in tachycardia with SR, as a slight deflection in the tachycardia QRS complex not seen in SR may represent the P wave.
- *P:R 2:1,3:1 or greater:* focal or macro-reentrant atrial tachycardia with AV nodal block.
- *P wave rate>250min–1:* this defines atrial flutter (macro-reentrant atrial tachycardia). Usually there will be 2 or 3:1 P:R ratio. In typical atrial flutter a characteristic saw tooth baseline is seen in the inferior leads.

4. Response to AV block (adenosine or carotid massage)

If a rapid p wave rate persists despite induced AV nodal block then the tachycardia is independent of the AV node i.e. macro-reentrant or focal atrial tachycardia and SNRT. If tachycardia is terminated by AV nodal block it is either AVRT or AVNRT (rarely junctional tachycardia). Focal atrial tachycardia and SNRT may also be terminated by adenosine, not due to AV nodal block, but because they are adenosine sensitive.

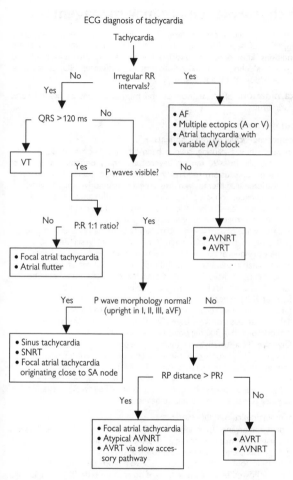

Fig 9.3 ECG diagnosis of tachycardia.

Tachycardia: emergency management

History: previous cardiac disease, palpitations, dizziness, chest pain, symptoms of heart failure and recent medication. Ask specifically about conditions known to be associated with certain cardiac arrhythmias (e.g. AF—alcohol, thyrotoxicosis, mitral valve disease, IHD, pericarditis; VT—previous MI, LV aneurysm).

Examination: BP, heart sounds and murmurs, signs of heart failure, carotid bruits.

Management

Haemodynamically unstable patients:

Tachyarrhythmias causing severe haemodynamic compromise (cardiac arrest, systolic BP <90 mmHg, severe pulmonary oedema, evidence of cerebral hypoperfusion) require urgent correction, usually with external defibrillation. Drug therapy requires time and haemodynamic stability.

- The only exception is a patient in chronic AF with an uncontrolled ventricular rate—Defibrillation is unlikely to cardiovert to SR. Rate control and treatment of precipitant is first-line.
- Sedate awake patients with midazolam (2.5–10 mg IV) ± diamorphine (2.5–5 mg IV + metoclopramide 10 mg IV) for analgesia. Beware respiratory depression and have flumazenil and naloxone to hand.
- Formal anaesthesia with propofol is preferred, but remember the patient may not have an empty stomach and precautions should be taken to prevent aspiration (e.g. cricoid pressure, ET intubation).
- Start at 200 J. synchronized shock and increase as required.
- If tachyarrhythmia recurs or is unresponsive try to correct $\downarrow P_aO_2$, $\uparrow P_aCO_2$, acidosis or $\downarrow K^+$. Give Mg^{2+} (8 mmol IV stat) and shock again. Amiodarone 150–300 mg bolus IV may also be used.
- Give specific antiarrhythmic therapy (see p614).
- If ongoing VT in context of cardiac arrest or recurrent VT episodes, causing haemodynamic compromise, requiring repeated DC cardioversions then iv amiodarone (300 mg iv bolus, followed by 1.2 g iv over 24 hours via central venous line). Follow Resuscitation Council periarrest arrhythmia guidelines[1].

Haemodynamically stable patients:

- Admit and arrange for continuous ECG monitoring and 12 lead ECG.
- Try vagotonic manoeuvres (e.g. Valsalva/carotid sinus massage).
- If diagnosis is clear introduce appropriate treatment.
- If there is doubt regarding diagnosis, give **adenosine** 6 mg as fast IV bolus followed by 5 ml saline flush. If no response, try 9, 12 and 18 mg in succession with continuous ECG rhythm strip.
- Definitive treatment should start as soon as diagnosis is known (p614). First episodes of AVNRT, AVRT, focal atrial tachycardia may need no further treatment. All other diagnoses and WPW should be referred to a cardiologist for further investigation and management.

---

1 Resuscitation Council (UK) guidelines www.resus.org.uk

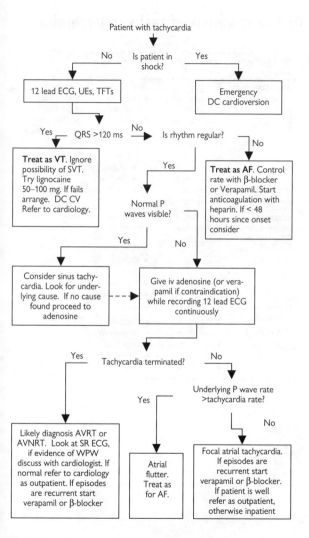

Fig 9.4 Guidelines to the safe management of arrhythmias in the A&E department (adapted from Barts and the London A+E guidelines).

Drug treatment of tachyarrhythmias

Sinus tachycardia	Look for cause. β-blockade if anxious		
Atrial fibrillation **Atrial flutter** **SVT** (see p378)	*Rate control (AV node)* • Digoxin • β-blockade • calcium blocker (e.g. verapamil)	*Version to SR.* • Flecainide • Amiodarone • Sotalol • Disopyramide • Synchronized DC shock	*Prevention* • Amiodarone • Sotalol • Quinidine • Procainamide
Junctional tachycardia (AVNRT) (see p382)	• Adenosine • β-blockade • Verapamil • (Vagal stimulation)	• Digoxin • Flecainide • Synchronized DC shock	
Accessory pathway tachycardias (i.e. AVRT) (see p382)	*At AV node* • Adenosine • β-blockade	*At accessory pathway* • Sotalol • Flecainide • Disopyramide • Quinidine • Amiodarone	*Termination only* • Synchronized DC shock
Ventricular tachycardia (see p390)	*Termination and Prevention* • Lignocaine • Procainamide • Amiodarone • Magnesium • DC shock	• Flecainide • Disopyramide • Propafenone • β-blockade	*Termination only* • Bretylium

Supraventricular tachycardia

This chapter deals with the diagnosis and pharmacological management of individual SVTs. Their mechanisms and ablation are discussed in detail in Chapter 10.

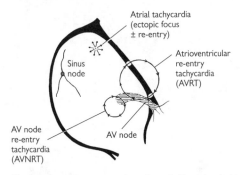

Fig. 9.5 Types of supraventricular tachycardia. Reproduced with permission from Ramrakha P, Moore K (2004). *Oxford Handbook of Acute Medicine*. 2nd ed. Oxford University Press: Oxford.

Sinus tachycardia

Defined as a sinus rate >100 this may be physiological (e.g. exercise or emotion) or pathological. Look for and treat underlying cause; anaemia, drug related (e.g. caffeine, cocaine, salbutamol, etc) hyperthyroidism, pain, hypoxia, pyrexia, or hypovolaemia. If no underlying cause found consider sinus node reentrant tachycardia (SNRT) or focal atrial tachycardia as alternative diagnoses. These will be paroxysmal in nature, have sudden onset or offset and are usually terminated by iv adenosine. If no underlying cause is found it may be termed *inappropriate sinus tachycardia*. β-blockers are useful for symptomatic persistent inappropriate sinus tachycardia and vital in controlling the sinus rate in hyperthyroidism, heart failure or post MI.

Sinus nodal reentrant tachycardia

This is a rare cause of narrow complex tachycardia due to a micro re-entry circuit within the SAN. ECG is identical to sinus tachycardia making diagnosis difficult. β-blockers or calcium channel antagonists are the first line treatment. Modification of the SA node by radiofrequency ablation (RFA) is reserved for drug refractory cases or those not wishing to take drugs.

Regular tachycardia

- Sinus tachycardia.
- Sinus node reentrant tachycardia.
- Atrial tachycardia (p380).
  - Focal atrial tachycardia.
  - Macro-reentrant atrial tachycardia (atrial flutter).
- Atrioventricular reentry tachycardia (AVRT) (i.e. with accessory path e.g. WPW) (p382).
- AV nodal reentry tachycardia (AVNRT) (p382).

Irregular tachycardia

- Atrial fibrillation (p384).
- Atrial flutter with variable block.
- Multifocal atrial tachycardia.
- Multifocal atrial tachycardia.

Atrial tachycardia

The term atrial tachycardia describes all regular atrial rhythms with a p rate >100 regardless of the mechanism, and this should be prefixed by either focal or macro-reentrant unless the mechanism is unknown.

Focal atrial tachycardia

This is due to an automatic focus of atrial cells firing faster than the SA node. The p wave morphology and axis during tachycardia can be used to predict the location of the source. They are characteristically paroxysmal with short bursts at a rate of 150–250, but may be incessant risking tachycardia induced cardiomyopathy. They occur in normal hearts but are also associated with many forms of cardiac disease. It may be terminated with iv adenosine.

Treatment is needed only for symptomatic patients or incessant tachycardia. β-blockers and calcium channel antagonists can be used to slow the atrial rate and the ventricular response by AV nodal blockade. Class 1c (flecainide and propafenone) or class 3 (amiodarone and sotalol) may suppress the tachycardia, but their use is limited by toxicity. RFA is the most effective therapy and is a cure.

Macro-reentrant atrial tachycardia (atrial flutter)

Atrial flutter (AFL) is an ECG definition of a p wave rate >240 and an absence of an isoelectric baseline between deflections. It is caused by a reentry circuit over large areas of the right or left atrium (see p429). The circuit is not influenced by adenosine and the AVN block reveals the underlying rhythm. It is usually (but not always) associated with structural heart disease. AFL exacerbates heart failure symptoms and if incessant will worsen LV function.

DC cardioversion effectively restores SR, but AFL often recurs. Drug therapy is not very effective. AVN blockade is difficult to achieve and the high doses of β-blockers, calcium channels antagonists and digoxin required may have unwanted side effects. Class 1c drugs are used to maintain SR, however propafenone and flecainide can paradoxically accelerate the ventricular rate in AFL by slowing the tachycardia rate down sufficiently to allow the AVN to conduct 1:1. They should always be used in combination with an AVN blocking agent. Amiodarone is an alternative agent, particularly if LV function is impaired.

RFA is the most effective way of maintaining SR and is a cure. If curative ablation is not possible and effective rate control is not possible with drugs, then ablation of the AV node and a pacemaker is a permanent palliative solution. Anticoagulation recommendations for patients with AFL are identical to those with AF.[1]

---

1 Blomstrom-Lundqvist C, Scheinman MM, Aliot EM *et al.* (2003). ACC/AHA/ESC guidelines for the management of patients with supraventricular arrhythmias *J Am Coll Cardiol* **42**:1493–1531.

Atrioventricular nodal reentrant tachycardia (AVNRT)

This is the commonest cause of a narrow complex tachycardia in patients with normal hearts, typically in young adults, commoner in women. They characteristically cause paroxysms of severe palpitations, with a pounding in the neck (due to reflux of blood into the jugular veins caused by the simultaneous atrial and ventricular contraction). It has a benign prognosis and may require no treatment. The ECG in SR is usually normal.

The tachycardia is terminated by iv adenosine or vagal manoeuvres. The underlying reentry circuit is entirely within the AV node and therefore can be controlled long term with β-blockers, verapamil or diltiazem. Alternative effective, but second line agents are flecainide, propafenone or sotalol. The first line treatment for recurrent symptomatic episodes however is RFA which is a cure. When symptoms are very infrequent a 'pill in the pocket' approach is sometimes helpful i.e. a large oral dose of, e.g., verapamil is taken to terminate the event.

Atrioventricular reentrant tachycardia (AVRT)

This is due to an AV re-entry circuit involving a connection other than the AV node. As these accessory pathways are congenital arrhythmias usually present much younger than AVNRT (infancy or childhood). Rapid paroxysmal palpitations are the usual symptom. It is usually a NCT (orthodromic) as the ventricle is activated via the AVN, however a BCT is also possible if the ventricle activates via the accessory pathway (antidromic). The prognosis may not be benign and specialist referral is mandatory. RFA is the treatment of choice. The most useful drugs are flecainide and propafenone which slow conduction in the accessory pathway without slowing the AV node. Verapamil, diltiazem and β-blockers should be used only when no ventricular preexcitation is present or when the accessory pathway is known to be safe.

Junctional tachycardia

This term should only be used for focal tachycardias that originate from the AV nodal tissue directly and are in fact rare in adult cardiology. Distinction from other forms of narrow complex tachycardia is only possible at the EP study. RFA is high risk as the AV may be damaged. Beta blockers and flecainide are effective.

Blomstrom-Lundqvist C, Scheinman MM, Aliot EM *et al.* (2003). ACC/AHA/ESC guidelines for the management of patients with supraventricular arrhythmias. *J Am Coll Cardiol* **42**: 1493–1531.

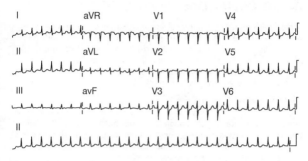

Fig. 9.6 Typical presenting ECG of AVNRT or AVRT.
A narrow complex tachycardia without visible P waves.

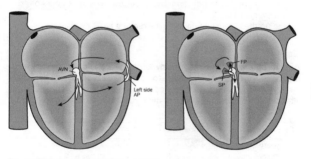

Fig. 9.7 Mechanism of AVNRT and AVRT
Both AVNRT and AVRT have reentry mechanisms. Orthodromic AVRT via a left
sided accessory pathway (AP) (above). Activation from A to V is down the atrio-
ventricular node (AVN), then across the ventricular myocardium and back from V
to A up the AP thus completing the circuit. The ventricle therefore is an essential
part of the circuit. Antidromic AVRT (not shown) would activate in the opposite
direction. Typical AVNRT (below) activates from the atrium to the AVN via the
slow pathway (SP) and from the AVN to the atrium via the fast pathway (FP) thus
completing the circuit. The ventricle is activated as a bystander via the bundle of His
and is not an essential part of the circuit. Atypical AVNRT (not shown) activates in
the opposite direction.

Atrial fibrillation

Atrial fibrillation (AF) is the most common sustained cardiac arrhythmia with a prevalence of 0.5–1% in the general population but 10 fold greater in those aged over 65. It is an atrial arrhythmia where uniform activation is replaced by chaos, such that coordinated contractile function is lost and the atria dilate. It is characterised by an ECG lacking any consistent p waves and a rapid, irregular ventricular rate.

Classification

Previously many terms have been used to prefix AF however now an international consensus on nomenclature has been reached.[1] This allows the correct selection of management options for patients. All episodes of AF lasting greater than 30s should be described as:-

- *First detected* or a *recurrent episode.*
- *Self terminating* or *not self terminating.*
- *Symptomatic* or *asymptomatic.*
- *Paroxysmal* (if self-terminating within 7 days).
- *Persistent* (if cardioverted to SR by any means or lasts >7 days regardless of how it terminates).
- *Permanent* (if it does not terminate or relapses within 24 hours of cardioversion).
- *Lone* (in the absence of underlying structural heart disease) or *idiopathic* (in the absence of any disease).

Causes

AF is a common end point for many forms of cardiac disease where atrial myocytes are damaged or subject to adverse stress generated by ischaemia, cyanosis, elevated intracavity or pericardial pressures. These changes alter the conduction properties of the myocardium facilitating fibrillation.

Common	Potentially reversible	Rare
• Hypertension.	• Alcohol binge.	• Congenital heart disease.
• Left ventricular failure (any cause).	• Hyperthyroidism.	• Autonomic 'vagal' overactivity.
• Coronary artery disease.	• Acute MI.	• Pericardial effusion.
• Mitral or tricuspid valve disease.	• Acute pericarditis.	• Cardiac metastases.
• HOCM.	• Myocarditis.	• Myocardial infiltrative diseases (e.g. amyloid).
	• Exacerbation of pulmonary disease.	• Atrial myxoma.
	• Pulmonary embolism.	
	• Cardiac surgery.	

Symptoms and signs

Palpitations, dyspnoea, fatigue, presyncope, syncope, and chest pains are common however, 30% of patients present with AF as an incidental finding only. Ambulatory monitoring reveals that even patients with symptomatic paroxysmal AF have many asymptomatic episodes. Physical findings are an irregular pulse (which if rapid will be faster at the apex than wrist), variable intensity of the first heart sound and absent 'a' waves in the JVP.

1 Levy S, Camm AJ, Saksena S, *et al.* (2003). International consensus on nomenclature and classification of atrial fibrillation. *J Cardiovasc Electrophysiol* **14:** 443–445.

Atrial fibrillation: investigations

A reversible cause should be identified early to allow appropriate treatment. The most important investigations are:

- *ECG:* irregular ventricular rate and absence of p waves. V rate depends on intact AV nodal function. In the presence of complete AV nodal block a slow regular ventricular escape rhythm is present. The QRS will be broad if there is aberrant conduction; ST-T wave changes may be due to rapid rate, digoxin or underlying cardiac disease.
- *CXR:* cardiomegaly, pulmonary oedema, intrathoracic precipitant, valve calcification (MS).
- *U&Es:* hypokalaemia, renal impairment.
- *Cardiac enzymes:* ?MI. Small rise after DC shock.
- *Thyroid function:* thyrotoxicosis may present as AF only.
- *Liver function tests.*
- *Drug levels:* especially if taking digoxin.
- Mg^{2+}, Ca^{2+}.
- *ABG:* if hypoxic, shocked or ?acidotic.
- *ECHO± TOE:* for LV function, valve lesions, pericardial effusion, and to exclude intracardiac thrombus prior to version to SR. LA size is an important predictor of likely future maintenance of SR.
- *Other investigations* depend on suspected precipitant.

Other investigations when patient stable

24 hour ambulatory monitor to assess heart rate control and look for episodes of symptomatic bradycardia, *CXR, exercise test (or other ischaemia stress test), coronary angiography.*

Management

Currently available antiarrhythmic drugs (AADs) are limited by their toxicity which explains why a strategy of rhythm control (electrical cardioversion and AADs) may be worse than rate control alone (AV nodal blocking agents). Also, rhythm control is associated with a higher rate of strokes, predominantly in patients who have stopped warfarin due to apparent maintenance of SR[1]. In view of this the cornerstones of AF management are controlling patients' symptoms and preventing thromboembolic complications, *not* restoration of SR.

Emergency management

If the patient is haemodynamically compromised then urgent external DC cardioversion under GA or sedation is needed. This is rarely necessary and usually rate control is sufficient to control symptoms. If symptoms persist despite rate control cardioversion can be attempted pharmacologically with flecainide (2 mg/kg, max 150 mg, infused via a peripheral line over 30 mins) or if LV impairment suspected, amiodarone (5 mg/kg, max 300 mg infused via a central line). Patients must be monitored throughout for possible ventricular arrhythmia and hypotension. If AF has been present for >48 hours, cardioversion should be preceded by a TOE to exclude atrial thrombus. All patients should be warfarinized for at least 4 weeks post cardioversion.

1 Wyse DG, Waldo AL, DiMarco JP et al. (2002). A comparison of rate control and rhythm control in patients with atrial fibrillation. *N Engl J Med* **347**: 1825–1833.

Atrial fibrillation: management

Rate control

Drugs: the first line agents are β-blockers or non dihydropyridine calcium-channel antagonists (verapamil or diltiazem), which are effective during both exercise and rest. Digoxin is effective at rest only and should be considered a second line agent.

Pace and ablate: where adequate rate or symptom control is not possible with drugs, or their side effects are not tolerated, a pacemaker is implanted and 6 weeks following this iatrogenic complete heart block induced with radiofrequency ablation. This brings dramatic symptom improvement however it is palliative only and patients are rendered pacing dependent. The life expectancy of patients with normal hearts is unchanged.[1]

Rhythm control

If symptoms are not improved by rate control alone, the restoration and maintenance of SR should be attempted. The trials of rate vs. rhythm control under represent younger patients (<65 years old) so in this group an aggressive strategy of rhythm control may be warranted regardless of symptoms.

Drugs: quinidine, flecainide, propafenone, disopyramide, and sotalol all are more effective than placebo in maintaining SR. They all can lead to long QT related VT/VF and are contraindicated in patients with impaired LV function. Amiodarone is the most effective drug; however its use is limited by non-cardiac side effects, not tolerated by up to 25%. If AV nodal function and QT interval are normal these drugs can safely be started out of hospital. QT interval should be monitored on a weekly basis until a target maintenance dose is reached.

Pacemakers: various pacemaker strategies are useful in maintaining SR. Atrial pacing modes (AAI or DDD) are mandatory as they reduce the AF burden.
• 'Vagal AF' is prevented by pacing.
• Sinoatrial node disease symptoms are improved by a 'block and pace' regimen i.e. rate controlling drugs for AF and pacing for bradycardic episodes.
• Trigger suppression. Atrial ectopy that initiates AF can be prevented by pacemakers with specific algorithms to pace the atrium just faster than the native rhythm or briefly pace rapidly following detection of an atrial ectopic.
• Multisite pacing. By reducing the intra and inter atrial activation time the tendency to AF is reduced.

Atrial defibrillators: by promptly cardioverting each episode of AF remodeling of the atria are prevented. AF episodes are reduced and quality of life improves, however even though shocks are low energy (1–2 J) they are painful. Careful patient selection is required.

Catheter and surgical ablation: see p432.

---

1 Ozcan C, Jahangir A, Friedman PA, *et al.* (2001). Long-term survival after ablation of the atrioventricular node and implantation of a permanent pacemaker in patients with atrial fibrillation. *N Engl J Med* **344:** 1043–1051.

Anticoagulation

Both aspirin (300 mg daily) and warfarin (INR >2) reduce strokes in AF. Decisions on whether to anticoagulate depend on the patients' overall stroke risk and no distinction should be made between paroxysmal, persistent or permanent.

Guidelines for anticoagulation in atrial fibrillation (modified from ACC/AHA/ESC guidelines for AF [§§])

Condition	Recommendation
<60 years old Normal heart (lone AF)	No therapy or aspirin (300 mg)
<60 years with heart disease Low risk for thromboembolism*	Aspirin (300 mg)
>60 years old Normal heart Low risk for thromboembolism*	Aspirin (300 mg)
>60 years old Coronary disease or Diabetes mellitus Low risk for thromboembolism*	Warfarin (INR 2–3)
>75 years old	Warfarin (INR 2–3)
Risk factors for thromboembolism* or thyrotoxicosis (any age)	Warfarin (INR 2–3)
Rheumatic heart disease Prosthetic heart valves Persistent atrial thrombus on TOE	Warfarin (INR 2.5–3.5 or higher)

*Risk factors for thromboembolism:
● Symptomatic LVF
● LV ejection fraction <35%
● ↑BP
● Previous thromboembolic event.

§§ Fuster V, Ryden LE, Asinger RW, *et al.* (2001). ACC/AHA/ESC Guidelines for the Management of Patients with atrial fibrillation. *Circulation* **104**: 2118–2150.

Ventricular tachycardia

This section deals with diagnosis and pharmacological management. Mechanisms and ablation are discussed in detail in Chapter 10.

The most important distinction is the presence of structural heart disease. Impaired LV function is the strongest predictor of a poor prognosis.

Normal heart VT (benign VT)

Right ventricular outflow tract (RVOT) tachycardia. This is due to automatic firing cells in the RVOT giving a characteristic ECG pattern of LBBB with a strongly inferior axis (see Fig. 9.8 opposite). Paroxysms of palpitation are related to exercise. The tachycardia is adenosine sensitive. Usually symptoms are well controlled by verapamil or β-blocker, but RFA is a successful curative option. Care must be taken to exclude arrhythmogenic right ventricular cardiomyopathy (ARVC) as the diagnosis, particularly if the ECG or Echo is not typical (see p312). LVOT tachycardia (RBBB + inferior axis) is also recognised.

Fasicular tachycardia. Its mechanism is uncertain however activation emerges from the left posterior fascicle. ECG typically shows RBBB with superior axis (see Fig. 9.9 opposite). It is sensitive to iv verapamil (which normally slows then terminates it) but not adenosine. Symptoms are well controlled with oral verapamil but RFA offers a cure.

VT with impaired LV function

Symptoms: palpitations, chest pain, presyncope, syncope, dyspnoea, pulmonary oedema, and sudden death all can occur. How well patients tolerate the arrhythmia depends on their LV function and the tachycardia rate.

Aetiology: any cause of impaired LV function can cause VT. Common causes are coronary artery disease, dilated cardiomyopathy and HOCM. They are due to reentry around areas of scarred or diseased myocardium. VT may rapidly deteriorate to VF and these patients die suddenly .

General management: it is essential to treat the underlying heart failure and cause (ACE inhibitors, β-blockers, diuretics, nitrates, statins). This not only reduces symptoms, but the incidence of arrhythmia.

Long term antiarrhythmic treatment: β-blockers reduce arrhythmia and SCD but the impact of other drugs is minimal and often harmful. Flecainide, propafenone and sotalol all *increase* mortality and should be avoided, except in patients with ICDs under supervision of an electrophysiologist. Amiodarone and mexilitine have a neutral impact on prognosis but may reduce the number of VT episodes in very symptomatic patients. RFA is only possible when VT is slow and haemodynamically well tolerated therefore limiting its use.

Preventing SCD: ICDs have dramatically improved survival for these patients.

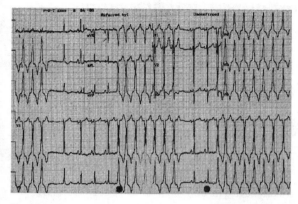

Fig. 9.8 Intermittent right ventricular outflow tract tachycardia and sinus rhythm. During the tachycardia beats notice the left bundle branch block appearance and the positivity in leads II, III and aVF indicating an inferior axis.

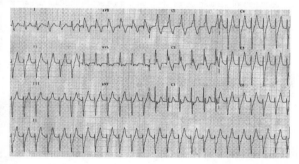

Fig. 9.9 12 lead ECG of fasicular tachycardia suggested by broad complex tachycardia with right bundle branch block appearance and superior axis.

Arrhythmogenic right ventricular cardiomyopathy (ARVC)

This is an unusual genetic disorder cause by fatty-fibro infiltration of RV myocardium due to an abnormality in ion channels. The scarring predisposes to VT of RV origin. The ECG in tachycardia has a LBBB appearance but in SR may be normal or have T wave inversion in V1–V3. It is a progressive disease, associated with worsening RV function (leading to symptoms of heart failure), arrhythmia and sudden death.

The diagnosis is indicated by typical ECG VT appearance and evidence on Echo (late) or MRI (early) of RV impairment, dilatation and fatty infiltration. RV biopsy is not necessary.

Drug management includes flecainide, sotalol, amiodarone and β-blockers however they have limited potential in preventing SCD. An ICD is warranted in high risk cases. Disarticulation of the RV from the LV (thus electrically isolating RV arrhythmias) has been used in difficult cases.

Brugada syndrome

This is an important different diagnosis of ARVC. It is an autosomal dominant condition of variable penetrance, with a defect in the SCN5A gene causing loss of function in the sodium channel. Patients are mainly found in Southeast Asia, mostly men (M:F 8:1). The heart is otherwise normal and the first manifestation may be VF or a very rapid, unstable VT. The hallmark feature is a RBBB appearance with ST elevation in leads V1–V3. A flecainide challenge will reveal the ECG abnormality if not already present. Perform serial ECGs after administration of flecainide 2 mg/kg body weight iv in 10 minutes, or procanamide 10 mg/kg iv in 10 minutes. The test is positive if an additional 1mm ST elevation appears in leads V1, V2 and V3. All positive individuals should undergo EP studies and further specialist evaluation. The only therapy is ICD to prevent SCD.

Bundle branch tachycardia

This is a reentry circuit when activation circuits up one bundle branch and down the other (in either direction). It only occurs in diseased ventricles with delayed conduction in the bundles. It is only confirmed during EP study and is treated with RFA.

Torsades de Pointes (TdP): see long QT syndrome (p394).

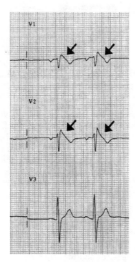

Fig. 9.10 Brugada ECG with flecanide challenge. A typical Brugada ECG with arrows marking the characteristic promiment coved ST-segment elevation in the right precordia leads, ≥2 mm at its peak folllowed by a negative T-wave with little or no isoelectric separation. Intravenous administration of either ajmaline (1 mg/min) or flecainide (2 mg/kg, max. 150 mg; in 10 minutes) exaggerate the ST changes or revals them if initially absent.[1]

1 Wilde AA, Antzelevitch C, Borggrefe M et al. Proposed Diagnostic Criteria for the Brugada Syndrome. Consenus Report. *Circulation*. 2002; 106:2514–2519.

Long QT syndrome

Long QT syndrome (LQTS) is a fascinating condition in which our understanding of the genes, molecular function of the myocyte, and clinical expression of the disease has evolved rapidly over recent years. The identification of genetic mutations that code for protein elements of specific ion channels has taught us more about the link between genotype and phenotype than any other cardiology disorder.

Pathology

LQTS is due to prolonged repolarization of the ventricular myocyte, which is manifest as a lengthened QT interval on the ECG and predisposes to ventricular tachycardia in the form of Torsades de Pointes (TdP), VF, and sudden cardiac death. The cardiac action potential is generated by at least 10 distinct but finely balanced ionic currents (principally gating the flow of Na^+, K^+ and Ca^{2+} ions across the cell membrane). A functional abnormality in any of these, whether acquired or genetic, that accentuates depolarizing currents or attenuates repolarizing currents, can potentially lead to LQTS.

Congenital LQTS

Two inherited forms of LQTS are well known. The commoner Romano–Ward syndrome (autosomal dominant with variable penetrance) that has no other phenotypic features and the much rarer Jervell Lange–Nielson syndrome (autosomal recessive) associated with deafness. A modern gene based classification however has now replaced these eponymous syndromes, and six chromosome loci (LQTS1–6) coding for 6 genes have been identified (see table opposite). Each genetic syndrome can also be characterized by distinct clinical features.

There is an interaction between congenital and acquired forms. Carriers of genetic abnormalities may not manifest the overt ECG changes, however if challenged by a QT prolonging drug such as erythromycin, they are at risk of developing Torsades and sudden death.

Acquired LQTS: (see table opposite)

Clinical features

The unmistakeable hallmark of LQTS is recurrent syncopal episodes precipitated by emotion or physical stress. The arrhythmia is Torsades de pointes, often preceded by a short–long–short cardiac cycles (Fig. 9.11 p397). This bradycardia related phenomena are more common in the acquired form. The clinical features of the congenital form are related to the specific genetic mutation (see table opposite). Unfortunately the first clinical event can be sudden cardiac death.

ECG: QTc values are typically >460 ms but may be as long as 600 ms. The T wave pattern may give a clue to the gene involved. In affected families a normal QT interval does not rule out genetic carrier status. The degree of QT prolongation varies across the ventricle so QT dispersion, if measured, is also greater.

$$\text{Normal QTc} = \frac{QT}{\sqrt{(RR\ interval)}} = 0.38\text{–}0.46\ \sec\ (9\text{–}11\ \text{small squares})$$

Characteristics of currently identified congenital LQTS

LQTS	Mutation	Ion current*	Effect of mutation	Clinical features
I	KVLQT1 (CW11)	$I_{k (slow)}$	Loss of function.	Exercise related syncope.
II	HERG (CW7)	$I_{k(rapid)}$	Loss of function.	Syncope related to sudden and extreme emotional stress.
III	SCN5A (CW3)	I_{Na}	Gain of function.	Symptoms at rest rather than when excited. Young age and usually presents as sudden death.
IV	Ankyrin-B (CW4)	See below	Loss of function.	–
V	KCNE1 (CW21)	$I_{k(slow)}$	Loss of function.	–
VI	KCNE2 (CW21)	$I_{k(rapid)}$	Loss of function.	–

* Potassium currents (I_k) are repolarizing and the sodium currents (I_{Na}) depolarizing. The ankyrin-B gene codes not for an ion channel but for a cellular structural protein that binds sodium ion channels (Splawski I, Shen J, Timothy KW et al. (2000). Spectrum of mutations in Long-QT syndrome genes. *Circulation* **102**: 1178–1185).

Common causes of acquired LQTS*

Drugs*	
Antiarrhythmics	Quinidine, procainamide, disopyramide, flecainide, propafenone, sotalol, ibutilide, dofetilide, amiodarone (rare).
Antimicrobials	Erythromycin, clarithromycin, trimethprim, ketoconazole, itraconazole, chloroquine.
Antihistamines	Terfenadine.
Other drugs	Amitriptyline, fluvoxamine, chlorpromazine, domperidone, cisapride, glibenclamide.
Electrolyte imbalance	Hypokalaemia, hypomagnesaemia, hypocalcaemia.
Severe bradycardia	Complete heart block, sino atrial node disease, hypothyroidism, hypothermia.

*Note this is not a comprehensive list and LQTS is the commonest single reason for new drugs being withdrawn. When a patient is known to be at risk from LQTS or there is concern that interaction may occur with other QT prolonging drugs, all drugs and potential interactions.

Long QT syndrome: management

Usually episodes of Torsades de pointes (TDP) are short lived and terminate spontaneously, however a prolonged episode causing cardiovascular compromise needs immediate DC cardioversion. For recurrent bursts or following a cardiac arrest; iv magnesium bolus and infusion, followed by urgent temporary pacing (at rate 90–110) if necessary. An isoprenaline infusion can be commenced while waiting to pace.

Acquired

The underlying cause should be identified and reversed. Stop offending drugs. Give Mg before getting blood results. K^+ can be checked rapidly with a blood gas analyser, replace if less than 4 mmol/l, aim to achieve high normal levels. Long term treatment is not usually necessary however a permanent pacemaker is required if non reversible heart block was the cause.

Congenital

As most events are triggered by sudden increases of sympathetic activity treatment is aimed at preventing this. The first choice is β-blockade. Propanolol reduces events in symptomatic patients. If full β-blockade cannot be achieved or not tolerated, surgical left cardiac denervation is an alternative.

Cardiac pacing is useful to alleviate the β-blocker-induced bradycardia and where pauses have been identified to precipitate symptoms (LQT3). Pacing is never the sole treatment in congenital LQTS. ICDs should only be used with careful consideration ie for patients at high risk of SCD or where a resuscitated cardiac arrest was the first event. ICDs prevent SCD but not TDP, and recurrent distressing shocks for non-sustained episodes can ruin a patient's life. Careful patient selection, concomitant use of β-blockers and shrewd device programming minimises inappropriate therapies.

Asymptomatic patient

Screening of affected families reveals patients with LQTS who have never had symptoms. Most patients do not die from LQTS but all are at risk (13% incidence of fatal events over a lifetime if untreated). A balance must be struck between life long treatment with side effects and the spectre of sudden death.

Predicting risk is extremely difficult but is helped by knowledge of the genetic abnormality, if known. A recent study has suggested commencing treatment in LQT1 if QTc >500 ms (men + women); LQT2 all men and women if QTc >500 ms, LQT3 all patients. All need individual counselling.

Priori SG, Schwartz PJ, Napolitano C et al. (2003). Risk Stratification in the Long-QT Syndrome. N Engl J Med **348**: 1866–1874.

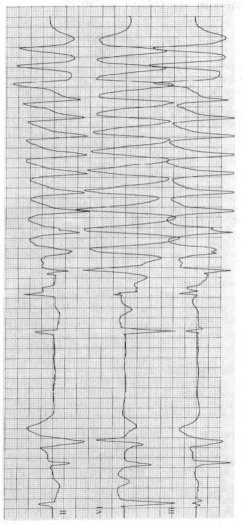

Fig. 9.11 Torsades de pointes. A continuous tracing from 3 leads of a patient monitored on CCU. The first complex is a sinus beat followed by 2 ectopics. There is then a long pause (2s) followed by another sinus beat.

Arrhythmia in special situations

Paediatrics

Arrhythmia may occur at any stage in the paediatric population from fetal life to adolescence.

Fetus and neonate

AVRT and atrial flutter are the usual cause of tachycardia. If persistent *hydrops fetalis* may result. The majority of AVRT resolves spontaneously in utero or by one year of age, although recurrences later in life may occur. Ablation is rarely necessary. Congenital heart block occurs mediated by maternal anti-Ro/SSA antibodies and if severe may also cause hydrops fetalis. This always persists after birth and usually requires permanent pacing, although timing depends on the stability of the subsidiary pacemaker.

Infancy and childhood

AVRT is the usual (80%) cause of tachycardia. AVNRT is rare in infancy, but becomes increasingly common in teenage years. Focal atrial tachycardias and a specific form of AVRT mediated by a slow atrial septal accessory pathway (persistent junctional reciprocating tachycardia) both lead to incessant tachycardia and profound ventricular dysfunction (tachycardia cardiomyopathy). This completely resolves with successful therapy. Radiofrequency ablation is now commonly performed in older children, and may also be used in refractory arrhythmias in neonates and young infants when necessary.

Congenital heart disease

Arrhythmias in association with congenital cardiac lesions are poorly tolerated, and if uncontrolled may lead to a rapid decline in ventricular function and cardiac output.

Supra ventricular tachycardia

These are a major cause of both morbidity and mortality in congenital heart disease. Accessory pathways are associated with Ebstein's anomaly and congenitally corrected transposition of the great arteries and this results in AVRT. Macro-reentrant-atrial tachycardia is common late following the Mustard or Fontan procedure. This is notoriously difficult to control with medication, and although ablation (either percutaneous or surgical) is commonly successful acutely, arrhythmia recurrence is a problem.

Ventricular tachycardia

VT is seen in Ebstein's anomaly and following repair of tetralogy of Fallot. Treatment may involve either radiofrequency ablation or an implantable cardiac defibrillator (ICD).

Pregnancy

The haemodynamic and hormonal changes associated with pregnancy may unmask arrhythmic substrates for the first time, or exacerbate preexisting arrhythmic conditions. Gestational palpitations are common, and most frequently an increased awareness of physiological tachycardia. If new ventricular arrhythmias occur, peripartum cardiomyopathy should be actively excluded.

Permanent pacemakers

Introduction

Permanent pacemakers can pace and sense in one, two, and/or even three chambers of the heart. There are two types of lead, unipolar which has one electrode in the heart, the other being the casing of the pulse generator or bipolar where there are two closely spaced electrodes in the heart.

International codes

This is a three letter identification code describing the basic function of the pacing system. 1st letter is the chamber(s) paced and the 2nd letter is the chamber(s) sensed. V = ventricle, A = atrium, D = dual (i.e. A+V). The 3rd letter is how the device responds to a sensed event. I = inhibits, T = triggers, D = dual (ie I+T) and O = nothing. Often a fourth letter is used to describe added features of the device e.g. R = rate response.

Implantation

Most pacemakers are implanted transvenously using the cephalic or subclavian vein. An incision is made about 2 cm below the clavicle across the deltopectoral groove. The cephalic vein is isolated and is often of sufficient calibre to accept two pacing wires. Alternatively a guide wire can be introduced followed by introducer sheaths to provide access. Sometimes the cephalic is not suitable and the leads have to be introduced via puncture of the subclavian vein using the Seldinger technique. The ventricular lead is then placed in the RV apex most commonly, in the RV outflow tract or on the septum requiring an active fixation lead. The atrial lead is placed in the right atrial appendage ideally but anywhere in the RA with adequate pacing parameters is acceptable but is likely to require an active fixation lead.

Acceptable pacing parameters for new leads		
	Atrium	Ventricle
Threshold*	<1.5 V	<1.0 V
Sensitivity	>1.5 mV	>4.0 mV
Slew rate	>0.2 V/sec	>0.5 V/sec
Impedance	400–1000 ohms	400–1000 ohms

* Using a pulse width of 0.5 ms.

After both leads are placed in acceptable positions they are then secured and attached to the pulse generator which is placed either subcutaneously or beneath the pectoral muscles.

Indications for permanent pacing

Definite indications
- Symptomatic complete heart block
  - Bradycardia with symptoms
  - Pauses >3 seconds
- Symptomatic 2nd degree heart block
- Bifasicular block with intermittent 3rd degree, 2nd degree block or alternating bundle branch block
- Trifasicular block with intermittent 3rd degree or 2nd degree block
- Symptomatic sinus node dysfunction
- Symptomatic chronotropic incompetence
- Carotid sinus hypersentivity
- Sustained VT caused by pauses
- Conditions that requuire drugs that result in symptomatic bradycardia.

Relative indications
- Asymptomatic 3rd degree or 2nd degree (type II) block
- Sinus node dysfunction where symptom-ECG correlation not available
- High risk patients with long QT syndrome
- Chronic chronotropic incompetence (HRC30)
- Neurocardiogenic syncope with significant bradycardia on tilt testing
- Symptomatic HCM with outflow gradient.

Adapted from ACC/AHA/'NASPE 2002 Guidelines. *Circulation* 106: 2145–2161.

Which pacing modality?

The vast majority of patients should have an atrial-based pacing (ie either AAI or DDD). Ventricular-only pacing leads to a greater incidence of AF and potential pacemaker syndrome.

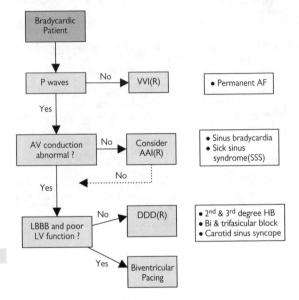

Complications of pacing

Pacemaker syndrome

This tends to occur in patients with normal or near normal LV function and intact VA conduction during VVI pacing. Symptoms include; presyncope, syncope, lightheadedness, fatigue, exercise intolerance, malaise, lethargy, dyspnoea, headache, chest pain, non-specific symptoms.

Loss of AV synchrony can decrease cardiac output by 20% at rest. There is atrial contraction against a closed mitral and tricuspid valve leading to cannon waves. There is activation of atrial stretch receptors with release of atrial natriuretic peptide. The treatment is to restore AV synchrony either by reducing the pacing rate or inserting an atrial lead.

Endless loop tachycardia (pacemaker-mediated tachycardia)

This occurs in dual chamber pacing (VDD, DDD, or DDDR) and is caused by inappropriate sensing of retrograde p waves and hence triggering a ventricular response. The treatment is to increase the post-ventricular atrial refractory period (PVARP) so as not to sense the retrograde p wave.

Other tachycardias

Atrial flutter or fibrillation can cause rapid ventricular pacing in dual chamber systems by sensing the atrial rate. To overcome this, the pacemaker can either mode-switch to VVI or be reprogrammed to DDI so that the atrial rate can not be tracked.

Interference

MRI: generally contraindicated in a patient with a pacemaker as can cause serious malfunction.

Radiation therapy: can damage pacemaker electronics or result in erosion of the generator. The radiation dose is cumulative. Shielding is mandatory. Pulse generator may need to be replaced.

Diathermy: pacemaker needs to be checked before and after surgery as the electronics of the generator can be damaged. Should be reprogrammed to a non-sensing mode (VOO) prior to surgery or have a magnet applied during diathermy to force the device to pace (see below).

Magnet response

When the pacemaker is within a sufficiently strong magnetic field it reverts to its magnet mode. This is non-sensing fixed pacing at the devices 'magnet rate' usually 70–80 min^{-1}, i.e. DOO (dual chamber) or VOO/AOO (single chamber).

Pacing clinic

The device is interrogated every 6–12 months. The battery voltage is measured and below a critical level the elective replacement indicator (ERI) activates. There is approximately 6 months between ERI and the dangerous EOL (end-of-life). The lead(s) function is assessed by checking pacing threshold, sensitivity (the size of sensed electrogram detected) and pacing impedance. Any change in these parameters could indicate a problem e.g. a low impedance suggests an internal insulation break, whilst a high impedance might suggest a conductor problem.

Modern devices store the time and duration in changes of pacemaker function which is helpful for arrhythmia detection. Some can also store electrograms which help in the diagnosis of arrhythmias and pacemaker malfunction.

Pacemakers for chronic heart failure

Cardiac resynchronization therapy (CRT)

CRT is a novel treatment for symptomatic heart failure (NYHA Class III-IV). In patients with a ventricular conduction delay (LBBB) the coordination of wall motion in the left ventricle is improved by pacing the lateral LV (via the coronary sinus) and septum (via the RV) simultaneously. This improves cardiac output and symptoms. Ventricular filling is improved by shortening the AV delay.

Current indications
- NYHA Class III–IV heart failure.
- Established on optimal medical therapy.
- Sinus rhythm.
- QRS duration >130 ms.
- LVEF ≤35%.
- LVEDD ≥55 mm.

Electrical vs mechanical dyssynchrony

Looking at QRS width on a 12-lead ECG is simple and widely available but is a very crude tool for assessing mechanical dyssynchrony and is probably why as many as 30% of patients in clinical trials have not responded. However LBBB is more prevalent in CHF and associated with increased mortality.

Mechanical dyssynchrony consists of:
- Atrio-ventricular dyssynchrony (PR >120 ms).
- Interventricular dyssynchrony (delay between RV and LV contraction).
- Intraventricular dyssynchrony (differences in regional wall motion).

There are various ways to assess mechanical dyssynchrony including the 12-lead ECG, tagged MRI (expensive), radionuclide ventriculography and echocardiography which is probably the most useful due to its availability and simplicity. Interventricular dyssynchrony can be measured by the difference in the aortic and pulmonary pre-ejection times (measured from the beginning of the QRS to aortic or pulmonary valve opening). A significant difference is 40 ms. Intraventricular dyssynchrony can be assessed by tissue doppler imaging (TDI) looking at the time to peak systolic contraction in different segments of the LV, in particular the difference between the septum and the lateral wall. Strain rate in different segments and colour TDI can reveal significant intraventricular dyssynchrony.

Implantation

The RA and RV leads are inserted by conventional techniques as described earlier. The coronary sinus (CS) is the preferred route for pacing the left ventricle. Normally a venogram of the CS is performed using an occlusive balloon in the RAO, PA, and LAO views and a suitable lateral or posterolateral vein identified. The unipolar or bipolar LV lead is then inserted either with a stylet or using the over the wire (OTW) technique in to a stable position with acceptable pacing parameters and no diaphragmatic stimulation. With increasing evidence for the prevention of sudden cardiac death in heart failure patients most biventricular pacemakers will include a defibrillator.

Future directions

There is evidence of mechanical dyssynchrony in patients with heart failure and a narrow QRS who may benefit from CRT.

Patients who have had AV nodal ablation for symptomatic AF have a better exercise tolerance with biventricular pacing rather than RV pacing alone. Pacing the apex of the RV is not the optimal site for ventricular function and high septal or His pacing may improve haemodynamics.

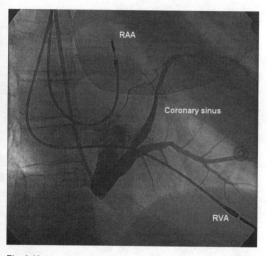

Fig. 9.12 Location of the coronary sinus prior to placing a left ventricular lead. A fluoroscopic image of the heart from the RAO projection. There is an active fixation lead in the conventional right atrial appendage (RAA) and a lead in the right ventricular apex. Dye has been injected from below retrogradely up the CS to demonstrate the lateral left ventricular branches, from where pacing stimuli can capture the ventricle.

Invasive electrophysiology

Mechanism of tachycardias

Knowledge of how arrhythmia are initiated and perpetuated is fundamental to understanding the techniques described in this chapter.

The electrical wavefront

The excitable impulse is generated at the cell membrane by the action potential. As one cell depolarizes it causes a reduction in negativity of the resting potential in the adjacent cell such that it this cell also reaches the threshold potential and depolarizes. The shape, orientation and presence of gap junctions between myocardial cells allow rapid progression of this depolarization which can be described as an electrical *wavefront*. After a cell has depolarized it cannot depolarize again until a fixed period of recovery time has passed, the *refractory period*. Cells that are able to depolarize are *excitable* and those that cannot are *refractory*.

In SR the source of these wavefronts is the SA node, and they may be modulated between the atrium and ventricle by the AV node. They are initiated (and therefore heart rate controlled) by regulation from the autonomic nervous system and circulating cathecholamines. This control is lost in tachyarrhythmia and heart rates are inappropriate.

Conduction block

A wavefront will propagate as long as there are excitable cells in its path. Anatomical barriers such as the mitral valve annulus, vena cava, aorta etc. do not contain myocardial cells and therefore the progression of wavefronts is halted there. This is described as *fixed conduction block*, as block is always present. Dead cells are another important source of fixed conduction block e.g. the left ventricular scar of a MI.

Functional conduction block describes when block is only present under certain conditions. An example is myocardial ischaemia which may alter the electrical properties of myocytes such that they do not conduct. It is also functional block that prevents a wavefront turning back on itself, as the cells behind the leading edge are temporarily refractory and force the wavefront to continue in one direction. Other causes of functional block are: cyanosis, myocardial stretch, rate of wavefront, and direction of wavefront.

Arrhythmia mechanism

3 distinct mechanisms are described:
- Enhanced Automaticity.
- Reentry.
- Triggered activity.

The first 2 account for nearly all clinical tachycardias and their characteristics are compared in the table opposite .

Characteristics of automatic and reentry tachycardias*

	Automatic	**Reentry**
Autonomic sensitivity? (e.g. to exercise, emotion)	Often	Unusual*
Reproducible induction and termination by programmed pacing?	No	Yes
Entrainment of the tachycardia by pacing (p)?	No	Yes
Induced by atropine/ isoprenaline infusion?	Yes	May augment induction by pacing*
Related to metabolic causes	Often	Unusual
Onset/offset	May be gradual (warm up and down)	Sudden
Specific tachycardias caused	Inappropriate sinus tachycardia, focal atrial tachycardia, focal AF, junctional tachycardia	SNRT, macroreentrant atrial tachycardia, AF, AVNRT, AVRT, VT

* The conduction properties of, e.g. the AV node, are influenced by autonomic tone.
Spontaneous or drug induced changes in this may then influence the development of reentry
tachycardias such as AV-nodal reentry tachycardia (AVNRT). AF (atrial fibrillation); SNRT
(sinus node reentrant tachycardia); AVRT (atrioventricular reentrant tachycardia); VT
(ventricular tachycardia).

Mechanism of arrhythmias

Enhanced automacity

If a nidus of myocardial cells depolarizes faster (rapid phase 4 of the action potential) than the SA node they will act as the source of wavefronts that conduct through the heart. May be atrial or ventricular but if occur in the atria they will override the SA node. As they occur from a single site they are often termed *focal*. Common sites are where myocardial cells suddenly change shape/size or under abnormal pressures such as; junction of veins/atrium (SVC,PVs), crista terminalis, CS, AV node area, mitral/tricuspid ring, ventricular outflow tracts.

Reentry

Accounts for >75% of clinical arrhythmias. Caused by a perpetually propagating wavefront that it is constantly meeting excitable myocardium. For reentry to occur at least 2 distinct pathways must exist around an area of conduction block. This is best described using the example of VT due to reentry around a LV myocardial scar (see Fig. 10.1 opposite).

(1) A myocardial scar acts as an area of block, around which a normal sinus wavefront passes via normal myocardium (A) and slowly through it via diseased myocardium (B)—hence 2 distinct pathways.

(2) The sinus beat is followed closely by a ventricular ectopic, which is conducted around A normally but is blocked in B which is still refractory following the last sinus beat.

(3) The distal end of B however is now excitable and the wavefront passes backwards up B which has had time to fully recover by the time it reaches the proximal end. Conduction is sufficiently slow up B that now A is excitable again and the wavefront can pass down A.

Thus a reentry wavefront has been formed that is constantly meeting excitable myocardium.

Triggered activity

This has features of both the above mechanisms. They are caused by spontaneous (hence automatic) *after depolarizations* (ADs) occurring late in phase 3 (*early ADs*) or in phase 4 (*delayed ADs*) of the action potential. These ADs however are often triggered by premature beats and are therefore are inducible (like reentry) If these ADs reach the threshold level then a single or burst of action potentials is set off. The ADs can be induced experimentally by ischaemia, QT prolonging drugs, cell injury, or low potassium. This mechanism underlies torsades de pointes and arrhythmias due to digoxin toxicity.

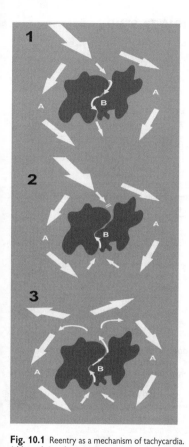

Fig. 10.1 Reentry as a mechanism of tachycardia.
1 Normal sinus beat passing around and through scar.
2 Ectopic beat passing around but blocked through scar.
3 Reentry circuit of tachycardia.
(Dark grey represents scar, light grey normal myocardium, and white arrows represent electrical wavefronts.)

The electrophysiology study

The EP study is most useful for the diagnosis of tachycardia. When this has already been documented or is strongly suspected then it is usually the first part of a combined procedure with catheter ablation to cure the arrhythmia. Note in EP it is usual to discuss cycle lengths (in ms) rather than heart rates e.g. 60/min=1000 ms, 100/min=600 ms, 150/min=400 ms.

Mapping electrical activity in the heart

EP is wrongly considered to be complex. Fundamentally it is just recording of the heart's electrical signals either during sinus rhythm, arrhythmia or in response to pacing at specific sites. The ECG provides a great deal of this information and so a full 12 lead ECG is recorded throughout the procedure.

The intracardiac electrogram (ICegram)

The ECG summates the entire cardiac activation. By placing 2 mm electrodes directly on the heart's endocardial surface the electrical activity at precise locations is known. The ICegram is therefore much narrower than the ECG and is best appreciated at 100 mms^{-1} sweep speed, four times faster than a standard ECG recording.

Either the potential difference between two closely spaced electrodes (a bipolar electrogram) or between 1 electrode and infinity (a unipolar electrogram) can be recorded. The unipolar electrogram is more accurate regarding direction and location of electrical activity however it is subject to much greater interference. Note a pacing current can be passed through any of these electrodes. Standard catheter location is shown in Fig. 10.2.

Pacing protocols

Pacing in the EP study is done in a predefined manner termed *programmed stimulation*. This has three forms:

- *Incremental pacing*: the pacing interval is started just below the sinus interval and lowered in 10 ms steps until block occurs or a predetermined lower limit (often 300 ms) is reached.
- *Extrastimulus pacing*: following a train of 8 paced beats at a fixed cycle length, a further paced beat (the extra stimulus) is introduced at a shorter coupling interval (the time between the last stimulus of the drive and the first extrastimulus). The stimuli of the drive train are conventionally termed S1, the first extra stimulus S2, the second extrastimulus S3 and so on. Extrastimuli can also be introduced after sensed heart beats ('sensed extras').
- *Burst pacing*: pacing at a fixed cycle length for a predetermined time.

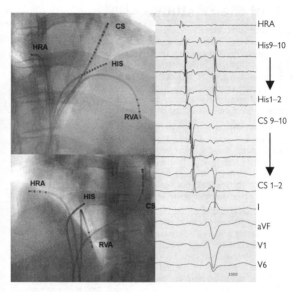

Fig. 10.2 Standard positions of catheters in the EP study and intracardiac electrograms at those sites.

Catheters have been passed up into the right heart from sheaths in the femoral veins under fluoroscopic guidance. These images from the right anterior oblique (above) and left anterior oblique (below) demonstrate the standard positions at the high right atrium (HRA) close to the SA node, on the His bundle (HIS), at the RV apex (RVA) and a catheter passed through the os of the coronary sinus (CS) which wraps around the left posterior atrio ventricular groove. From this position IC egrams are recorded from the left atrium and ventricle. This catheter is often inserted via the left or right subclavian veins.

The intracardiac electrocardiograms are conventionally ordered HRA, His, CS, and RV (not displayed here), with an ECG lead at the bottom. On each catheter bipoles are then ordered proximal to distal. In SR then activation is seen to start at the HRA pass across the His and then along the CS catheter proximally to distally. Earliest ventricular activation is at the RVA (where the Purkinje fibres insert).

Normal *sinus intervals* are PA 25–55 ms, AH = 50–105 ms, HV 35–55 ms, QRS <120 ms, corrected QT <440 ms men, <460 ms women.

Uses of the EP study

Sinus node function

The *corrected sinus node recovery time* and *sinoatrial conduction time* are both measures of SAN function. Unfortunately however they are unreliable tests as SAN function is greatly influenced by autonomic tone, drugs and observer error. SAN dysfunction is best assessed with ambulatory monitoring and exercise testing. It is very rare that invasive EP testing would contribute to the decision to give a patient a permanent pacemaker and therefore it is not part of our routine procedure.

AV conduction

Heart block: the degree of heart block is assessed via the ECG which can also indicate the level (i.e. either at the AV node itself or in the His Purkinje system, infra nodal). The level of block is ascertained easily in the EP study. The AH time is prolonged in nodal and the HV time in infranodal block. The AH (but not the HV) time may be shortened by exercise, isoprenaline or atropine and prolonged by vagal manoeuvres.

AV nodal function: this is assessed both anterogradely (A to V) and retrogradely (V to A), using both incremental and extrastimulus pacing. By incremental pacing at the HRA, conduction is observed in the His and RVA until block occurs. The longest pacing interval at which block occurs is the anterograde Wenckebach cycle length (WCL). Normal values are <500 ms however this increases with age and autonomic influences. The retrograde WCL is also measured however absent VA conduction can be normal. From the HRA extrastimulus pacing is performed. As the coupling interval between S1 and S2 is reduced, AV conduction is observed. The longest S1S2 interval at which AV block occurs is the anterograde AVN effective refractory period (ERP). This is measured at drive trains of 600 and 400 ms. If VA conduction is present the retrograde AVNERP is measured.

Decremental conduction: this is the key physiological property of the AV node. As the interval between successive impulses passing through the AV node decreases the conduction velocity within the AV node also decreases. In AV conduction this is manifest as a prolongation of the AH (and AV) interval as the atrial pacing interval decreases. This phenomena can be observed during incremental and extrastimulus pacing. During extrastimus pacing if the AH interval is plotted against the S1S2 (=A1A2) then an anterograde conduction curve can be plotted.

Dual AV nodal physiology: it is possible in many patients (but not all) to identify two electrical connections between the atrial myocardium surrounding the compact AV node and the node itself, which have different conduction properties. The *slow pathway* has slower conduction velocity but a shorter ERP than the *fast pathway*. This is observed by plotting an anterograde conduction curve. For longer A1A2 intervals AV conduction is preferentially via the fast pathway, however once the fast pathway ERP is reached conduction is via the slow pathway and consequently the AH time suddenly prolongs. This is called an AH interval *jump* and is defined as a lengthening of the AH by >50 ms, following reduction in the A1A2 interval of 10 ms. Dual AV nodal pathways is the substrate for AVNRT.

A standard basic electrophysiology study

Pacing protocol	Measure	Comments
1. Sinus rhythm	Basic sinus intervals (PA, AH, HV, QRS, corrected QT)	Is there AV conduction block?
2. Incremental ventricular pacing (IVP)	RWCL	Is VA conduction present? If so, is atrial activation normal and decremental?
3. Incremental atrial pacing (IAP)	AWCL	Is AV conduction decremental? Is prexcitation manifest during pacing?
4. Extrastimulus pacing from atrium at 600 and 400 ms	Anterograde AVNERP at 600 and 400 ms	Is AV conduction decremental? Is prexcitation manifest during pacing? Is there dual AV nodal physiology?
5. Extrastimulus pacing from ventricle at 600 and 400 ms	Retrograde AVNERP at 600 and 400 ms	Is VA conduction present? If so, is atrial activation normal and decremental?
6. Arrhythmia induction from atrium. Use 2–4 extrastimuli, sensed extra stimuli, burst pacing.	.	Note pacing protocol that induces arrhythmia. Is it reproducible? Compare arrhythmia induced to clinical arrhythmia.
7. If VT suspected perform Wellen's protocol	VERP at 600 and 400 ms	
8. Repeat steps 2–7 during isoprenaline infusion		Essential for tachycardias with enhanced automaticity mechanism.

Note: RWCL (retrograde Wenckebach cycle length), AWCL (anterograde Wenckebach cycle length), AVNERP (atrio ventricular nodal effective refractory period).

Identifying abnormal AV connections

In normal hearts there is only one connection between the atrium and ventricle, the AV node. Activation of the atrium (during V pacing) or ventricle (during A pacing or SR) should therefore start at the AV node. Accessory pathways (AP) do not decrement. Their presence can be identified then by both abnormal activation patterns and conduction physiology using incremental and extrastimulus pacing.

Atrial pacing: as the AV node decrements, a greater proportion of ventricular activation will occur via the AP. Thus non decremental AV conduction times and broadening of the QRS complex will be observed as the pacing interval shortens. Note: If the effective refractory period (ERP) of the AP is shorter than the ERP of the AV node then the QRS will suddenly narrow and the AV time suddenly prolong when the AP blocks.

Ventricular pacing: the normal order of atrial activation is His then CS (proximal to distal) and finally the HRA, termed *concentric* activation. If the atrium is activating via an AP an *eccentric* activation pattern is observed. The site of the earliest atrial activation will localise the AP. Non decremental VA conduction is also seen.

Induction of arrhythmia

The presence of an AP, dual AV nodal physiology or a known ventricular scar provides the substrate for a tachycardia but does not necessarily imply it will occur. A diagnosis can only be confirmed by inducing the tachycardia.

In addition to the pacing techniques described, burst pacing, extrastimulus pacing with multiple extrastimuli, and sensed extras are deployed. If this fails pacing manoeuvres can be repeated during an isoprenaline infusion (1–4 mcg min^{-1}) or boluses (1–2 mcg). This is particularly important for tachycardias with an enhance automaticity mechanism. 'Aggressive' induction protocols increase the likelihood of inducing an unwanted arrhythmia such as AF or VF.

Once a tachycardia is initiated, it is useful to compare it with a 12 lead ECG recorded during symptoms to ensure this is the clinical arrhythmia. How individual tachycardias are diagnosed and treated is considered in subsequent chapters.

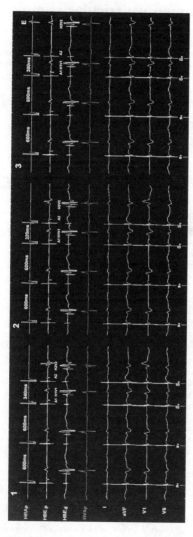

Fig. 10.3 Example of A–H interval jump during extrastimulation.

Programmed ventricular stimulation

An EP study focusing on induction of ventricular arrhythmias (the VT stimulation study) has previously been used to risk stratify for sudden cardiac death (SCD), to decide on the effectiveness of antiarrhythmic drugs in suppressing VT, and the need for an ICD. Evidence has now accumulated however that it is of little predictive value, and that decisions regarding ICD prescription should be based on other risk factors, particularly LV function. The EP study can be useful prior to ICD implant for other reasons:
- To aid programming of device:
  - Is VT well haemodynamically tolerated?
  - Is it easily terminated with overdrive pacing?
  - Is there VA conduction? During V pacing or VT?
- To assess suitability for VT ablation (e.g. bundle branch VT).
- Are other arrhythmias present and easily induced?

Programmed ventricular stimulation is performed using the protocol devised by Wellen's or a modification thereof (see below).

Clinical indications

- Documented symptomatic tachycardia (as first stage of diagnostic and ablation procedure).
- Risk stratification for sudden cardiac death.
- Suspected but not documented symptomatic tachycardia (diagnostic only).
- Wolff–Parkinson–White syndrome.
- Unexplained syncope (suspicious of arrhythmic cause).
- Symptomatic SAN or AVN heart block suspected but never documented (rare).

Protocol for programmed ventricular stimulation:
- From RV apex, extrastimulus pacing, reduce the coupling interval until refractory:
    1 extrastimulus during SR
        2 extrastimuli during SR
        1 extrastimulus following 8 paced beats at 600 ms
        2 extra stimuli following 8 paced beats 600 ms
        1 extrastimulus following 8 paced beats at 400 ms
        2 extra stimuli following 8 paced beats400 ms
        3 extrastimuli during SR 0 ms
        2 extra stimuli following 8 paced beats at 600 ms
        3 extrastimuli following 8 paced beats at 400 ms
- If no ventricular arrhythmia induced, repeat from RV outflow tract

---

Thus the pacing protocol becomes gradually more aggressive. The more aggressive the induction protocol the more non-specific the result. The most useful result is induction of a sustained monmorphic VT with one or two extrastimuli. This indicates a poptential substrate for ventricular arrhythmias. Non-sustained VT, polymorphic VT and VF are all non-specific results.

New technologies

EP procedures have become increasingly complex (e.g. for AF or congenital heart disease) and require greater radiation exposure. Both of these problems have been overcome by non-fluoroscopic, 3-dimensional mapping systems. A computer-generated image of the cardiac chamber of interest is formed and onto this the electrical activation in the heart and the EP catheter location is superimposed (see Fig. 10.4). In some cases it is now possible to perform a complete EP study and ablation without the use of X-ray. Also, 3-D CT or MR images of the patient can be imported and used as a guide.

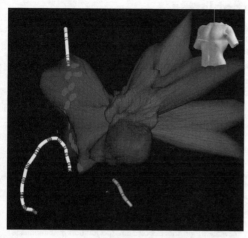

Fig. 10.4 An Ensite NavX image of the left atrium. The torso demonstrates this is a LAO projection. The catheter positions are located without the use of X-ray.

Catheter ablation

In medical terms ablation is the removal of tissue. As many tachycardias depend on discreet foci or pathways to be sustained they are amenable to cure by destruction of these areas.

Energy sources for ablation

Radiofrequency (RF) energy

Cells are destroyed by heating > 50°C. The RF generator delivers an alternating current of 500–750 KHz between the active catheter electrode and a large indifferent electrode placed on the patient's skin. The ions within cells immediately adjacent to the catheter are agitated and generate heat (resisitive heating). The heating power generated in this way dramatically decreases as the distance form the catheter increases. The remaining heat is conducted away to the surrounding tissue. A lesion of ~5 mm depth is formed after 30–60 s, which is sufficient to destroy the full thickness of atrial myocardium. Catheters are 7 Fr with tip electrodes of 4 mm length as standard or 8mm where longer lesions needed.

If the temperature approaches 100°C boiling of cell water occurs generating steam which escapes either by exploding through the endocardium causing a large lesion (cavitation) or the pericardium (perforation ± tamponade). Temperature is monitored at the tip of the catheter and power delivery automatically limited to prevent such overheating. The generator allows the power, temperature and duration of each RF delivery to be adjusted.

Cooled RF

The tip of the catheter is cooled during RF by the flow of blood, so the hottest part of an RF lesion is 1 mm beneath the surface. Stasis of flow occurs as the lesion is formed, hence the temperature rises, limiting the amount of power that is delivered and therefore size of the lesion. Normal saline passed through a lumen in the tip of the catheter at a rate of 10–30 ml/hr continuously cools the catheter, allows higher powers and bigger lesions to be formed. This is needed where the myocardium is thick e.g. left ventricle (VT) or Eustachian ridge (typical atrial flutter). Low flow (2 ml/hr) RF ablation is useful to keep the tip of the catheter free of thrombus, reducing stroke risk during RF in the LA or LV.

Cryoablation

Completely contained within the specialized ablation catheter, liquid nitrous oxide released into the tip, rapidly vaporizes and removes heat the tissue in contact with the catheter. The gas is rapidly recycled back to the catheter console. The tissue temperature (monitored at the tip of the catheter) falls to −30°C at which stage there is reversible loss of cell function. If an appropriate response is seen (e.g. loss of preexcitation during AP ablation) then the tissue is further cooled to −60°C for 4 minutes to cause permanent destruction. The formation of ice adheres the catheter to the tissue making it very stable. If however an adverse change is seen (e.g. AVN block) at −30°C, then the tissue can be rewarmed.

Other

Other energy sources under investigation are; microwave, ultrasound and laser.

Catheter ablation: complications

SVTs (other than AF) are cured in >90% of cases with ablation. For AVNRT >97%. Registry data demonstrates significant complications occur in 2–3% of cases, however this varies with specific procedures.

Major complications

- *Death* (0.1–0.3%).
- *Stroke* (0.2%). Risk higher for left-sided procedures. Minimize risk by: pre-op TOE, intra-operative heparin guided by activated clotting time, post-operative anticoagulation (aspirin or warfarin), irrigated catheters, continuous pressured heparinised saline administration through left sided sheaths, cryoablation.
- *Cardiac tamponade* (0.5–1%). Risk higher if trans-septal puncture performed, but can occur even during diagnostic procedure. BP is monitored throughout the procedure and in any hypotensive episode tamponade suspected. EP lab should be equipped with hand held echo machine and emergency pericardial aspiration sets.
- *AV nodal block* (1%). High risk for septal accessory pathway (AP) or AVNRT (slow pathway) ablation. During RF continuously image catheter position and atrial and ventricular electrograms. If AV, VA block or catheter movement occurs STOP. Cryoablation may be preferred for high risk cases.
- *Coronary artery spasm/MI.* Transient ST elevation and chest pain may occur without any long term effect due to spasm.
- *Pneumothorax.* Only if subclavian approach used for catheters (coronary sinus).
- *X-ray exposure.* EP cases may be prolonged. Deterministic effects such as skin damage can be avoided with care to fluoroscopy technique. Women of fertile age should be counselled and have pregnancy tests if necessary. Non-fluoroscopic catheter location (Carto, LocaLisa, Ensite NavX) is increasing.

Minor complications

- *Bruising/haematoma.* Common at puncture site if anticoagulation used.
- *Chest pain.* Occurs transiently during energy delivery, iv opiates, or benzodiazepines may be necessary.
- *Vasovagal episode.* Often during initial percutaneous sheath insertion. Ensure patient has iv cannula prior to entering the lab.

Atrial tachyarrhythmias: mechanism

All regular atrial tachyarrhythmias should be named mechanistically i.e. either focal atrial tachycardia or macroreentrant atrial tachycardia (which includes atrial flutter).

Focal atrial tachycardia

Atrial cells with enhanced automaticity fire faster than the SA node. Common foci are the crista terminalis, PV–LA junction, vena cavae–RA junction, triangle of Koch.

Macroreentrant atrial tachycardia

Commonest form is *typical atrial flutter*. This is an ECG diagnosis i.e. P wave rate >240 min^{-1}. There is a reentry circuit contained within the RA, rotating anticlockwise around the tricuspid valve (see Fig. 10.5). The opposite of this is *reverse typical flutter*.

Reentry circuits are also found in the left atrium, following cardiac surgery or in congenital heart disease. These have varying circuits that need to be carefully mapped before ablation can be performed.

Atrial fibrillation

The chaotic electrical wavefronts are seen because the atria do not activate uniformly. Two mechanisms account for this:

Focal: a single source of wavefronts emerge from either; cells of enhanced automaticity (like an atrial tachycardia located in a PV) or a single small reentry circuit (microreentry) that depolarize so rapidly the rest of the atria cannot conduct them uniformly and the wavefronts break up to give multiple wavefronts (=fibrillatory conduction). This is usually the mechanism of paroxysmal AF and these foci are considered triggers of AF.

Multiple reentry: this underlies permanent AF. 4–6 separate reentry circuits of constantly varying course and velocity rotate around the atria colliding with each other and anatomical structures such as veins and valves. They are self-perpetuating. The larger the atria, the more room these wavefronts have to rotate and more likely they will be sustained.

As any episode of AF persists the greater the atrial dilation due to mechanical stunning (remodelling), explaining the natural progression of AF from paroxysmal to persistent to permanent. *'AF begets AF'.*

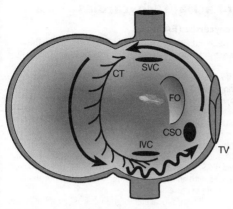

Fig. 10.5 Mechanism of typical atrial flutter. A diagram of the RA with the anterior surface cut open and swung out to the left. The arrow represents the wavefront passing up the septum, over the roof of the RA, anterior to the crista terminalis (CT) and then passing through between the inferior vena cava (IVC) and tricuspid valve (TV) = the RA isthmus. Conduction is slowed in this area. Fossa ovalis (FO), Superior vena cava (SVC).

Ablation of atrial tachycardias

Focal atrial tachycardia (FAT)

- Tachycardia must be induced and sustained to map location in the atria of earliest activation (the focus) and this may need an isoprenaline infusion.
- The hallmark of AT is dissociation of the atrial electrograms from ventricular during tachycardia. This may occur spontaneously (AV block) or it may be necessary to pace the ventricle faster than the atrium.
- ECG may indicate origin (+ve I & aVL, −ve V1 = high lateral RA; −ve II, III & aVF=LA or RA posteroseptal; +ve I, aVL & V1= right PVs; −ve I & aVL, +ve V1= left PVs,).
- Catheters in RA and CS will identify whether LA or RA activates first. Beware: FAT from RSPV may give appearance of having an RA origin. RA is easily mapped with an ablation catheter via the IVC, but the LA requires a transeptal puncture.
- A successful site usually has a local electrogram at least 30 ms ahead of the onset of the pwave.
- Success rates are >90%.

Typical atrial flutter

- The reentry circuit can be interrupted by creating a series of ablation lesions adjacent to one another so that a line of conduction block is created between the inferior vena cava and tricuspid valve (see Fig. 10.5 p429 and Fig. 10.6 opposite). This is therefore a purely anatomical procedure that can be performed in SR or tachycardia.
- The TV annulus is usually mapped with a 20 pole catheter.
- Success is proved by showing that there is conduction block in both directions across the RA isthmus (bidirectional block).
- Acute success occurs in 90% of cases with a 10% relapse.
- 30% of patients who undergo atrial flutter ablation later develop AF.

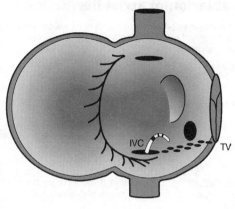

Fig. 10.6 Ablation of typical atrial flutter. An ablation catheter is passed up from the IVC, and a series of burns made in the RA isthmus to join the TV to the IVC with a line of scar. In this way no activation can pass through and the reentry circuit of typical atrial flutter is broken. (See Fig. 10.5 on p429 for landmarks on the diagram.)

Catheter ablation of atrial fibrillation

There are 2 main strategies to prevent recurrences of AF—abolishing the focal triggers, and changing the atrial substrate such that multiple reentry circuits cannot be sustained.

Single focal trigger: e.g. focal AT from PV. This is selectively ablated in same way as described above. This is rarely a cure of AF as there often multiple triggers.

Abolish all potential triggers: all four PVs are isolated. This is done in 2 ways:
- Selectively ablating all the electrical connections between the LA and each PV (electrical isolation, see Fig. 10.7A). An important risk is PV stenosis (3%) which causes progressive dyspnoea and is very difficult to manage.
- Creating a line of conduction block well outside the ostia of the veins (anatomical isolation, see Fig 10.7B opposite), isolating not just the vein but the LA tissue adjacent to the veins. The risk of PV stenosis is virtually eliminated.

In some centres it is common to also ablate electrical signals in the superior vena cava and coronary sinus. For paroxysmal AF clinical success rates using this technique are 60–70% in published series.

Linear ablation: the LA and RA can be compartmentalized by creating long lines of ablation within them. These interrupt the multiple reentry circuits and hence AF cannot be sustained. This treatment was pioneered by the cardiac surgeons performing the surgical maze with great success; however improvements in catheter technology and non-fluoroscopic location systems (e.g. Carto or Ensite NavX) have made it feasible to do this percutaneously.

This treatment is suitable for symptomatic patients with persistent or permanent AF. In addition to isolating the PVs, lines are drawn across the roof of the LA, between the LIPV and MV, the RA isthmus and between the SVC and IVC. Success rates are lower than for paroxysmal AF. Procedures are long (4 hours) and carry a risk of stroke higher than standard ablation.

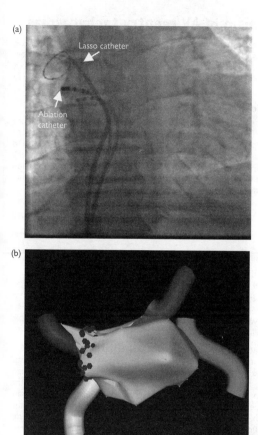

Fig. 10.7 (a) Electrical isolation of the left superior pulmonary vein. A lasso catheter is placed well up inside the vein to record pulmonary vein potentials. The ablation catheter is back at the mouth of the vein. Where potentials are found linking the pulmonary vein to the surrounding LA, energy is applied. The procedure continues until no potentials are recorded in the vein or potential are dissociated. (b) Anatomical isolation of the right superior pulmonary vein. This is a Carto image of the LA from the front with the four pulmonary veins posterior. Lesions can be seen well outside the vein therefore not risking pulmonary vein stenoisis, however no attempt is made to demonstrate electrical isolation.

Mechanism of AV reentry tachycardias

In young patients with paroxysmal regular narrow complex tachycardia the diagnosis is either AVNRT or AVRT. The mechanism of both is reentry (see Figs. 9.7 p383). The substrate for AVNRT is dual AVN pathways and for AVRT the presence of an AP. Occasionally an atrial tachycardia may give an identical ECG appearance.

Diagnostic testing

4 standard catheters are positioned (see Fig. 10.2 p415) and an EPS carried out (see table p417). Look for evidence of dual AVN physiology and presence of an AP. If tachycardia is induced, atrial activation is observed to see whether it is via the AVN (AVNRT) or an AP (AVRT). Look closely for AVN block, BB block, and at the onset and termination of tachycardia. HSVPBs are introduced to identify whether an AP is mediating the tachycardia (AVRT).

AV block

If AVN block occurs, but tachycardia persists, it is almost always an atrial tachycardia.

Onset

- AVN jump immediately followed by tachycardia: AVNRT.
- Loss of preexcitation followed by tachycardia: AVRT.

Termination

- Last tachycardia complex atrial (block in AVN): AVNRT or AVRT (almost certainly not atrial tachycardia).
- Last tachycardia complex ventricular: atrial tachycardia (AVNRT or AVRT still possible).

His synchronous ventricular premature beats (HSVPBs)

The aim is to introduce an ventricular paced beat exactly coincidental with the His potential during tachycardia, to see whether the ventricle is an essential component of the reentry circuit (Fig. 10.8). To do this the cycle length of the tachycardia is measured and a single sensed extrastimulus is delivered from the catheter in the RV at 20 ms less than the cycle length. This is repeated, reducing the coupling interval by 10 ms each time, until it is clear the sensed extra is pre-His. Tachycardia is then terminated and the electrograms analysed.

Analysis (Fig. 10.8): the HH and AA intervals are measured to ensure a stable tachycardia. The paced VPB must be synchronus with the His potential. The AA interval before and after the HSVPB are measured. If the subsequent A is premature this implies that the atrium *must* have been activated via an AP (as we know the His bundle is refractory due the presence of the potential) and that the ventricle is part of the reentry circuit hence AVRT. If the A is not advanced it suggests this is AVNRT.

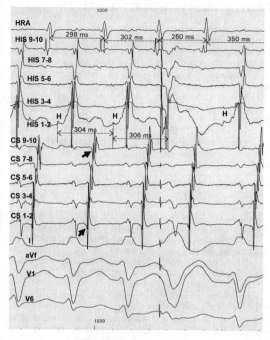

Fig. 10.8 HSVPBs resetting tachycardia. From top to bottom; intracardiac electrograms from High right atrium, His bundle catheter (proximal to distal), CS catheter (proximal to distal), and 4 surface ECG leads. The tachycardia cycle length is approximately 300 ms. During tachycardia the earliest atrial activation is at the distal coronary sinus (lateral left atrium)—see arrows. A sensed extra (the HSVPB) is introduced just ahead of the His potential (H). The next atrial complex is advanced (see cycle lengths measured at the HRA). This strongly suggests an AVRT mediated by a left lateral pathway.

AV reentry tachycardias: ablation

AVRT

Ablation must be performed during ventricular pacing or AVRT to identify the location of the AP (unless it is manifest on the resting ECG i.e. WPW). The earliest atrial activation is looked for with an almost continuous V then A electrogram. Its general location is found by bracketing it with a diagnostic catheter on the valve annulus i.e. the CS catheter on the left side or a multipolar catheter on the right side (see Fig. 10.9). The precise location is then found with the ablation catheter. A true annular site is needed for success so an equal sized atrial and ventricular component on the mapping catheter is looked for. Left sided APs are approached either retrogradely (via the aortic valve and LV) or anterogradely (trans-septal puncture).

AVNRT

The target is the slow AVN pathway (see Fig. 10.9B). This is found inferior to the His bundle, close to the mouth of the CS. The presence of a slow pathway signal (bump and spike) with a small A and large V component should be seen. Energy is delivered and usually transient slow junctional escape beats are seen as the cells die. If the catheter moves or any AV or VA block occurs ablation is stopped immediately. If the lesion is therapeutic a full EP study is then repeated to test and ensure no AVN damage. A successful procedural outcome is the inability to induce tachycardia and complete loss of dual AV nodal physiology. Conventionally the presence of a jump and a single echo beat is permitted providing tachycardia cannot be induced. If isoprenaline was needed to induce tachycardia it must also be used during testing.

Following ablation full EP testing is repeated. VA conduction should be absent or via the AVN (concentric). If VA conduction persists adenosine boluses are given to demonstrate both VA and AV block.

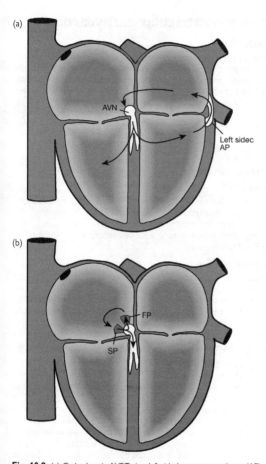

Fig. 10.9 (a) Orthodromic AVRT via a left sided accessory pathway (AP).
Activation from A to V is down the atrioventricular node (AVN), then across the
ventricular myocardium and back from V to A up the AP thus completing the circuit.
The ventricle therefore is an essential part of the circuit. Antidromic AVRT (not
shown) would activate in the opposite direction. A left sided AP as shown above
would be accessed by a trans-septal puncture or retrogradely (via Ao valve and LV).
(a) Typical AVNRT activates from the atrium to the AVN via the slow pathway (SP)
and from the AVN to the atrium via the fast pathway (FP) thus completing the
circuit. The ventricle is activated as a bystander via the bundle of His and is not an
essential part of the circuit. Atypical AVNRT (not shown) activates in the opposite
direction. Ablation targets the slow pathway.

Ablation of ventricular tachycardia

Clinical indications

Only a small percentage of patients with VT in structural heart disease are suitable for ablation. It needs to be well tolerated (see Fig. 10.10), ideally of a single morphology. In this group success rates of 70% are expected. Ablation should be offered to patients whose VT is well tolerated and one of the below:

- Recurrent symptomatic paroxysms.
- To reduce the number of therapies delivered by an AICD.
- Incessant VT.
- VT in normal hearts: ablation offers a cure for these patients (>90% cure). RVOT and fascicular tachycardia are mapped during VT looking for the earliest ventricular activation. Ablation here terminates VT.

Mechanism of VT

In structural heart disease VT almost always has a reentry mechanism. Scarred ventricular myocardium (due to ischaemia, cardiomyopathy etc) provides the substrate for reentry as described previously. A stable reentry circuit can break down in to chaotic activation, VF hence the link between VT and sudden death.

Mapping reentry VT

To successfully map the reentry circuit the patient must be in VT (activation mapping). Thus the VT needs to be haemodynamically well-tolerated. Remote defibrillation paddles are attached to the patient so that if VF or hypotensive VT occurs it can be immediately cardioverted. The aim is to identify the critical diastolic pathway at which the circuit is most susceptible to destruction. This is achieved by entrainment mapping.

Entrainment of VT

This can only be performed on tachycardias with a reentry mechanism. The ablation catheter is moved around the ventricle to sites where the circuit is expected (i.e. adjacent to areas of scar). By pacing with this catheter at a rate just faster than the tachycardia cycle length, a VT is entrained if it is following the same circuit but at a faster rate. If the ECG during pacing is a 12/12 lead match to the clinical VT then this is concealed entrainment. This implies the pacing catheter is within the critical portion of the circuit. To confirm this when pacing is stopped the return cycle length (the time form the final paced beat to the next activation at the catheter) should be almost identical to the TCL.

Ablation technique

The standard steps of a VT ablation are:

- Induce VT (Wellen's). Ensure similar to clinical VT and well tolerated.
- Map VT to identify critical diastolic pathway:
  - Very early local electrogram occurring mid diastole (50–150 ms ahead of ECG).
  - Concealed entrainment during pacing.
  - Return cycle length (=post pacing interval) < tachycardia cycle length + 30 ms.

- Deliver energy at site meeting criteria above.
- If VT terminated, attempt to reinduce again.

Failed ablation

If conventional ablation fails alternative approaches are:
- Arrhythmia cardiac surgery.
- Ablate the epicardial surface of the heart by delivering the catheter via the pericardium (as for a pericardial aspiration).
- Alcohol ablation via a small terminal coronary branch subtending the scarred area supporting reentry. Hence give the patient a controlled, small MI that destroys the critical portion of the re-entry circuit.

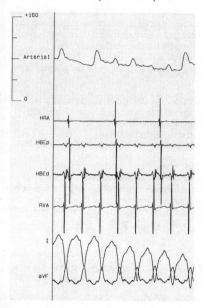

Fig. 10.10 An induced VT at a cycle length of 320 ms (187 min⁻¹). From top to bottom a tracing of arterial pressure, high right atrial ICegram, proximal then distal His bundle ICegram, RV ICegram, then 2 suface ECG leads. There is no V to A conduction at this rate and the atrium is dissociated form the ventricle. Despite the rapid rate the systolic BP is maintained at 100 mmHg, enabling the VT to be mapped if necessary.

Accessory pathways (Wolff–Parkinson–White syndrome)

Definitions and ECG

The atria and ventricles are separated by the fibrous annuli of the TV on the right and MV on the left. The AV node is the only electrical connection in normal hearts. Abnormal accessory pathways can occur at any position along these annuli and are named accordingly (see Fig. 10.11). They may conduct in one or both directions. They are the substrate for AVRT to occur.

If an AP conducts anterogradely (A to V) it will be manifest on the ECG as pre-excitation (short PR interval and delta wave). The morphology of the delta wave predicts the location of the accessory pathway. An AP that conducts only retrogradely is described as concealed.

Wolff–Parkinson–White syndrome strictly refers to APs which are both manifest as pre-excitation on the resting ECG and cause tachycardia.

Tachycardias

An AP can be associated with tachycardia by several mechanisms:
• Orthodromic AVRT (commonest, accounts for 95% of AP mediated tachycardias)—narrow complex tachycardia.
• Antidromic AVRT—broad complex tachycardia.
• Bystander—SVT of another aetiology that conducts down the AP.

Prognosis

AF in the presence of an AP can be dangerous as the ventricle is not protected by the decremental behavior of the AV node. This can precipitate VF and sudden death. If patients are discovered incidentally, and are truly asymptomatic, then sudden death is extremely rare (2 deaths in 600 patients followed for 3–20 years). Invasive EP can be used to risk stratify patients.

A worse prognosis is predicted by:
• Invasive EP testing.
  • Anterograde ERP of the AP <250 ms (the longest interval that will not conduct down the AP during atrial extrastimulus pacing or AF).
  • Inducible AVRT.
  • Multiple APs.
• Symptomatic tachycardia.
• Ebstein's anomaly.

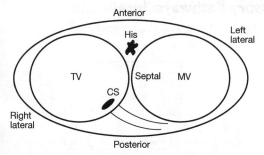

Fig. 10.11 Tricuspid (TV) and mitral valve (MV) annuli. Accessory pathways can be positioned anywhere on the annuli. They are named anatomically i.e. anterior, left antero-lateral, left lateral, left posterolateral etc. Anteroseptal pathways are close to the His bundle and AV node and are termed parahisian.

Accessory Pathways: localization

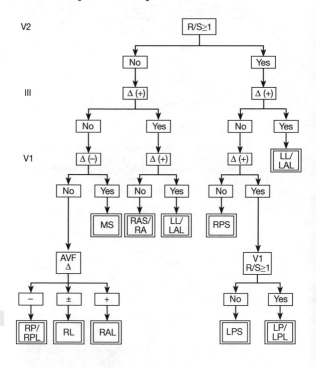

Algorithm to locate the accessory pathway from the ECG with prexcitation.
Δ = delta wave; Reprinted from Chiang et al (1995). *American Journal of Cardiology* **76**(1):40–46, with permission.

Accessory pathways: management

Ablation

APs can be cured by catheter ablation and this is first line treatment for symptomatic patients. A catheter is moved around the MV or TV annulus until the AP is located by finding the exact point of:

- Earliest ventricular activation during SR or atrial pacing.
- Earliest atrial activation during ventricular pacing.
- Earliest atrial activation during orthodromic AVRT.

Acute success is >90%. The complication rate is very low (death 0–0.2%, AV nodal block <1%). For paraHisian AP the risk of AV nodal block is higher and cryoablation used if available. Left sided pathways can be approached via the femoral artery, aorta, and left ventricle, or from the RA by a transeptal puncture.

All symptomatic patients (with tachycardias) should be offered ablation. Asymptomatic young patients (<35 yrs) or those in a high risk profession (pilots, divers etc) should be considered for invasive EP testing and ablation. However, risk of sudden death must be balanced against the 2% serious complication rate of ablating the pathway (particularly if left sided or paraHisian).

Pharmacological

Flecainide and propafenone slow conduction in the AP without affecting the AV node and are the preferred agents. Drugs that slow AV nodal conduction only (verapamil and digoxin) should not be used unless invasive EP has demonstrated that the AP does not conduct anterogradely (or conducts only very slowly).

Unusual pathways

Mahaim pathways: these are APs between the RA and RV (atrioventricular) or RA and right bundle branch (atriofasicular). Unlike ordinary APs they exhibit AV nodal properties of decremental conduction and sensitivity to adenosine. They only conduct anterogradely and mediate an AVRT with a broad complex LBBB appearance. They are successfully treated by catheter ablation.

Implantable cardioverter defibrillators

Mirowski implanted the first defibrillator in 1980 to manage sudden cardiac death. Since then there has been dramatic improvement in technology, and randomized control trial evidence to support their use. Initial implants used epicardial leads and required surgical implantation. The generators were large and placed in abdominal pockets. Nowadays the devices are implanted transvenously and the generators placed in the pectoral region. They employ a series of complex sensing algorithms for detection and use various tiered therapy to minimize myocardial injury.

Components

A pulse generator consists of a lithium silver vanadium oxide battery, an aluminum electrolytic capacitor and sensing circuitry which can sense local electrograms and filter out noise like skeletal myopotentials. Defibrillators have a least one lead in the RV for pacing/sensing and defibrillation. There may be a second lead in the SVC or a dual coil lead to lower defibrillation threshold. An atrial lead can be implanted for dual chamber pacemaker indications or to help with detection/discrimination of arrhythmias.

Detection

Most leads sense between the tip of the lead and an electrode anywhere along the length of the shocking coil (integrated bipolar sensing). Potential problems are with noise, far-field sensing, or post-shock undersensing. True bipolar sensing between a ring and tip electrode is more reliable but requires the lead to have three conductors.

Basic detection of VT involves heart rate, above which therapy will be delivered. Modern devices can be programmed to have multiple detection zones each with their own specific therapies. Rate detection is very reliable but susceptible to inappropriate therapies like sinus tachycardia or poorly-controlled atrial fibrillation. This is where medical therapy like β-blockers is very important to help prevent this.

To decrease inappropriate shocks various *detection enhancements* are included in modern devices. These include rate stability (looking at variations in R–R intervals to recognize AF), electrogram morphology (to distinguish a normal QRS, including BBB from the QRS when in VT) and sudden onset criteria (gradual onset of sinus tachycardia). The most useful algorithm however is to have an atrial lead so the device can analyse the timing of simultaneous atrial electrograms. The trade off of improved detection means that therapy for VT is inhibited. Most devices include 'sustained rate duration' as a back up which ensure delivery of therapy if the tachycardia is sustained. As a default these detection algorithms do not apply in the programmed VF zone.

Indications for ICD implantation

Definite indications

- Cardiac Arrest due to VF or VT with no reversible cause.
- Spontaneous sustained VT in a patient with structural heart disease.
- Syncope with haemodynamically significant sustained VT or VF induced at EP study.
- Nonsustained VT in patients with coronary artery disease, prior MI, LV dysfunction.
- Inducible VF or VT at EP study in a patient with coronary artery disease.
- Spontaneous sustained VT in patients without structural heart disease.
- Patients with LV ejection fraction ≤30%, at least one month post MI and three months post CABG

Relative indications

- Cardiac Arrest presumed to be due to VF when EP testing is precluded by other medical conditions.
- Symptoms attributable to sustained VT in patients awaiting cardiac transplantation.
- Familial or inherited conditions with a high risk of life-threatening VT i.e. long-QT syndrome or HCM.
- Nonsustained VT in patients with CAD, prior MI, LV dysfunction and inducible sustained VT or VF at EP study.
- Recurrent syncope in the presence of impaired LV function and inducible VT at EP study.
- Syncope of unexplained aetiology or FHx of unexplained sudden cardiac death in association with Brugada Syndrome.
- Syncope in patients with advanced structural heart disease in which thorough invasive and noninvasive investigation has failed to find a cause.
- Incessant VT or VF.
- NYHA Class IV drug-refractory CHF in patients not suitable for cardiac transplant.

Adapted from ACC/AHA/NASPE 2002 Guidelines (2002) *Circulation* **106**: 2145–2161.

ICD therapies

Antitachycardia pacing (ATP)

Two most common methods of ATP are rate adaptive burst pacing and autodecremental or ramp pacing. With rate adaptive burst pacing the device is programmed to deliver a set number of pulses (6–12) at a cycle length that is a programmed percentage of the tachycardia cycle length (i.e. 81% of the TCL). The sequences may be repeated with a decrementing cycle length. In ramp pacing the initial coupling interval is also a % of the TCL but each subsequent coupling interval decrements by a set amount (i.e. 10 ms). Again this sequence can be repeated. Generally modern devices can be programmed to have one to three VT zones with multiple tiers of therapy. One manufacturer allows for a fast VT zone in the VF zone which allows painless ATP to treat fast VT instead of cardioversion.

Defibrillation

Most ICDs deliver a maximum energy of 25–36 via their capacitors as a biphasic waveform from the tip of the RV lead to the pulse generator which is an 'active can'. The shocking vector travels superiorly from the RV including most of the IVS and LV. Sometimes a third electrode is needed as either a separate SVC coil or a dual coil RV lead to improve the defibrillation threshold (DFT) and the device can shock either between both coils or between the can and either coil. Very rarely now days, a subcutaneous patch is needed and is placed in the left axillary region.

Low energy defibrillation

Devices can also deliver low energy cardioversions when the tachycardia is generally <180 bpm which has some efficacy but patients feel shocks above 1 J and has not been shown to be better than ATP.

Defibrillation threshold (DFT) testing

Unless contraindicated should be tested at implant. Goal is for the DFT to be less than the maximum output of the device, ideally 10 J. VF is induced via rapid burst pacing, T-wave shock, or using AC current (unpleasant) whilst the patent is sedated. Appropriate VF detection and device charge time as well as the DFT can be evaluated.

ICD: trouble shooting and follow-up

Complications of ICD implantation

Early	Late
• Infection.	• Infection.
• Haemopneumothorax.	• Pain.
• Cardiac perforation.	• Erosion.
• Haemorrhage and pocket	• Lead/insulation break.
haematoma.	• Lead displacement.
• Vascular injury.	• Twiddler's syndrome.
• Venous thrombosis.	
• Lead displacement or damage.	
• VT.	
• Heart block.	

Follow-up

Oversensing leading to therapy (e.g. T wave sensing, electrical noise from lead fractures, atrial activity). Can programme sensitivity to prevent T wave sensing. Lead fractures require replacement and atrial leads help distinguish atrial activity.

Undersensing more serious but less common. May not detect VT or VF. More likely with Unipolar systems. May indicate lead displacement, inflammation or fibrosis at the lead tip.

Drug interactions

- Increased defibrillation threshold—Class I antiarrhythmics and amiodarone.
- Decreased defibrillation threshold—sotalol.
- Antiarrhythmics may slow VT below the detection threshold, affect the ability of ATP to terminate the tachycardia, or cause incessant VT. They may impair ventricular function and cause bradycardia requiring pacing. May also affect the pacing threshold for bradycardia.

Congenital heart disease

Introduction

Congenital heart disease (CHD) is one of the commonest congenital defects, occurring in approximately 0.6–0.8% of newborns i.e. there are about 5000 newborns with CHD each year in the UK. Advances in therapy have led to a dramatic improvement in outcome such that over 85% of infants, even with complex CHD, are expected to reach adolescence and early adulthood. As a result of the success of paediatric cardiology and surgery *there will soon be more adults than children with CHD*. In addition, there are patients with structural or valvular CHD who may present late during adulthood. It is estimated that there are approximately 1600 new patients per annum with moderate to complex CHD, of whom 800 might benefit from specialist follow-up in the UK. Most of these patients have had palliative or reparative rather than corrective surgery and further cardiac operations will be necessary for many.

Role of specialist CHD centres
- Initial assessment of adults with known or suspected CHD.
- Surgical and non-surgical interventions e.g. transcatheter closure ASD.
- Continuing care of patients with moderate and complex CHD.
- Advice and ongoing support for non-cardiac surgery and pregnancy.
- Training new specialists and evidence based clinical decision making.
- Provide feedback of late results to refine early treatment.

Paediatric to adult care transition
A smooth transition from the paediatric to the adult CHD specialist is essential. This should be tailored to the individual patient with in-built flexibility. Transfer to the adult unit should occur at around eighteen years of age. Patient education about the diagnosis and specific health behaviour, including contraception/pregnancy planning, should be included. Patient passports which include detailed diagrams of the individual cardiac defect and relevant information on topics such as exercise and need for antibiotic prophylaxis should be prepared for each patient.

No patient with CHD should reach adulthood without a clear management plan

Treat adult congenital heart disease with respect. Many problems or errors arise Percutaneous transcatheter interventions for CHD (2) from arrogance or ignorance. The patients may often know more about their condition and its management than the 'emergency' medical team he/she consult; therefore be patient and listen. Patients are often accompanied by a parent/s even well into late teens/second or third decade. They can prove a great source of information and help; keep them on your side. Increasingly in the UK adult congenital heart physicians are available for advice, either via e-mail or telephone. None will refuse a call for help. **Get to know your local specialist centre!**

Disease complexity and hierarchy of care for the adult with congenital heart disease

Level 1

Exclusive care by specialist unit e.g. Eisenmenger syndrome, Fontan repairs, transposition of the great arteries, any condition with atresia in the name, Marfan.

Level 2

Shared care with 'interested' adult cardiologist e.g. coarctation of the aorta, atrial septal defect, Tetralogy of Fallot.

Level 3

Ongoing management in general adult cardiology unit e.g. mild pulmonary valve stenosis, post-operative atrial/ventricular septal defect.

Information sources on adult congenital heart disease **1.** Management of grown up congenital heart disease. European society of cardiology task force report. *European Heart Journal* 2003:**24**;1035–1084. **2.** British cardiac society report **3.** Canadian taskforce report.

Congenital heart disease in adults

Acyanotic lesions

- Atrial septal defect p470.
- Ventricular septal defect p470.
- Complete atrioventricular septal defect p470.
- Pulmonary stenosis p470.
- Left ventricular outflow tract obstruction p472.
- Coarctation of the aorta p472.
- Anomalous pulmonary venous drainage p472.
- Ebstein's anomaly of the tricuspid valve p476.

Cyanotic lesions

- Transposition of the great arteries p474.
- Tetralogy of Fallot p474.
- Fontan patients p472.
- Congenitally corrected transposition of the great arteries p474.
- Severe Ebstein's anomaly of the tricuspid valve: p474.

Assessment of patients with CHD

History
- Family history of CHD.
- Exposure to teratogens/toxins during pregnancy.
- CHD suspected during pregnancy or at birth. (Ask the mother!!)
- History of prolonged childhood illnesses.
- Prior interventions.
  - Any previous hospitalizations for catheter or surgical-based interventions.
  - Names of previous paediatric cardiologists and surgeons as well as unit in which surgery, if any, was performed.
- Dental hygiene.

Current symptoms
- Shortness of breath on exertion?
- Ability to climb stairs, hills, walk on the flat, and distance covered?
- Breathless on lying down?
- Chest pain?
  - Precipitating/relieving factors?
  - Any associated symptoms?
- Syncopal episodes?
- Palpitations?
  - Onset, duration.
  - Associated pre-syncope/chest pain?
  - Ask patient to tap out rate and rhythm of palpitations.
- Assess ability index.

General inspection
- Chart the patient's height, weight, and blood pressure against standard reference charts.
- Does the patient have an obvious syndrome?
  - Down's syndrome (1/3 associated with CHD, especially atrioventricualr septal defect)?
  - William's syndrome (supravalvar aortic and pulmonary stenosis)?
  - Noonan's syndrome (dysplastic pulmonary valvular stenosis, hypertrophic cardiomyopathy)?
  - Turner's syndrome (coarctation of the aorta/aortic valve stenosis)?
- Is the patient anaemic or jaundiced?
- Are there any features to suggest infective endocarditis?
- Is there evidence of poor oral hygiene with dental caries or infected gums?
- Any tattoos or body piercing?

Systematic approach to auscultation of CHD patient

1. Listen to the heart sounds.

- *First heart sound*
  - The first heart sound is usually heard as a single sound but since mitral closure is loudest, it is best heard at the apex.
  - A loud first heart sound may be heard in mitral stenosis or sometimes with an atrial septal defect.
  - Soft first heart sounds are a feature of poor myocardial contractility or a long PR interval.

- *Second heart sound*
  - Fixed splitting in the presence of a significant atrial septal defect and is best appreciated in the high or mid left sternal border.
  - Accentuated in the presence of pulmonary hypertension.
  - Widely split following repair of tetralogy of Fallot, the second heart sound is reflecting the right bundle branch block, characteristic of the post-operative electrocardiogram.

2. Check for systolic/diastolic murmurs.

(Draw an imaginary line between the nipples).

- *Murmurs loudest above nipple line*
  - Ejection systolic in type.
  - Arise from the right or left ventricular outflow tract.
  - If associated with a carotid or suprasternal thrill, usually from the left ventricular outflow tract.
  - If an ejection click is heard, the murmur is valvar in origin.
  - Ejection click of aortic valve stenosis is best heard at the apex.
  - Ejection systolic murmur best heard in the interscapular region and associated with a left thoracotomy may indicate turbulence across a prior coarctation repair.

- *Murmurs loudest below nipple line*
  - Pan-systolic and arise from mitral/tricuspid regurgitation or from a ventricular septal defect.
  - A 'to and fro' murmur best heard at the upper left sternal edge following cardiac surgery usually results from combined right ventricular outflow tract obstruction and pulmonary regurgitation.
  - The mid-systolic click and systolic murmur of mitral valve prolapse is best heard with the patient standing up.
  - A continuous murmur arises from an arterial duct, systemic to pulmonary shunt or arterio-venous fistulas.

Measure height, weight, blood pressure, and oxygen saturation in all patients. 12 lead ECG is essential at every visit.

Electrocardiogram

- Rate and rhythm: consider atrial flutter with variable block if constant rate of 120 or 150/minute—easily confused with 'sinus rhythm'. Atrial tachycardias are especially common after all forms of atrial surgery e.g. intra-atrial repair for transposition of the great arteries.
- Look for signs of chamber enlargement—atrial or ventricular hypertrophy.
- Assess presence/absence of bundle branch block.
- Measure duration of QRS in all post-operative tetralogy of Fallot patients: QRS duration >180 ms associated with higher risk of arrhythmias, right heart dilatation and late sudden death.
- If tachycardia suspected, record 12 lead ECG during administration of intravenous adenosine.

Role of exercise testing

- Assess heart rate and blood pressure response to exercise (blunted response in important aortic valve stenosis).
- Compare upper and lower limb BP following coarctation repair.
- Monitor oxygen saturation by pulse oximetry to improve risk stratification in cyanosed patients.
- Also, improves counselling and planning for pregnancy.
- Formal cardiopulmonary exercise testing reserved for decision making retiming of surgical or catheter-based intervention.
- Can help distinguish limitation due to lack of aerobic fitness and assess maximal effort.

Chest X-ray

- Cheap and invaluable investigation in CHD.
- Identify right–left orientation to assess cardiac and visceral positions.
- Assessment of the bronchial branching permits diagnosis of isomeric cardiac defects e.g. symmetric morphologic right bronchi characteristic of right atrial isomerism (usually associated with complex CHD—common right atria, a common atrio-ventricular orifice, a great artery arising form one ventricular chamber and total anomalous pulmonary venous connection).
- Identify situs inversus (mirror image anatomy with liver on the left and stomach bubble on the right with cardiac apex in right chest). Consider Kartagener syndrome. Discordance between position of the apex and visceral situs usually associated with CHD.
- Record cardiothoracic ratio in the notes. Look for rib notching related to collateral blood supply in severe coarctation of the aorta. Assess pulmonary vasculature (see p459).

CXR assessment of pulmonary vasculature in CHD patients

Increased vascularity
- Left to right shunt (ASD, VSD).
- Pulmonary oedema.
- Obstructed pulmonary venous drainage.

Decreased vascularity
- Right ventricular outflow obstruction e.g. Isolated severe pulmonary stenosis, following tetralogy repair.
- Pulmonary hypertension.

Unilateral increased pulmonary vascular markings
- Consider ipsilateral systemic to pulmonary arterial shunt.
- Over-perfused major arterial pulmonary collateral artery.
- Obstructed pulmonary venous drainage e.g. following Mustard/ Senning intra-atrial repair for transposition of the great arteries.

Imaging modalities in CHD

Echocardiography
- Most useful investigation in CHD but only when directed by detailed history taking and clinical examination.
- This should be performed by an experienced examiner with detailed knowledge of all aspects of congenital heart disease.
- There is no substitute for sequential data and a protocol for regular, standardized analysis is required.
- Imaging in adults may be limited by poor echogenic windows.

Magnetic resonance imaging
- Ideal for the assessment of extra-cardiac pulmonary arterial and venous trees.
- Accurate quantification of valvar regurgitation e.g. assessment of pulmonary regurgitation and right ventricular function following repair of tetralogy of Fallot.
- Its utility is limited by scarcity of expert radiologists in the field of congenital heart disease.

Cardiac catheterization
- This still has its place in quantifying shunts and obtaining accurate haemodynamic data.
- Increasingly this is carried out to facilitate percutaneous transcatheter procedures such as occlusion of atrial septal defects.
- With an ageing population, many patients with CHD need to undergo coronary angiography as combined surgical procedures may be required.

Specific signs in patients with CHD

Inspection

Cyanosis or clubbing?

Oxygen saturation should always be measured by pulse oximetry. Central cyanosis is an indication of arterial desaturation and is noted when more than 5 g/dl of reduced haemoglobin is circulating. Thus it is dependent in part on the total haemoglobin concentration and may be missing in a patient with significant desaturation but who is anaemic. Differential cyanosis implies flow of deoxygenated blood from the pulmonary trunk into the aorta distal to the left subclavian artery e.g. non-restrictive patent arterial duct with pulmonary vascular disease and right to left shunt.

Previous operation scars?

Lift patient's arms and look for evidence of thoracotomy scars. Is the apex beat displaced or even in the right chest? Assess co-morbidity e.g. scoliosis and respiratory dysfunction related to prior lateral thoracotomy.

Jugular venous pulse

This can give information about conduction effects and arrhythmias, waveform and pressure. Increased resistance to atrial filling results in an exaggerated 'a' wave which may occur in isolated severe pulmonary stenosis or in tricuspid atresia. Episodic 'cannon' waves occur in cases of heart block when the atrium contracts against a closed tricuspid valve. A prominent 'v' wave is characteristic of tricuspid regurgitation.

Palpation

- Feel all the pulses including the femorals. Coarctation of the aorta is a clinical diagnosis.
- Check the blood pressure in upper and lower limbs, palpating the posterior tibial artery with cuff inflated around the calf.
- Bounding pulses are characteristic of severe aortic regurgitation, patent arterial duct or presence of a surgical systemic to pulmonary arterial shunt (Blalock–Taussig).
- An increase in the right brachial pulse may reflect the Coanda effect of supravalvar stenosis in patients with William's syndrome. Thrills may be felt in the femoral vessels reflecting arteriovenous malformation following prior cardiac catheterization.
- Check the position of the apex beat. Also, check that the liver and stomach are in the correct position. Situs inversus with the apex in the right chest is the mirror image of normal. 95% of patients with mirror image dextrocardia have no coexisting congenital cardiac disease. Situs solitus with apex in the right chest is invariably associated with CHD, often complex and unpredictable.
- A parasternal heave represents right ventricular overactivity, most marked when there is both pressure and volume overload of the chamber, such as following repair of tetralogy of Fallot.
- A palpable second sound in the upper left intercostals space is detected when pulmonary hypertension is present.

Surgical operations for CHD

Congenital heart surgery in adolescents and adults should only be undertaken in specialist centres. There are three categories:

- Patients who have not undergone prior operations.
- Patients who have undergone previous palliative operations.
- Patients who have undergone previous reparative procedures.

Re-do sternotomy, preservation of myocardial performance, attention to pulmonary bed vascular abnormalities and aorto-pulmonary collaterals require careful prior planning and close cooperation between surgeon, cardiac anaesthetist, cardiologist, and intensive care team

Blalock–Taussig shunt

Systemic to pulmonary arterial shunt using a subclavian arterial flap (Classical) or Gore-Tex® tube (Modified) to increase pulmonary blood flow and improve oxygenation in cyanotic congenital heart disease. This is a palliative procedure which has superseded earlier operations such as Waterston shunt (ascending aorta to right pulmonary artery) or Pott's shunt (descending aorta to left pulmonary artery).

Coarctation of the aorta

Relieved by either a subclavian flap approach or direct end-to-end anastomosis. Occasionally, a bypass graft is required in adult patients from ascending to descending aorta.

Glenn shunt

The superior vena cava is anastomosed to the ipsilateral pulmonary artery as a means of improving oxygenation in infants or young children. This is usually confined to patients with 'single' ventricles and univentricular circulations. In its classical from the right pulmonary artery was detached from the main pulmonary artery. The bi-directional Glenn shunt was fashioned such that blood from the superior vena cava entered both pulmonary arteries.

Tetralogy of Fallot

Closure of the ventricular septal defect with a patch of pericardium or Goretex® and relief of the right ventricular outflow tract obstruction by trans-annular patching, valvectomy or placing a homograft/conduit between right ventricle and pulmonary artery.

Rastelli operation

Usually undertaken in patients with complex CHD, for example transposition of the great arteries with large ventricular septal defect. The VSD is closed by a large patch in such a way as to connect the left ventricle to the aorta and a conduit or homograft connects the right ventricle to the pulmonary artery.

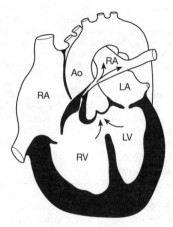

Fig. 11.1 Picture of Tetralogy of Fallot.

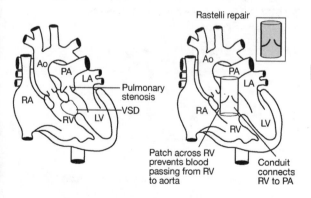

Fig. 11.2 Picture of Rastelli operation.

Ross operation

An alternative to aortic valve replacement which may be attractive to younger patients, especially females. The diseased aortic valve is removed with the coronary arteries detached. The patient's own pulmonary valve is resected and placed in the aortic position with the coronaries reattached. A homograft is placed between the right ventricle and the pulmonary artery.

Fontan operation

This represents the definitive palliation for patients with effectively univentricular circulations such as mitral or tricuspid atresia. Blood from the superior and inferior vena cava is directed to the pulmonary arteries without the benefit of a sub-pulmonary ventricle. Oxygenated blood returns to the systemic ventricle and is then pumped to the aorta.

Mustard/Senning operations

Life-saving innovations for treatment of patients with transposition of the great arteries which involved intra-atrial redirection of oxygenated and de-oxygenated blood to the systemic and pulmonary systems respectively. The right ventricle served as the systemic sub-aortic ventricle. Largely abandoned because of late problems with arrhythmias, pathway obstruction, and ventricular failure.

Arterial switch

This has largely superseded the Mustard/Senning procedure. The aorta and pulmonary artery are relocated to their original positions with re-anastomosis of the coronary arteries to the neo-aorta.

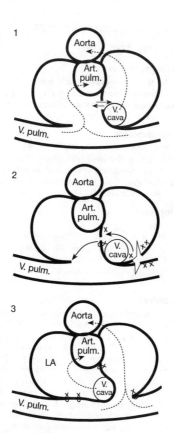

Fig. 11.3 Picture of Senning operation.

Redrawn from Koustantinov, IE et al. (2004). Atrial Switch operation: past, present, and future. *Annals of Thoracic Surgery*, **77**: 2250–8, with permission.

Percutaneous transcatheter interventions for CHD

Balloon atrial septostomy

Life-saving intervention in neonates with transposition of the great arteries in which an atrial communication is created by tearing a hole in the atrial septum using a balloon catheter. This can be performed at the bedside under echocardiographic control.

Pulmonary valvuloplasty

The procedure of choice for patients with pulmonary valvar stenosis of all ages. Less successful if the valve is dysplastic (Noonan's syndrome). The pulmonary valve annulus is measured by echocardiography or angiography and a balloon (100–120%) diameter is used. One of the most effective transcatheter interventions.

Aortic valvuloplasty

Limited use in adults. If the aortic valve is pliable but not calcified, balloon dilatation may defer the need for definitive surgery but usually at the expense of aortic regurgitation. The balloon size should not exceed the size of the aorta at the site of the valve attachment. An antegrade approach via a trans-septal puncture is advised to reduce the incidence of valve damage.

Atrial septal defect

Most secundum atrial septal defects are amenable to percutaneous closure. The Amplatzer® septal occluding device is made of Nitinol (a nickel titanium alloy with inherent shape memory) and comprises two discs with a self centering waist. The defect is balloon sized under transoesophageal echocardiographic guidance. Defects up to 40 mm in size can be closed providing there are sufficient rims (>5 mm) to the pulmonary veins and the attachment of the mitral valve. This is not suitable for any atrial defects other than those of the secundum variety i.e. sinus venosus defects or partial atrioventricular septal defects. Procedural complications are rare in expert hands. Anti-platelet agents are administered for three to six months until the device has completely endothelialised. Transient headaches are common in the weeks following closure but serious complications are rare. These include transient ischaemic episodes/stroke, atrial arrhythmias and embolization of the device. Remember that concomitant electrophysiological procedures may need to be undertaken in patients with significant atrial arrhythmias.

Ventricular septal defects

Indications for closing defects in adults are limited. Occasionally, 'small' defects can produce volume overload of the left ventricle over time and require closure. Such defects may be amenable to transcatheter occlusion using the Amplatzer® peri-membranous or muscular occluding devices. This should only be undertaken in specialist centres. Complete heart block and device embolization have been described.

Coarctation of the aorta

Surgical correction in the adult is a major challenge with its associated risk of paraplegia. Both native and re-coarctation of the aorta can now be successfully treated by transcatheter balloon dilatation and stenting. Covered stents may be required for native coarctation to reduce incidence of dissection and rupture. Remember that the aorta in these patients is especially friable and that an aortopathy commonly coexists. Magnetic resonance imaging is invaluable in patient selection and for selecting stent size. This intervention should only be undertaken in specialist centres where expert surgical help is readily available. Remember that balloon dilatation of previous patch aortoplasty carries the highest risk of aortic rupture. Lifelong surveillance is necessary to detect aneurysm formation.

Patent arterial duct

May occasionally present in later life. If small or medium-sized with no pulmonary hypertension, most can be successfully occluded with a variety of transcatheter occluding devices or coils.

Pulmonary valve implantation

Percutaneous transcatheter implantation of a bovine jugular venous valve mounted within a platinum-iridium stent into the right ventricular outflow tract is now possible. This procedure, if it stands the test of time, will revolutionise our approach to management of patients with pulmonary regurgitation following right heart congenital surgery offering as it does a non-surgical approach. It may not be long before an implantable valve which can be used in the systemic circulation becomes available.

Specific management issues

Complications of cyanotic CHD

Chronic hypoxaemia results in an increased red cell mass and total blood volume. This compensatory mechanism may initially enhance oxygen delivery; however, symptoms of hyperviscosity may develop.

- Symptoms of hyper-viscosity: headaches, visual disturbances (blurred or double vision), impaired alertness, fatigue, paraesthesia, tinnitus, myalgia, muscle weakness, restless legs. Transient ischaemic events or stroke.
- Measure haemoglobin and red cell indices; most patients have a compensated erythropoesis with a stable haemoglobin.
- Therapeutic phlebotomy should be reserved for symptomatic patients e.g. haemoglobin >20 g/dl or haematocrit >65%. Symptoms may be relieved by removal of 500 ml (maximum) of blood with concomitant fluid replacement of dextrose or saline. Phlebotomy should be performed no more than 2 times per annum as it increases the risk of stroke by causing iron deficiency. Intravenous line filters should always be used.

Iron deficiency in a polycythaemic patient should be aggressively treated with oral iron supplementation (ferrous sulphate 600 mg/day), recheck haemoglobin 8–10 days later.

Skin

- Severe acne is common in cyanotic congenital heart disease.
- It can act as a source of infection and endocarditis.
- Treat aggressively.

Gallstones

- Common in cyanosed patients.
- Bilirubin is a product of haemoglobin breakdown.
- Suspect if patient presents with severe abdominal pain/discomfort.

Renal function

- Reduced glomerular filtration rate.
- Increased levels of creatinine.
- Abnormalities in clearance of uric acid frequently accompanies chronic cyanosis and gout, sometimes frank, may result.
- Cautious use of contrast in angiography and always pre-hydrate.

Non-cardiac surgery

- Should be undertaken in specialist centres and care delivered by multi-disciplinary team.
- Local anaesthesia if possible; otherwise cardiac anaesthetist with experience in congenital heart disease.
- Consider preoperative phlebotomy if haemoglobin >20 g/dl or haematocrit >65%.
- Endocarditis prophylaxis and air line filters should be employed.

Pregnancy

The majority of women with CHD can tolerate pregnancy

But

- Congenital heart disease is now the major cause of maternal cardiac death in developed countries All need specialist counselling **before** embarking on pregnancy.
- Cardiologists are woefully ill-prepared to give such advice; paediatric cardiologists less so!
- All young women of child-bearing age should undergo a detailed clinical and haemodynamic assessment which should include a formal exercise test and detailed cross-sectional echocardiography with emphasis on systemic ventricular function.
- All women with complex CHD should be closely monitored in specialist centres where delivery should take place. Multidisciplinary input is essential.
- Pregnancy is contraindicated in some CHD patients.

Arrhythmia

- An important cause of morbidity and mortality and major cause for hospitalization of CHD patients. It may lead to significant haemodynamic deterioration and is poorly tolerated.
- May be due to:
  - Underlying cardiac defect e.g. atrial isomerism.
  - Part of natural history e.g. haemodynamic changes such as chamber enlargement or scarring.
  - Residual postoperative abnormalities.

Management

Specialist advice is essential New presentation demands a complete haemodynamic assessment including electrophysiological investigation. Correction of any underlying postoperative haemodynamic abnormality may be one of the most important therapeutic interventions.

- Record a 12 lead electrocardiogram.
- Administer intravenous adenosine whilst recording the ECG. The mode of termination of the tachyarrhythmia may give very useful information on its aetiology e.g. pre-excitation.
- Urgent direct current cardioversion may be required if haemodynamic compromise present. Ideally, transoesophageal echocardiography should rule out intracardiac thrombus. If the patient is on warfarin, always check the INR as well as the serum electrolytes prior to cardioversion.

Women with CHD in whom pregnancy is contraindicated

- Pulmonary hypertension
  - e.g. Eisenmenger syndrome (50% maternal and fetal mortality; maternal death may occur up to two weeks post-partum).
- Heart failure secondary to failing fontan circulation.
- Women with severe cyanosis and polycythaemia.
  - If saturation is less than 80% at rest and haemoglobin is greater than 18 g/dl, there is a greater incidence of miscarriage and intrauterine growth retardation.

Atrial septal defect

One of the commonest lesions presenting for the first time in adult life. Often missed as clinical signs of fixed splitting of the second heart sound can be difficult to appreciate. May present for the first time with new onset atrial flutter or fibrillation. Consider the need for electrophysiological interventions e.g. Maze procedure for atrial fibrillation. Shunting trends to increase with ageing as the left ventricle stiffens. Closure is indicated in all symptomatic patients…few are truly asymptomatic when assessed by cardiopulmonary testing! There is no upper age limit. The vast majority of secundum defects are amenable to transcatheter closure. Pulmonary hypertension needs to be excluded. Atrial arrhythmias are one of the common late medical problems. All other types such as sinus venosus defect (defect in upper atrial septum associated with overriding of the superior vena cava and anomalous right pulmonary venous drainage) and partial atrio-ventricular septal defect require surgical closure. A sinus venosus defect represents a major surgical challenge involving redirection of the anomalous pulmonary vein(s). Risk of endocarditis is very low. Antibiotic prophylaxis is not indicated.

Ventricular septal defect

Majority are small as usually repaired in childhood. Eisenmenger syndrome (pulmonary vascular disease associated with reverse, right-to-left shunting via intracardiac communication—VSD, ASD, PDA) is becoming increasingly rare. Should be closed if significant shunt, previous endocarditis, development of aortic regurgitation, or right ventricular outflow tract obstruction. It is always important to demonstrate reversibility of pulmonary hypertension prior to intervention. May be amenable to surgical or transcatheter closure. Ventricular arrhythmias may occur late during follow up. Antibiotic prophylaxis is indicated in all patients.

Atrioventricular septal defect

Common defect in patients with Down syndrome. If unoperated, pulmonary vascular disease (Eisenmenger syndrome) develops. Left atrioventricular valve regurgitation/stenosis are the major determinants of need for further interventions. Valve replacement may be necessary. Endocarditis prophylaxis is indicated in all.

Pulmonary stenosis

May present for first time in adult life. This can be successfully treated by balloon valvuloplasty, which should be undertaken if the valve gradient exceeds 30 mmHg on Doppler echocardiography. Surgery is reserved for calcified and dysplastic valves. The outlook is excellent. The risk of endocarditis is low.

Left ventricular outflow tract (LVOT) obstruction

Aortic valve stenosis is especially common in association with a bicuspid valve. This is a complex lesion and an aortopathy is commonly present. There is a risk of aortic dilation and dissection. The degree of stenosis or regurgitation may increase over time. Effort intolerance, chest pain, or syncope especially with exertion need to be taken seriously and intervention considered. It may occasionally be amenable to balloon valvuloplasty but more commonly requires surgical intervention. Aortic valve replacement (lifelong anticoagulation) or homograft insertion/Ross operation (no anticoagulation but potential need for further interventions, critically operator-dependent) can be offered. Sub-aortic stenosis is uncommon (no ejection click) and requires surgical resection if severe or patient symptomatic. Recurrence is possible. Supravalvar stenosis is commonly seen in patients with William's syndrome. It may be associated with multiple stenoses in the origins of the coronary arteries and the aortic arch arterial branches. Reconstructive surgery is complex.

Coarctation of the aorta

Most patients seen in adult clinics will have already undergone surgery. Some may present for the first time with hypertension. Always feel the femoral pulses! Consider Turner's syndrome in female patients. Coarctation of the aorta is a complex lesion usually associated with a bicuspid aortic valve (ejection click at the apex) and aortopathy. During follow up, upper (right arm) and lower limb blood pressure should be recorded and evidence of left ventricular hypertrophy on electrocardiogram and cross-sectional echocardiography should be noted. Re-coarctation may occur over time and should be suspected if there are reduced femoral pulses or radio-femoral delay on examination. Doppler echocardiography can help by revealing an increased systolic velocity signal with forward flow through the site of re-coarctation during diastole. Magnetic resonance imaging with three dimensional reconstruction is the imaging modality of choice. Transcatheter balloon dilatation and stenting is feasible in many patients thus avoiding the risks of thoracic aortic surgery. Lifelong surveillance is necessary to rule out aneurysm formation or recurrence. Antibiotic prophylaxis is indicated.

Anomalous pulmonary venous drainage

Many patients will undergo surgery in early childhood. This may occur in association with Scimitar syndrome. If the patient is symptomatic (shortness of breath, arrhythmia) and there is evidence of right heart volume overload, for example on the cross sectional echocardiogram, consider surgery. There is a low risk of endocarditis.

Transposition of the great arteries

The aorta arises from the right ventricle and the pulmonary artery from the left ventricle. It is the commonest cyanotic cardiac lesion presenting in the first few days of life. In the absence of mixing at cardiac or great arterial level, this condition is uniformly lethal. The majority of adult survivors have undergone intra-atrial repair by Mustard or Senning procedure. These produced excellent early survival but significant late morbidity and mortality. Common late problems are atrial arrhythmias (flutter/fibrillation), venous baffle narrowing, and right ventricular failure with tricuspid regurgitation. Arrhythmias are poorly tolerated and prompt restoration to sinus rhythm is essential. Baffle stenosis can be relieved by transcatheter balloon dilatation/stenting. Ventricular failure requires intensive medical therapy but ultimately may necessitate cardiac transplantation. Patients who have undergone the arterial switch procedure are now reaching early adulthood. Problems with coronary arterial stenoses at the site of re-anastomosis to the neo-aorta have been identified in some. Antibiotic prophylaxis is required.

Tetralogy of Fallot

This comprises a large non-restrictive VSD, over-riding aorta, right ventricular outflow tract (RVOT) obstruction, and right ventricular hypertrophy. This is the commonest cyanotic cardiac lesion presenting outside the neonatal period. If it presents with critical cyanosis in the neonatal period, the patient may undergo a palliative Blalock–Taussig shunt prior to complete repair in early childhood. Many centres now opt for definitive repair even in the first few months of life. The vast majority of adults will have undergone some form of repair with surgical closure of the septal defect and relief of the RVOT obstruction. Arrhythmias are an inevitable consequence of surgery (scarring, ventriculotomy, and pulmonary regurgitation). Late arrhythmias (both atrial and ventricular) and sudden death occur. Pulmonary regurgitation, ignored for many years as a benign condition, is now known to be one of the most important causes of morbidity and mortality in patients following RVOT surgery. The QRS duration >180 ms on the ECG has been used as a marker for patients at risk of arrhythmia and late sudden death. Patients should be assessed by exercise testing and MRI. A percutaneous approach to pulmonary valve implantation is now available using a bovine jugular venous valve mounted within a platinum-iridium stent and is suitable for patients with severe pulmonary regurgitation and outflow tracts <20 mm in size. Branch pulmonary arterial stenoses should be treated aggressively by catheter intervention. Surgical insertion of a homograft valve is currently performed with peri-operative mortality less than 1% in specialist centres. The majority of such conduits need replacing within a 10 year period i.e. need for multiple re-operations. Aortic regurgitation may also occur. Endocarditis prophylaxis is indicated in all patients.

Fontan patients

This is the definitive palliation for patients born with 'single ventricle' physiology in which all the systemic venous return is directed back to the lungs without the benefit of a sub-pulmonary ventricle e.g. mitral/ tricuspid/pulmonary/aortic atresia. It produces excellent early and mid-term survival but late failure occurs even in the most carefully selected candidates. The late problems comprise atrial arrhythmias including sinus node dysfunction and heart block, atrio-ventricular valve regurgitation, ventricular failure, venous obstruction, and protein-losing enteropathy (<50% 5 year survival). The failing Fontan is a major challenge and transplantation or conversion to a more streamlined modification with concomitant arrhythmia surgery should be considered. All patients require endocarditis prophylaxis.

Congenitally corrected transposition of the great arteries

Cyanosis present if associated ventricular septal defect and pulmonary stenosis or if pulmonary vascular disease if VSD and no PS. Rare lesion with normal survival in some if isolated lesion. Ongoing risk of complete heart block (2% per annum). Atrio-ventricular valve regurgitation in association with systemic right ventricular failure is a major long term problem.

Ebstein's anomaly of the tricuspid valve

This condition is associated with apical displacement of the tricuspid valve and is associated with atrial communication. Cyanosis occurs via right-to-left shunt at atrial level. A wide spectrum of presentation depending on severity of tricuspid valve regurgitation and associated anomalies. In infancy this presents with heart failure and cyanosis, and prognosis is poor. In the older child or young adult the murmur may be an incidental finding, and mild forms can be asymptomatic. Atrial arrhythmias are common and associated with pre-excitation (accessory pathways). Intervention is warranted if symptomatic with heart failure, severe tricuspid regurgitation arrhythmias. Tricuspid valve replacement/repair can be offered. Inter-atrial communications causing cyanosis/paradoxical emboli can be closed percutaneously if haemodynamic assessment permits.

Extra-cardiac complications

- **Polycythaemia:** chronic hypoxia stimulates erythropoietin production and erythrocytosis. The 'ideal' Hb level is ~17–18 g/dl; some centres advocate venesection to control the haematocrit and prevent hyperviscosity syndrome. Follow local guidelines. Generally consider phlebotomy only if moderate or severe symptoms of hyperviscosity are present and haematocrit >65%. Remove 500 ml of blood over 30–45 minutes and replace volume simultaneously with 500–1000 ml saline, or salt-free dextran (if heart failure). Avoid abrupt changes in circulating volume. If hyperviscosity symptoms are the result of acute dehydration or iron deficiency venesection is not required and patient must be rehydrated and/or treated with iron.
- **Renal disease and gout:** hypoxia affects glomerular and tubular function resulting in proteinuria, reduced urate excretion, increased urate reabsorption, and reduced creatinine clearance. Overt renal failure is uncommon. Try to avoid dehydration, diuretics, radiographic contrast. Asymptomatic hyperuricaemia does not need treatment. Colchicine and steroids are first line agents for treatment of acute gout. NSAIDs should be avoided.
- **Sepsis:** patients are more prone to infection. Skin acne is common with poor healing of scars. Skin stitches for operative procedures should be left in for 7–10 days longer than normal. Dental hygiene is very important due to the risk of endocarditis. Any site of sepsis may result in cerebral abscesses from metastatic infection or septic emboli.
- **Thrombosis and bleeding:** are multifactorial and are caused by a combination of abnormal platelet function, coagulation abnormalities and polycythaemia. PT and aPTT values may be elevated and secondary to a fall in factor V, VII, VIII and X. Both, arterial ± venous thromboses and haemorrhagic complications (e.g. petechiae, epistaxes, haemoptyses) can occur. Dehydration or oral contraceptives are risk factors for thrombotic events. Spontaneous bleeding is generally self-limiting. In the context of severe bleeding general measures are effective including platalet transfusion, FFP, cryoprecipitate and Vitamin K. Aspirin and other NSAIDs should generally be avoided to decrease chances of spontaneous bruising/bleeding.
- **Primary pulmonary problems** include infection, infarction, and haemorrhage from ruptured arterioles or capillaries.
- **Stroke:** can be both thrombotic as well as haemorrhagic. Arterial thrombosis, embolic events (paradoxical emboli in R→L shunt) and injudicious phlebotomy lead to spontaneous thrombosis. Haemostasis problems especially when combined with NSAIDs or formal anticoagulation can lead to haemorrhagic stroke. Any injured brain tissue is also a nidus for intracranial infection/abscess formation.
- **Complications secondary to drugs, investigations, surgery:** avoid abrupt changes in blood pressure or systemic resistance. Contrast agents may provoke systemic vasodilatation and cause acute decompensation. They may also precipitate renal failure. Before cardiac surgery, try to optimize haematocrit and haemostasis controlled phlebotomy and replacement with dextran. High-flow

oxygen is important before and after surgery. Extreme precaution with IV lines.

- **Arthralgia:** is mainly due to hypertrophic osteoarthropathy. In patients with R→L shunt megakaryocytes bypass the pulmonary circulation and become trapped in systemic vascular beds, promoting new bone formation.
- **Haemoptysis** is common. Most episodes are self-limiting and precipitated by infection. Differentiation from pulmonary embolism may be difficult. Try to keep the patient calm and ensure adequate BP control. Give high flow oxygen by mask. If there is clinical suspicion of infection (fever, sputum production, leukocytosis, raised CRP, etc.) start broad-spectrum antibiotics. VQ scan may help in the diagnosis of pulmonary embolism but is often equivocal. Avoid aspirin and NSAIDs as these exacerbate the intrinsic platelet abnormalities. There is anecdotal evidence for the use of low dose IV heparin, Dextran 40 (500 ml iv infusion q4-6h), acrid (Arvin® — reduces plasma fibrinogen by cleaving fibrin), or low dose warfarin therapy for reducing thrombotic tendency in these patients. Severe pulmonary haemorrhage may respond to aprotinin or tranexamic acid.
- **Breathlessness** may be due to pulmonary oedema or hypoxia (increased shunt) secondary to chest infection or pulmonary infarction. Do not give large doses of diuretics or nitrates as this will drop systemic pressures and may precipitate acute collapse. Compare chest X-ray to previous films to try to assess if there is radiological evidence of pulmonary oedema. The JVP in patients with cyanotic CHD is typically high and should not be used as a sole marker of heart failure. Overall patients need a higher filling pressure to maintain pulmonary blood flow. Give high flow oxygen by mask. Start antibiotics if there is a clinical suspicion of infection. Give oral diuretics if there is evidence of pulmonary oedema or severe right heart failure. Monitor haematocrit and renal function closely for signs of over-diuresis.
- **Effort syncope** should prompt a search for arrhythmias in particular VT (Holter monitor), severe valve disease, or signs of overt heart failure. Treat as appropriate.
- **Chest pain** may be secondary to pulmonary embolism or infarction (spontaneous thrombosis), pneumonia, ischaemic heart disease, or musculoskeletal causes. It requires careful evaluation with conventional diagnostic modalities already described.

Multisystem disorders

Libman–Sacks endocarditis

Associations

- Systemic lupus erythematosus.
- Primary and secondary anti-phospholipid antibody syndrome.

Epidemiology

- 50% of fatal systemic lupus erythematosus cases post-mortem. Up to 43% of cases with echocardiography.
- 6–10% of primary anti-phospholipid antibody syndrome cases with echocardiography.
- Young, African/Caribbean women typically.

Pathology

- Classically sterile, verrucous vegetations on the ventricular aspect. Diffuse leaflet thickening is thought to be the chronic, healed stage.
- Commonly mitral and aortic valves. Other valves and endocardial surfaces also affected.
- Usually valve regurgitation; stenosis rare.
- Uncertain whether association with antiphospholipid antibodies is causal. Antigens are negatively-charged phospholipids in endothelial cell membranes. Prevalence and severity of valve disease similar whether antibodies are present or not.
- Sites of endothelial damage due to turbulence and jet impaction may act as foci for thromboses and further damage.
- Valve thickening and regurgitation more common after chronic steroid therapy and in older patients.

Clinical features

- Usually asymptomatic with a normal cardiovascular examination.
- General lupus features like a malar rash, arthritis, sweats, and alopecia.
- Recurrent miscarriage, arterial and venous thromboses and thrombo-cytopaenia suggest anti-phospholipid antibody syndrome.
- Symptoms and signs due to heart failure and valve disease.

Imaging findings in lupus

- Valve abnormalities in 28–74% of cases. Vegetations in 4–43% of cases particularly those with anti-phospholipid antibodies. Thickening in 19–52% of cases with associated regurgitation in 73%.
- Pericardial effusion or thickening, left ventricular hypertrophy (due to hypertension), left ventricular dilatation, left ventricular segmental dysfunction, left ventricular global dysfunction, and pulmonary hypertension.

Imaging findings in primary anti-phospholipid antibody syndrome

- Valve abnormalities in 30–32% of cases particularly those with peripheral arterial thromboses. Vegetations in 6–10% and thickening in 10–24%.
- Regurgitation in 10–24% of cases.

Blood tests
- Blood cultures to exclude infective endocarditis.
- Full blood count, clotting profile, autoantibody screen.

Treatment
- No specific therapy.
- Treat underlying conditions and complications.
- Antibiotic chemoprophylaxis for bacteraemia-prone procedures e.g. dental work.

Prognosis in lupus
- Cardiovascular death ranked third in lupus patients.
- Combined incidence of heart failure, valve replacement, thromboembolism, and infective endocarditis is 22%.

Marfan syndrome

Epidemiology
- One of the commonest single gene mutation diseases. Incidence 1 in 5,000 to 1 in 10,000 persons.
- No known geographical, racial, or gender predilections.
- Diagnosed prenatally through to adulthood.

Pathology
- Autosomal dominant point mutations in fibrillin-1 gene on chromosome 15. Over 200 described.
- Fibrillin-1 glycoprotein is an integral component of microfibrils in connective tissues.
- Structural integrity of ocular, skeletal, cardiovascular, and other tissues compromised.
- Phenotype is highly variable due to varying genotype expression.

Ghent criteria for diagnosis
- Index case—no contributory family or genetic history, major criteria in at least two different organ systems plus involvement of a third organ system. Alternatively, contributory family or genetic history, one major organ system criterion plus involvement of second organ system.
- Relative of index case—major criterion in family history, major criterion in organ system plus involvement of a second organ system.

Imaging
- Radiographs, CT, and MRI scans to assess axial skeleton, hip joints, hands, and feet.
- Echocardiography and MRI scan to assess the mitral and aortic valves, aortic root, and ascending aorta. If measured aortic root dimension is greater than that expected from a nomogram by 1.18 times, there is root dilation.
- Slit-lamp examination looking for retinal detachment, superolateral lens dislocation, cataracts, severe myopia, and open-angle glaucoma. Globe ultrasound and keratometry to assess the cornea.

Genetic testing
This has a limited role in diagnosis, and is used primarily to diagnose family members if a mutation is known. Linkage analysis can be applied in families with several affected relatives.

Treatment
- β-blockers (possibly calcium channel blockers) delay and attenuate aortic root dilation.
- Antibiotic chemoprophylaxis for bacteraemia-prone procedures.
- Surgery for aortic root and valve disease, skeletal and ocular complications.
- Gentle exercise.

Prognosis
- Life expectancy about two-thirds of normal.
- Cardiovascular death in over 90% of cases due to aortic dissection or heart failure.

Ghent criteria for Marfan's syndrome

Skeletal system involvement
(two major or one major and two minor criteria)

Major criteria	Minor criteria
1. Pectus carinatum,	1. Moderately severe pectus excavatum
2. Pectus excavatum requiring surgery,	2. Joint hypermobility
3. Reduced upper to lower segment ratio or arm span to height ratio >1.05,	3. High arched palate with teeth crowding
4. Wrist and thumb signs,	4. Facial appearance (dolichocephaly, malar hypoplasia, down-slanting palpabral fissures, retrognathia) or
5. Scoliosis exceeding 20° or spondylolisthesis,	
6. Elbow extension <170°,	5. Enophthalmos.
7. Medial displacement of medial malleolus causing pes planus or	
8. Protrusio acetabulae.	

Ocular system involvement (one major or two minor criteria)

Major criteria	Minor criteria
1. Ectopia lentis.	1. Abnormally flat cornea,
	2. Axial globe lengthening
	3. Iris or ciliary muscle hypoplasia.

Cardiovascular system involvement
(one major or one minor criterion only).

Major criteria	Minor criteria
1. Ascending aortic dilation involving at least the sinuses of Valsalva with or without aortic regurgitation and	1. Mitral valve prolapse with or without mitral regurgitation,
	2. Main pulmonary artery dilation,
2. Ascending aortic dissection.	3. Mitral annulus calcification
	4. Descending thoracic or abdominal aortic dilation or dissection.

Pulmonary system involvement (requires one minor criterion)

1. Spontaneous pneumothorax or apical blebs.

Skin and integument involvement (requires one of the following)):

1. Striae atrophicae without marked weight change, pregnancy or repetitive stress or
2. Recurrent or incisional herniae

Dural involvement (one major criterion)

1. lumbosacral dural ectasia.

A contributory **family or genetic history** (one major criterion)

1. Parent, child, or sibling meeting diagnostic criteria independently,
2. Known fibrillin-1 mutation or
3. Presence of haplotype around fibrillin-1 inherited by descendent known to be associated with unequivocally diagnosed Marfan syndrome in the family.

Ehlers–Danlos Syndrome

Epidemiology
- 1 in 5,000 live births. Incidence about 1 in 400,000.
- Typically presents between childhood and early adulthood.
- No racial or gender bias known.

Pathology
- Inherited (autosomal dominant or recessive and X-linked recessive) defects in synthesis and metabolism of different types of collagen producing connective tissue defects.
- New form recently described due to deficiency of Tenascin-X (extracellular matrix protein) with normal collagen.
- Six different subtypes described: classic, hypermobile, vascular, kyphoscoliosis, arthrochalasia, and dermatosparaxis. Much overlap between types in up to 50% cases.
- Increased tissue elasticity with decreased strength and poor healing.

Clinical features
- Typically joint hypermobility, skin hyperextensibility, tissue fragility, and poor wound healing. Classically get 'cigarette paper' scarring over knees.
- Mitral valve prolapse typically seen in classic, hypermobile, and vascular forms. Minority patients progress to severe mitral regurgitation requiring surgery. Recent echocardiographic studies suggest cardiac defects may be less frequent than previously thought, although coronary artery aneurysm can be devastating.
- Also see aortic root ectasia with dilated sinuses of Valsalva. Rarely severe or progressive and aortic root replacement is exceptional.
- Vascular form also exhibits prominent veins, low weight, short stature, spontaneous pneumothorax and rupture of medium and large-sized arteries and bowel perforation. Joints affected less frequently. Skin is fragile but not hyperextensible.
- Differential diagnoses include Marfan Syndrome, Menkes Kinky Hair Disease, Williams Syndrome, Stickler Syndrome, Cutis Laxa, and pseudoxanthoma elasticum.

Treatment
- No specific medical therapy. High-dose vitamin C may provide some benefit but no controlled studies.
- Patient education and preventive strategies. Avoid excess and repetitive lifting, contact sports.
- Avoid suturing wounds if possible.
- Regular eye and dental assessments.
- Antibiotic chemoprophylaxis for mitral valve prolapse.
- Genetic counselling. Limited role for genetic testing.

Prognosis
- Increased mortality in vascular form. Median age 50 years with death from spontaneous arterial and gastrointestinal rupture.
- Other forms usually have normal life expectancy with increased morbidity from recurrent dislocations, poor wound healing and scarring.

Kawasaki disease

Epidemiology
- UK incidence between 1999–2000 around 8.1 cases per 100,000 children.
- More than 90% of cases in children under 10 years age. Peak incidence 18–24 months in USA and 6–12 months in Japan. Commoner in males, and children of Japanese descent.

Pathology
- Aetiology unknown but likely to be infectious. Possible agents include *Parvovirus B19*, meningococcus, *Coxiella burnetii*, bacterial toxin-mediated superantigens, HIV, *Mycoplasma pneumoniae*, adenovirus, *Klebsiella pneumoniae*, *Parainfluenza* type 3 virus, rotavirus, measles, and human lymphotropic virus.
- Other determinants may be genetic and immunological factors, vectors, and passive maternal immunity.
- Generalized vasculitis most severe in medium-sized arteries affecting all layers of the wall. Smooth muscle necrosis with splitting of internal and external elastic laminae and aneurysm formation.
- Subsequent vessel fibrosis, stenosis, thrombosis and aneurysm rupture.

Clinical features
- *Acute stage* (days 1–11) characterized by high fever, irritability, non-exudative bilateral conjunctivitis (90%), iritis (70%), perianal erythema (70%), acral erythema and oedema that impede ambulation, strawberry tongue, lip fissures, hepatic, renal and gastrointestinal dysfunction, myocarditis, pericarditis, and cervical lymphadenopathy (75%).
- *Subacute stage* (days 11–30) characterized by persistent irritability, anorexia, conjunctival injection, decreased temperature, thrombocytosis, acral desquamation and aneurysm formation.
- *Convalescent/chronic phase* (after 30 days) characterized by aneurysm expansion, possible myocardial infarction, and resolution of smaller aneurysms (60% of cases).

Diagnosis requires exclusion of other illnesses with similar clinical signs, fever lasting more than 5 days, and 4 out of: polymorphous rash, bilateral conjunctival injection, mucous membrane changes (diffuse injection of oral and pharyngeal mucosa, erythema or fissuring of the lips, and strawberry tongue), acute, non-purulent cervical lymphadenopathy (one lymph node must be >1.5 cm), and extremity changes (erythema of palms or soles, indurative oedema of hands or feet and membranous desquamation of the fingertips).

Other features include heart failure, mitral regurgitation, aseptic meningitis, facial palsy, stroke, arthralgias or arthritis, pleural effusion, pulmonary infiltrates, meatitis, vulvitis, urethritis, extremity gangrene, pustules, and erythema multiforme-like lesions.

Imaging

- Echocardiogram at baseline, 3 weeks, and 1 month after bloods have normalized. Look for coronary artery aneurysms and evidence of valvulitis, myocarditis and pericarditis.
- Diffuse coronary dilation seen in 50% of cases by day 10.
- Alternative is magnetic resonance angiography.

Bloods

- Normocytic anaemia, granulocytosis, thrombocytosis (weeks 2–3), and thrombocytopaenia (with severe coronary disease).
- Elevated ESR, CRP, α 1-antitrypsin and serum complement (may be normal).
- Mild transaminitis (40%) and raised bilirubin (10%).

Treatment

- Intravenous gammaglobulin.
- Aspirin (small aneurysms). Dipyridamole (large aneurysms). Consider anticoagulation.
- In hospital until apyrexial and inflammatory markers normalized.
- Influenza vaccine if long term aspirin therapy.

Prognosis

- Mortality 0.1–2%. Cardiac complications in 25% if untreated.
- Recurrence rate 1–3%.

Takayasu arteritis

Epidemiology
- Global incidence of 2.6 cases per million population annually. UK incidence of 0.15 cases per million population annually.
- Common in south-east Asia where it is associated with TB.
- Typically affects women (80–90% of cases) in their second and third decade.

Pathology
- Idiopathic, segmental, granulomatous vasculitis of large and medium-sized arteries particularly involving the aorta and its branches, the pulmonary arteries, and consequently all major organs.
- Subsequent arterial stenosis (90% of cases), occlusion, thrombosis and aneurysm formation (27% of cases) produces end-organ ischaemia. Heart failure due to hypertension, myocarditis and aortic regurgitation is common.
- Associated with HLA-A10, B5, Bw52, DR2 and DR4 in Japan and Korea, but HLA-B22 in the USA.

Clinical features
- *Systemic:* fever, night sweats, fatigue, weight loss, myalgia, arthralgia or arthritis, rash (erythema nodosum, pyoderma gangrenosum or lupoid), headaches, dizziness, and syncope.
- *Local:* heart failure, angina, hypertension (may be paroxysmal), stroke, transient ischaemic attack, visual disturbances, carotidynia, abdominal pain, limb claudication, asymmetric pulses (common), absent pulses (rare), post-stenotic dilations producing bounding pulses (common), and bruits (over subclavian arteries and aorta).
- *Pregnancy* does not affect the vasculitis. May have problems with haemodynamic monitoring, malignant hypertension, pre-eclampsia and foetal complications.

Imaging
- Angiography showing stenoses, occlusions or aneurysms of the aorta and its primary branches or large arteries in the proximal upper or lower extremities. Changes are focal or segmental and not due to atherosclerosis, fibromuscular dysplasia, or similar causes. (American College of Rheumatology, 1990).
- Magnetic resonance imaging, magnetic resonance angiography, and computed tomography useful for serial examinations and diagnosis in the early stages. Show mural thickening and thrombi of aorta and stenoses. Distal vessels not imaged as well. Contrast may reveal pre-stenotic inflammatory lesions that may be missed on angiography.
- Echocardiogram to assess ventricles, aortic root and valve.

Bloods
- No specific markers.
- Normochromic normocytic anaemia (50% of cases), mild leucocytosis, thrombocytosis, and elevated ESR (more than 50 mm initially).
- Transaminitis, hypoalbuminaemia, negative ANA and positive rheumatoid factor (15% of cases).

Treatment

- High-dose steroids for 4–6 weeks until ESR normalized.
- If steroid-resistant or relapses consider weekly intravenous methylprednisolone or methotrexate, daily or monthly intravenous cyclophosphamide, cyclosporine (renal toxicity and hypertension), azathioprine, or mycophenolate mofetil.
- Antihypertensives, antiplatelet drugs, and anticoagulants.
- Balloon angioplasty and stenting, bypass surgery, and replacement with synthetic grafts.

Prognosis

- Determined by severity of vascular and end-organ damage.
- 60% of patients respond to steroids but 40% relapse. Survival can be up to 95% at 15 years.

Polyarteritis nodosa and other systemic vasculitides

Epidemiology
- 4–9 cases per million population per year.
- Typically affects men between the ages of 40–70 years.

Pathology
- Usually involves small and medium-sized muscular arteries.
- Fibrinoid necrotizing vasculitis beginning in the tunica media and spreading to the intima and adventitia. Immune complex mediated.
- Sequelae: aneurysm formation, haemorrhage and thrombosis.
- Macroscopic ('classic') form affects kidneys (80–90%), heart (<70% and excluding pulmonary arteries), gastrointestinal tract (50–70%), liver (50–60%), spleen (45%) and pancreas (25–35%). Microvasculature typically spared.
- Microscopic ('microscopic polyangiitis') form also involves the microvasculature, typically glomeruli and pulmonary capillaries.

Clinical features
- Fever, malaise, weight loss (>50% cases).
- Arthralgia, arthritis, tender subcutaneous nodules (15% cases), abdominal pain, nausea and vomiting (>60% cases), retinopathy, gastrointestinal haemorrhage (6% cases), bowel perforation (5% cases), and infarction (1.4% cases).
- Renal failure, hypertension, myocardial infarction, heart failure, and pericarditis.
- Unique features of Churg–Strauss syndrome include allergic rhinitis, polyposis, recurrent bronchitis and asthma. Heart involved in 85% cases causing pericardial effusion, perimyocarditis, restrictive cardiomyopathy with systolic and diastolic dysfunction.
- Wegener's granulomatosis rarely causes pericarditis and coronary arteritis (10–20% cases antemortem). Can cause myocardial infarction and sudden death.

Imaging
- Selective angiography remains gold standard.
- Saccular microaneurysms (2–5 mm diameter) seen in 60–80% cases. Usually at least 10 per single visceral circulation. Typically at branching points and bifurcations.
- Also find vessel ectasia and irregularity, segmental stenoses, occlusions, and hypervascularity.
- Similar appearances also found in vasculitis associated with rheumatoid disease, SLE and Churg–Strauss syndrome.

Bloods
- Elevated ESR, positive anti-neutrophilic cytoplasmic antibodies (ANCA), hypergammaglobulinaemia, and hepatitis B surface antigenaemia (30% cases).
- Churg–Strauss syndrome characterized by peripheral blood eosinophilia (90% untreated cases), high serum IgE levels and positive rheumatoid factor (70% cases). Hepatitis B surface antigen usually negative.

Treatment and prognosis
- High-dose steroids and cyclophosphamide produce remission in 90% cases.
- Relapse rate up to 40%.
- 5-year survival if untreated is 15% with death from progressive renal failure or gastrointestinal complications.
- Morbidity and mortality in Churg–Strauss syndrome mainly due to severe asthma, heart failure, and gastrointestinal complications. Prognosis is similar to polyarteritis nodosa.

Ankylosing spondylitis

Epidemiology
- Incidence 0.1–1% in general population and 1–2% amongst HLA-B27 positive individuals.
- Usually seen in northern Europeans with onset during late adolescence and early adulthood. Juvenile onset (before 16 years) especially amongst Native Americans, Mexicans, and in developing countries.
- Three times commoner in males.

Pathology
- Chronic multisystem inflammatory disease. Other seronegative spondyloarthropathies include reactive arthritis (Reiter's syndrome), juvenile chronic arthritis, and those in association with psoriasis and inflammatory bowel disease.
- Strong association with HLA-B27 and a genetic predisposition. 10–20% of first-degree relatives positive for HLA-B27 develop the disease.
- Typically affects ligament and capsule attachments to bone in sacroiliac joints and axial skeleton-enthesitis. Culminates in joint erosion, fibrosis, and ossification producing vertebral fusion.
- Cardiac involvement usually manifests late but occasionally precedes overt joint disease.
- Aortic regurgitation (1–10% cases) causes: 1) ascending aortitis (1–10% cases) causing thickening, stiffness and dilation of aorta. 2) Aortic valve fibrosis causing cusp thickening, nodularity and shortening.
- Fibrosis of aortic and mitral valve junction producing subaortic bump on echocardiography.
- Anterior mitral valve leaflet thickening rarely causing mitral regurgitation.
- Pericarditis (<1% of cases).
- Myocardial fibrosis causing systolic and diastolic dysfunction on echocardiography. May progress to dilated cardiomyopathy. Myocardial function may be further compromised by secondary amyloidosis.
- Atrioventricular node conduction problems with complete heart block.

Clinical features
- Fever and weight loss.
- Insidious low back pain progressing proximally in relapsing-remitting pattern.
- Chronic pain and morning stiffness (>70% cases); fatigue (65% cases); reduced mobility (47% cases).
- Depression (20% cases, especially females) and neurological deficits.
- Acute unilateral iritis (25–30% cases).
- Chest tightness and breathlessness from restricted chest movements.

Imaging
- Erosions and sclerosis of sacroiliac joints.
- Squared-off vertebral bodies and syndesmophytes culminating in the bamboo spine.

Bloods

- No diagnostic tests.
- Elevated ESR and CRP (75% cases).

Treatment

- Non-steroidal anti-inflammatory drugs and sulphasalazine.
- Specialist treatment for complications. May require spinal or cardiac surgery.
- Genetic counselling.

Prognosis

- Disease of the aorta and valves more frequent with increasing disease duration. May be progressive or resolve.
- Death can be due to cardiac complications like complete heart block.

Polymyositis and dermatomyositis

- Cardiac involvement is frequent but usually subclinical. 15% cases are symptomatic and 55% noted on echocardiography.
- T cell-mediated cytotoxicity against muscle fibres in polymyositis. Complement-mediated lysis of cell membranes with vascular smooth muscle hyperplasia, coagulation and infarction in dermatomyositis. This produces a small vessel and capillary vasculopathy that does not cause significant deterioration in ventricular function.
- 25% cases have myocarditis at post-mortem with microscopic interstitial fibrosis, non-specific inflammatory infiltrates, and necrosis. Ventricular function is usually preserved.
- Conducting tissues are particularly affected producing non-specific ST and T wave changes, atrial arrhythmias, atrioventricular, and bundle branch block. These are more commonly seen in children.
- Pericarditis is rare and seen in 25% of cases on echocardiography.
- Coronary vasospasm may occur and provocation testing has demonstrated endothelial dysfunction with vasoconstriction in response to intracoronary acetylcholine.
- Cor pulmonale may occur secondary to primary lung disease and pulmonary hypertension.
- Overt cardiac complications should be treated using steroids, immunosuppressive drugs and calcium channel blockers.
- Cardiac complications are an important cause of death together with malignancy and lung problems.

Rheumatoid disease

- Multisystem disease characterised by a symmetrical, deforming, peripheral arthropathy.
- Prevalence 1%. Typically affects females with peak onset in the fifth decade.
- Cardiac involvement seen in 60% of cases echocardiographically with 10–15% symptomatic. Directly related to severity of joint disease and the presence of nodules.
- 50% of cases have a subclinical fibrinous pericarditis with effusions seen in 40% of cases on echocardiography. 1–2% of cases are symptomatic. Usually independent of disease duration and may precede it. Cardiac tamponade and constrictive pericarditis are rare. Usually responds to treatment with steroids and disease-modifying drugs.
- More than 50% of patients with subcutaneous nodules have myocardial and endocardial nodular granulomas. Rarely compromise cardiac function through mitral valve deformity and regurgitation or conduction problems like first degree (commonest), left bundle branch, and complete heart blocks.
- 20% of patients with severe disease have a diffuse myocarditis with non-specific inflammatory infiltrates, myocyte necrosis and fibrosis that may cause biventricular failure, arrhythmias and conduction problems. Ventricular function may also be compromised by secondary amyloidosis.
- Coronary arteritis noted in 20% of cases postmortem. Rarely causes angina and infarction.
- Non-specific valvitis producing fibrotic, hyalinized valves with occasional incompetence. Aortic valve affected more commonly than mitral.

Cardiology in developing countries

Burden of cardiovascular disease in developing countries

Approximately 80% of the world's people reside in developing countries. Although cardiovascular diseases (CVD) occur throughout the world, their form and the burden change as a country undergoes economic development. Developing countries begin with a disease burden dominated by infectious, perinatal, and nutritional diseases and, in the process of development, make the transition to one dominated by noncommunicable disease (NCD), particularly CVD. The four stages of transition are shown in the table on p501.

Many developing countries have a triple burden of disease, encompassing disorders that characterize the first three phases of the epidemiologic transition.

In 2000, CVD accounted for 16.7 million deaths globally; 31% of all global deaths are due to CVD. Coronary heart disease (CHD) and stroke account for 71% of CVD deaths. Low and middle income countries contribute 78% of all CVD deaths, and 86% of disability-adjusted life years (DALY) loss attributed to CVD. The relative importance of CHD and stroke vary across regions and countries. For example, more than twice as many deaths from stroke occurred in the developing countries as in developed countries.

NCDs rank first in most developing countries, in developed countries, and worldwide as a cause of death. CVD accounts for about half of all NCD deaths. In 1990, CVDs were the leading cause of death for all major geographic regions of the developing world except India and sub-Saharan Africa.

There is an early age of CVD deaths in developing countries compared to developed countries. In 1990, the proportion of CVD deaths occurring below the age of 70 years was 26.5% in developed countries, compared to 46.7% in developing countries. Therefore, the contribution of the developing countries to the global burden of CVD, in terms of disability adjusted life years (DALY) lost, was nearly 3 times higher than that of developed countries.

Rheumatic heart disease (RHD) is the most common cause of CVD in children and young adults in developing countries. At least 12 million persons are estimated to be to be affected with RHD globally. More than 2 million require repeated hospitalization and 1 million will need heart surgery over the next 20 years. Annually, 500,000 deaths occur as a result of RHD, and many poor persons, who are preferentially affected, are disabled because of lack of access to the expensive medical and surgical care demanded by the disease. The prevalence of RHD in developing countries ranges from 1 to 10 per 1000 and the incidence of rheumatic fever ranges from 10 to 100 per 100,000, with a high rate of recurrence.

Deaths caused by cardiovascular disease at different stages of development—1990 (Howson et al., 1998)

Stage of development	Deaths from CVD (% of total)	Predominant CVDs	Regional examples
Age of pestilence and famine.	5–10%	Rheumatic heart disease; tuberculous pericarditis; and infectious and nutritional cardiomyopathies.	Sub-Saharan Africa; rural India; and South America.
Age of receding pandemics.	10–35%	As above, plus hypertensive heart disease, haemorrhagic stroke, and renal failure.	China; urban South Africa.
Age of degenerative and man-made diseases.	35–55%	All forms of stroke; ischaemic heart disease at relatively young ages.	Urban India; formerly socialist economies.
Age of delayed degenerative diseases.	<50%	Stroke and ischaemic heart disease at older ages.	Western Europe; North America; Australia; New Zealand.

Managing with limited resources

The management of CVD is often technology-intensive and expensive. Procedures for diagnosis or therapy, drugs, hospitalization, and frequent consultations with healthcare providers all contribute to the high cost. The high expenditure on tertiary care in most developing countries probably has a large contribution from CVD. This may divert scarce resources from developmental needs and from the unfinished agenda of infectious and nutritional disorders. Thus there is an urgent need for cost-effective preventive strategies and case management approaches that are based on the best available evidence, and generalized to the context of each developing country.

Infectious disease and the heart

Numerous infectious diseases may involve the endocardium (see Chapter 3), myocardium (see Chapter 7), and the pericardium (see Chapter 8). This section deals with a miscellaneous group of infectious diseases that are of particular relevance to cardiology practice in developing countries, i.e., HIV infection, Chagas' disease, diphtheria, syphilis, and tetanus. Although occasional examples have been reported, myocardial involvement is so rare as to be of little clinical significance in tuberculosis (apart from pericarditis), typhoid fever, scrub typhus, poliomyelitis, infective hepatitis, virus pneumonias, and other respiratory tract infections.

Diphtheria

Cardiac damage in diphtheria is due to a circulating exotoxin that inhibits protein synthesis in target tissues, with a high degree of affinity for the conduction system. Myocarditis occurs in up to 25% of cases of diphtheria and carries a mortality of approximately 60%. Pathological examination shows a flabby dilated heart with a 'streaky' appearance of the myocardium. Microscopy reveals characteristic fatty infiltration of the myocytes, and other features of myocarditis.

Clinical features
Sinus tachycardia, gallop rhythm, cardiomegaly, and hypotension typically appear in the second week of illness.

Investigations
The ECG abnormalities are useful in diagnosis and fall under two headings:
- Tracings showing evidence of diffuse myocardial damage: low voltage, prolongation of the QT interval, and T wave flattening or inversion.
- Tracings showing evidence of damage to the conduction system with all degrees of atrioventricular block. The development of bundle branch block or complete heart block is a particularly ominous finding and the reported mortality rates vary from 54 to 100% despite the insertion of transvenous pacing. The presence of myocardial damage is confirmed by marked elevation of serum transaminase level; a high level is associated with poor prognosis.

The **ECG** eventually returns to normal (in those cases that survive) but conduction abnormalities may persist for years.

Treatment
This involves supportive measures for heart failure, antibiotics (procaine penicillin G 600,000 U IM 12 hourly for 10 days or erythromycin 250–500 mg po 6 hourly for 7 days) to prevent secondary infection and eliminate the diphtheria organisms in the throat, and temporary pacing in cases of atrioventricular heart block. Antitoxic serum should not be given at this stage because the exotoxin is already fixed and because of the risk of fatal serum reactions. Intubation and ventilation may be required for those patients with evidence of respiratory failure.

HIV and the cardiovascular system

The clinical effects of HIV on the heart are relatively uncommon relative to the impact of HIV infection on the lungs, gastrointestinal tract, central nervous system, and the skin. There are similarities in the pattern of cardiovascular disease involvement in people living in developed and developing countries, but differences in the causative organisms implicated. The main presentations are (1) pericardial effusion, (2) cardiomyopathy, (3) pulmonary hypertension, (4) large vessel aneurysms, and (5) metabolic complications associated with anti-retroviral drug use.

Pericardial effusion is one of the early presenting features of HIV infection in patients living in sub-Saharan Africa. Whereas in Western countries, a large effusion is usually idiopathic in 80% patients with AIDS, the disease is caused by tuberculosis in over 80% of Africans living with HIV. Purulent pericarditis is not uncommon, while involvement with Kaposi's sarcoma and B-cell lymphoma is rare. Treatment of tuberculous pericarditis is with standard anti-tuberculous regime similar to HIV-negative patients, and the short-term outcome is similar. The role of adjuvant steroids is uncertain.

Cardiomyopathy is found in 50% of acutely ill hospitalized patients, and in 15% of ambulatory asymptomatic patients living with HIV. Myocarditis is present in the majority of the cases. In Western series, the myocarditis is associated with cardiotropic virus, whereas in Africa preliminary data suggests that it may be associated with non-viral opportunistic infections such as Toxoplasmosis, Cryptococcosis, and *Mycobacterium avium intracellulare* infection. HIV-positive patients with cardiomyopathy should be considered for endomyocardial biopsy to exclude a treatable cause of myocarditis. Otherwise treat as for heart failure. Prognosis is poor with a median survival of 100 days without anti-retroviral drugs.

HIV-associated pulmonary hypertension is estimated to be 1/200, much higher than the 1/200,000 found in the general population. Primary pulmonary hypertension is found in 0.5% of hospitalized AIDS patients and is a cause of cor pulmonale and death. The pathogenesis is poorly understood.

HIV-related arterial aneurysm is a distinct clinical and pathological entity that is associated with advanced HIV disease. HIV-related aneurysms affect young patients (median age 30 years) with no risk factors for atherosclerosis, occur mainly in peripheral arteries (carotid, distal superficial femoral and popliteal sites), are usually multiple (1–10 per patient), and have been reported more frequently in Black patients than in White patients. The inflammatory process involves the *vasa vasorum* of the adventitia with sparing of the media and intima. The most frequent mode of presentation is that of a painful mass of increasing size. The diagnosis is confirmed by duplex sonography or computed tomography. Arterial angiography is performed to delineate the extent of aneurysm. Serological testing for syphilis, typhoid, HIV, and autoimmune disease is indicated. Treatment is by operative intervention for symptomatic aneurysm in patients with an acceptable surgical risk and anticipated life expectancy.

Drug-related cardiac disorders: the use of protease inhibitor anti-retroviral agents is associated with the following **metabolic abnormalities**: fat redistribution (lipodystrophy), increased total cholesterol and triglycerides, decrease in HDL, impaired glucose tolerance, and increased intra-abdominal fat. These changes translate to a small increase in the risk of myocardial infarction with the long-term use of protease inhibitors. It is prudent to avoid protease inhibitors in patients with other cardiovascular risk factors if possible, modify risk factors, and treat the metabolic complications when they arise according to standard guidelines.

Chagas' disease

Chagas' disease is a myocarditis of parasitic origin that is caused by the protozoan *Trypanosoma cruzi*. The disease is a major public health problem in South and Central America. 15–18 million people are infected with the parasite, and 65 million people are at risk. Chagas' disease is transmitted by contamination of the bite wound of the 'assassin' or 'kissing' reduviid bugs with the infected faeces of the insect.

Natural history: acute Chagas' disease occurs predominantly in children in less than 10% of infected cases; it is fatal in 10% of cases It is characterized by fever, lymphadenopathy, hepatosplenomegaly, and facial oedema. Acute myocarditis is common and may be fatal. Rarely, meningoencephalitis or convulsive seizures may occur, sometimes causing permanent mental or physical defects or death. Recovery is usual, however, and the disease is quiescent for the next 10 to 15 years (latent Chagas' disease). **Chronic Chagas' disease** may be asymptomatic, mild, or may be accompanied by cardiomyopathy, megaoesophagus, and megacolon, with a fatal outcome. The late manifestations probably result from lymphocyte-mediated destruction of muscle tissue and nerve ganglions during the acute stage of the disease. *Trypanosoma cruzi* may be found in degenerated muscle cells, especially in the right atrium.

Clinical features: the disease is characterized clinically by anginal chest pain, symptomatic conduction system disease; severe, protracted, congestive cardiac failure—often predominantly right-sided—is the rule in advanced cases. Bifascicular block is present in more than 80% of cases and death from asystole and arrhythmia is common. Autonomic dysfunction is common. Apical aneurysms and left ventricular dilatation increase the risk of thrombo-embolism and arrhythmias.

Diagnosis: Chagas' disease is identified by demonstration of trypanosomes in the peripheral blood or leishmanial forms in a lymph node biopsy, or by animal inoculation or culture, xenodiagnosis (i.e., the patient is bitten by reduviid bugs bred in the laboratory; the subsequent identification of parasites in the intestine of the insect is proof of infection in the human host), or serologic tests. The CXR shows cardiomegaly. The ECG is usually abnormal. The echocardiogram features in advanced cases are those of DCM; a left ventricular posterior wall hypokinesis and relatively preserved interventricular septum motion, associated with an apical aneurysm is typical. Radionuclide ventriculography may show ventricular wall motion abnormality in the absence overall depression of global ventricular function. Perfusion scanning with thallium-201 may show fixed defects (corresponding to areas of fibrosis) as well as evidence of reversible ischaemia. Gadolinium-contrast MRI can identify patients with more active myocardial disease

Treatment: there is no specific therapy for Chagas' disease. Prolonged administration of nifurtimox, a nitrofurazone derivative, may effect parasitologic cure, but chronic organ damage is irreversible. Heart failure, arrhythmias and thrombo-embolism are treated with the usual measures.

Prevention: reduviid bugs, the vectors for Chagas' disease, inhabit poorly constructed houses and outbuildings. Spraying with 5% γ-benzene hexachloride is most effective in controlling the vector. Patching wall cracks and cementing over dirt floors also help to eliminate the vectors.

Cardiovascular syphilis

Cardiovascular syphilis produces thoracic aneurysm, narrowing of the coronary ostia, or aortic valvular insufficiency that usually appears 10 to 25 years after the initial infection. Involvement of the myocardium is rare. The introduction of penicillin has made the disease less common, but it remains an important cause of cardiovascular disease in poor populations.

Coronary disease: angina pectoris, rarely myocardial infarction, cardiac aneurysm or sudden death may result from involvement of the coronary ostia. Aortic insufficiency is nearly always present. The condition should be suspected when angina pectoris is encountered in young men, and when severe angina is associated with disproportionately mild aortic insufficiency. Nitroglycerine is often less effective in relieving symptoms. Attacks of angina decubitus are not infrequent. The diagnosis is established by positive syphilis serology and coronary angiography. Successful surgical treatment may be achieved by endarterectomy of the coronary ostia or by bypass grafting.

Aortic insufficiency: the presenting symptoms may be those of coronary insufficiency or of left heart failure. The physical signs are the same as those of rheumatic aortic insufficiency. Pure insufficiency without any stenosis is the rule. Because of the unfolding and dilatation of the aorta, the murmurs are frequently better heard to the right of the sternum. Occasionally a musical ('cooing-dove') diastolic murmur is produced by eversion or detachment of an aortic cusp.

Syphilitic aortic aneurysm: this involves the ascending aorta and the arch with equal frequency. Less commonly, the descending aorta is involved, and least commonly the abdominal aorta. It is not unusual for the aorta to be involved at more than one site in the same patient. Syphilitic aneurysms are usually saccular (vs. fusiform aneurysms of atherosclerosis). Syphilitic aneurysms can rupture, but never dissect. The clinical presentation is dependent on compression of adjacent structures and therefore varies with the portion of the aorta involved.

An aneurysm may be suspected clinically by unequal pulses and blood pressures in the upper limbs or by the presence of a tracheal tug. Not infrequently, an aneurysm is first detected by CXR, and must be distinguished from other masses. Linear calcification of the aneurysmal sac and expansile pulsation on fluoroscopy are helpful signs when present. Aortic angiography is required for diagnosis.

Treatment: Benzathine penicillin G should be given in doses of 2.4 million units weekly for three successive weeks. When there is penicillin allergy, tetracycline 500 mg four times per day for 1 month may be administered.

Types of aneurysms associated with syphilis

Ascending aorta aneurysms (the 'aneurysms of signs')

- Compression of superior vena cava—distended non-pulsatile neck veins with oedema in their drainage area.
- Compression of the right main bronchus—lung complications.
- Compression of the right ventricular outflow tract—signs of pulmonary stenosis.
- Erosion of the sternum—superficial pulsating mass.

Aortic arch aneurysms (the 'aneurysms of symptoms')

- Large airway compression—dry 'brassy' cough, dyspnoea.
- Recurrent laryngeal nerve compression—hoarseness.
- Oesophageal compression—dysphagia.
- Compression of the sympathetic chain—Horner's syndrome.
- Erosion of the vertebrae and compression of nerves—deep seated continuous bone and root pain.

Tetanus

Tetanus is caused by the endotoxin (tetanospasmin) from the anaerobic organism *Clostridium tetani*. Portal of entry is usually a severe or untreated wound, often a neglected burn, or, occasionally, a septic incomplete abortion. In a few cases (15–30%) the portal of entry is never isolated. Public health immunization programmes with tetanus toxoid have dramatically reduced the incidence of neonatal tetanus in many parts of the world, but there is still a significant number of cases in adults.

Features of special importance in the history are the period from injury to onset of symptoms and time interval between the onset of stiffness to the onset of spasms. In general, the shorter the period from injury to onset of symptoms and the shorter the time interval between symptoms and spasms, the more severe the tetanus will be.

The most useful classification of tetanus is simply:
• Mild—stiffness and mild spasms.
• Moderate—stiffness and/or spasms with dysphagia.
• Severe—severe recurrent spasms and dysphagia ± autonomic overactivity.

Sympathetic overactivity remains the major cause of death in patients with tetanus once early deaths from respiratory obstruction and the deaths from mechanical failure have been eliminated. The syndrome of sympathetic overactivity results in tachycardia, marked fluctuation of blood pressure (i.e., both hypo- and hypertensive changes), excessive salivation, and sweating. This fluid loss may result may result in dehydration. The effect on the heart can give rise to myocardial infarction.

A treatment approach that involves the use of extremely heavy sedation with intermittent positive pressure ventilation has proven to be successful in reducing mortality to 6% in our practice.

Beriberi (thiamine deficiency)

The coenzyme thiamine pyrophosphate (TPP) participates in carbohydrate metabolism through decarboxylation of α-keto acids. Thiamine also acts as coenzyme to the apoenzyme transketolase in the pentose monophosphate pathway for glucose. Thiamine deficiency may produce dry or wet beriberi. Dry beriberi manifests with peripheral neurologic and cerebral disturbances. The wet form is associated with cardiovascular manifestations.

Aetiology

Primary thiamine deficiency arises from inadequate intake, particularly in people subsisting on highly polished rice (e.g., in the Far East). Milling removes the husk, which contains most of the thiamine.

Secondary thiamine deficiency arises from (1) increased requirement, as in hyperthyroidism, pregnancy, lactation, and fever; (2) impaired absorption, as in long-continued diarrhoea; (3) impaired utilization, as in severe liver disease; and (4) increased urinary excretion, as in chronic furosemide therapy. A combination of decreased intake, impaired absorption and utilization, increased requirements, and possibly apoenzyme defect occurs in alcoholism. Highly concentrated dextrose infusions, coupled with low thiamine intake, may precipitate thiamine deficiency.

Cardiovascular (wet) beriberi

This takes 2 forms:

1. The most common is a high output state. Before heart failure supervenes, there is tachycardia, a wide pulse pressure, sweating, and a warm skin. With heart failure orthopnoea, pulmonary and peripheral oedema, and peripheral vasoconstriction causing cold and cyanosed extremities, occur.
2. Less common is a low output state (*Shoshin disease*). Severe hypotension, lactic acidosis, very low systemic vascular resistance, and absence of oedema characterize this. Death occurs within a few hours or days, unless appropriate treatment is given.

Even after several episodes of cardiovascular beriberi, permanent myocardial damage is extremely rare.

Infantile beriberi

This is seen in infants breast-fed by thiamine deficient mothers, usually between the 2nd and 4th month of life. Cardiac failure, aphonia, and absent deep tendon reflexes are characteristic.

Clinical features

The diagnosis of beriberi should always be considered in any case of heart failure in an alcoholic where the cause is not readily apparent. Neurologic symptoms such as paraesthesiae and weakness because of peripheral neuropathy, and Wernicke's encephalopathy are occasionally present.

Signs of a hyperkinetic circulatory state are manifested by warm hands, tachycardia, collapsing pulses, and raised jugular venous pressure. A wide pulse pressure with systolic hypertension is commonly found, but occasionally diastolic hypertension is also present initially, so that hypertensive heart failure may be suspected. The heart is almost invariably enlarged, with a gallop rhythm. Atrioventricular regurgitant murmurs may be present, and tricuspid insufficiency is particularly common. Occasionally, right-sided heart failure dominates the clinical picture and there is disproportionate oedema and hepatomegaly. In Shoshin beriberi, there is severe heart failure with low cardiac output, orthopnoea, systemic congestion, and oliguria.

Investigations

The **ECG** findings are of crucial value in diagnosis. The most common finding is a normal tracing, or one demonstrating right axis deviation with clockwise rotation, when the patient is most severely ill. Less commonly, the initial ECG shows T wave inversion over the left or right ventricular precordial leads. In either event, daily tracings will show serial changes, either over the right ventricle or left ventricle or both. Thus, when the patient has apparently recovered completely, the ECG may actually be at its worst, showing extensive and deep T wave inversion. The abnormal changes may persist for 24 hours, days, or even weeks following recovery, but complete return to normal is the rule.

CXR: radiologically, equally striking serial changes occur. Marked cardiomegaly with a prominent right ventricular outflow and hilar congestion rapidly returns to normal in a week or two following appropriate treatment.

Laboratory findings: erythrocyte transketolase activity is diminished before and increases after the addition of thiamine pyrophosphate (TPP effect); a TPP effect > 15% suggests thiamine deficiency. The blood sample must be taken before administration of thiamine in a heparin-coated vial and transported to the laboratory on ice. Elevated blood pyruvate and lactate, and diminished urinary thiamine excretion (< 50 μg/day) are also found.

Treatment

Thiamine 50–100 mg IV or IM immediately, and repeated daily for 1–2 weeks. The response to thiamine is usually prompt and complete. Marked diuresis, decrease in heart rate and size, and clearing of pulmonary congestion may occur in 12 to 48 hours. However, sudden death from pulmonary oedema may occur, so that it is prudent to treat with digitalis and diuretics at the outset.

Keshan disease (selenium deficiency)

Selenium is involved in the reoxidation of reduced glutathione and has close metabolic interrelationships with vitamin E. It is part of the enzyme glutathione peroxidase, which is thought to destroy peroxides derived from unsaturated fatty acids.

Deficiency has occurred in patients on long-term parenteral feeding. Several cases of fatal cardiomyopathy have been attributed to selenium deficiency. In China, a childhood cardiomyopathy known as Keshan disease, after the province in which it has been studied, has been attributed to selenium deficiency and protection claimed for prophylactic dosing with 150 µg selenium/day as selenomethionine.

Selenium levels have also been found to be low in some patients with HIV-associated cardiomyopathy, with a response to selenium supplementation.

Restrictive cardiomyopathy

Restrictive cardiomyopathy (see p310) is divided into a diffuse **non-obliterative** variety (e.g., amyloidosis, haemochromatosis) and an **obliterative** variety in which the endocardium and subendocardiun are fibrosed (e.g., endomyocardial fibrosis).

Variants of restrictive obliterative cardiomyopathy occur in temperate zones described as **Loeffler endocarditis** (p520), and in the tropical rainforest regions as **endomyocardial fibrosis (EMF)** (p518). Tropical endomyocardial fibrosis affects children in the very low socio-economic groups; it is not restricted to specific racial groups as Europeans living in the tropics have also been affected.

It has been suggested that Loeffler endocarditis and tropical EMF are part of a continuum of the same disease commencing with hypereosinophilia of whatever cause resulting in myocardial damage in three stages: a necrotic phase (eosinophilic myocarditis with arteritis i.e., Loeffler endocarditis) for the first few months of illness; a thrombotic phase with early thickening of the myocardium with thrombosis after about 1 year of presentation; and the late stage of fibrosis (i.e., EMF).

However, there are differences in the clinical presentation of tropical EMF and Loeffler endocarditis: i.e., geographic, age (Loeffler endocarditis affects middle aged men vs. tropical EMF which affects young people and children), pattern of ventricular involvement (tropical EMF affects mainly right ventricle vs. Loeffler endocarditis affects either ventricle), and a link with eosinophilia (Loeffler is associated with hypereosinophilia vs. link of tropical EMF with eosinophilia has not been established).

Endomyocardial fibrosis (EMF)

Pathophysiology

Fibrous tissue and the chordae adherent to the ventricular wall may bind down the papillary muscle. In the extreme stage when there is obliterative cardiomyopathy, the cavity of the ventricle is occupied entirely by fibrous tissue and superimposed thrombus. The disease may involve either or both ventricles and be complicated by pericarditis with effusion. High diastolic pressure giving rise to pulmonary and systemic venous congestion with atrioventricular valve incompetence.

Symptoms and signs

Typically, symptoms are suggestive of congestive cardiomyopathy, but signs resemble constrictive pericarditis (see p334). Like congestive cardiomyopathy, patient present with dyspnoea, orthopnoea, and peripheral oedema. Like constrictive pericarditis, pulsus paradoxus, a raised jugular venous pressure with rapid 'x' and 'y' descents, an early third heart sound, hepatomegaly, and ascites are present. In contradistinction to constrictive pericarditis, however, there is frequently a murmur of tricuspid and/or mitral regurgitation. Chronic, severe tricuspid regurgitation that is often seen in right-sided endomyocardial fibrosis may cause bilateral proptosis.

Diagnosis

ECG is usually non-specifically abnormal, showing low-voltage QRS complexes, ST-T wave abnormalities, and may indicate right atrial enlargement in the form of tall peaked P waves.

CXR may demonstrate an enlarged cardiac silhouette similar to a pericardial effusion.

Echocardiography shows increased ventricular wall thickness cavity obliteration; enlarge atria, with or without a small pericardial effusion.

Cardiac catheterization demonstrates the combination of restricted filling and incompetence of the atrioventricular valves. The right atrial pressure is elevated with prominent systolic waves and steep 'x' and 'y' descents. In severe obliterative cases, the pressures in the right atrium, right ventricle, and pulmonary arteries may be identical and an **intracardiac ECG** may be required to locate the position of the tricuspid and pulmonary valves. A dip and plateau ('square root') type of pressure pulse is frequently present in both ventricles. Ventriculography shows an enormously dilated right atrium and obliteration of the right ventricular apex. Endomyocardial biopsy of the right ventricle may be useful by demonstrating an excess fibrous tissue, a finding that is highly suggestive of endomyocardial fibrosis. The distinguishing clinical, echocardiographic, and haemodynamic features between restrictive cardiomyopathy and constrictive pericarditis are discussed under the section on constrictive pericarditis. However, in those forms of this syndrome where significant cardiomegaly is absent, a distinction from constrictive pericarditis may be impossible. The only means of making a diagnosis is then **exploratory thoracotomy**.

Prognosis and treatment

There is no specific treatment for endomyocardial fibrosis, and prognosis is poor (35–50% 2 year mortality). **Diuretics** must be used with caution because of their ability to lower preload upon which the noncompliant ventricles depend to maintain cardiac output. **Digitalis** is helpful in patients with atrial fibrillation. Afterload reducers may induce profound hypotension, and are usually of no value. Operative excision of the fibrotic endocardium (**endocardial resection**) and replacement of one or both atrioventricular valves may lead to symptomatic improvement, but is associated with a high peri-operative mortality (15–25%) and no survival benefit. **Cardiac transplantation** is the definitive treatment for EMF.

Loeffler endocarditis

Marked eosinophilia of any cause may be associated with endomyocardial disease but the cause of eosinophilia in most patients with Loeffler endocarditis is unknown. Typical patient is a man in his 4th decade who lives in a temperate climate and has the hypereosinophilic syndrome (i.e., persistent eosinophilia with ≥ 1500 eosiniphils/mm^3 for at least 6 months or until death, with organ involvement).

Pathology

Multi-organ disease involving the heart, lungs, bone marrow, and brain. Cardiac involvement is often biventricular, with mural endocardial thickening of the inflow portions and apex of ventricles. Histological features of eosinophilic myocarditis, mural thrombosis, and fibrotic thickening of the endocardium.

Symptoms and signs

Constitutional symptoms (fever, weight loss), cough, and rash. Overt symptoms and signs of congestive heart failure are found in 50% of patients. Cardiomegaly and the murmur of mitral regurgitation may be found even in patients without cardiac symptoms. Systemic embolism is frequent. Death is usually due to cardiac failure, often associated with renal, hepatic or respiratory failure.

Diagnosis

ECG most commonly shows non-specific ST-T wave changes, but atrial fibrillation and right bundle branch block are common.

CXR may reveal cardiomegaly and pulmonary congestion or pulmonary infiltrates. Echocardiogram shows localized thickening of the posterobasal left ventricular wall, with limited or absent motion of the posterior leaflet of the mitral valve; enlarged atria, atrioventricular valve regurgitation; and usually preserved systolic function.

Cardiac catheterization reveals the haemodynamic features of a restrictive cardiomyopathy and are indistinguishable from tropical EMF outlined above. The diagnosis is often confirmed by **endomyocardial biopsy.**

Management

Medical therapy during the course of Loeffler endocarditis and surgical therapy during later phases of fibrosis may have a positive effect on symptoms and survival. **Corticosteroids** are indicated for acute myocarditis together with **hydroxyurea** may improve survival. Some non-responders have responded to **interferon**. Routine cardiac therapy with diuretics, digitalis, afterload reduction, and anticoagulation are important adjuncts. Surgical therapy offers palliation of symptoms once the fibrotic stage has been reached.

Further reading

- Chesler E (1992). *Clinical cardiology.* Springer-Verlag: New York.
- Falase AO, Akinkugbe OO (2000). *A compendium of clinical medicine* 2nd ed. Spectrum Books Limited: Ibadan.
- Howson CP, Reddy KS, Ryan TJ, Bale JR (1998). *Control of cardiovascular diseases in developing countries: research, development, and institutional strengthening.* Institute of Medicine. National Academy Press: Washington, D.C.
- Magula NP, Mayosi BM (2003). Cardiac involvement in HIV-infected people living in Africa: a review. *Cardiovascular Journal of South Africa*, **14**, 231–237.
- Nair R, Robbs JV, Naidoo NG, Woolgar J (2000). Clinical profile of HIV-related aneurysms. *European Journal of Vascular and Endovascular Surgery*, **20**, 235–240.
- Potgieter PD (1990). Tetanus. In: Potgieter PD, Linton DM, eds. *Intensive care manual* pp 99–103. CTP Book Printers: Cape Town.
- Reddy KS (2002). Global perspective on cardiovascular disease. In Yusuf S, Cairns JA, Camm AJ, Fallen EL, Gersh BJ eds. *Evidence-based cardiology*, pp 91–102. BMJ Books: London.
- Berkow R, Fletcher AJ (1987). *The Merck Manual of Diagnosis and Therapy.* Merck Sharp & Dohme Research Laboratories: Rahway.
- Wynne J, Braunwald E (2001). The cardiomyopathies and myocarditides. In Braunwald E, Zipes DP, Libby P, eds. *Heart disease: a textbook of cardiovascular medicine*, pp. 1751–1806. W.B. Saunders Company: London.

Heart disease in pregnancy

Basic principles

Cardiac disease in pregnancy is rare in the UK, Europe, and the developed world, but common in developing countries. In the UK, rheumatic heart disease is now extremely rare in women of childbearing age and is confined to immigrants. Women with congenital heart disease, having undergone corrective or palliative surgery in childhood survive into adulthood, are encountered more frequently. These women may have complicated pregnancies. Women with metal prosthetic valves face difficult decisions regarding anticoagulation in pregnancy. Ischaemic heart disease is becoming more common in pregnancy as the mean age of pregnancy increases and the smoking epidemic continues. Dissection of the aorta and its branches occurs more commonly in pregnancy and pregnancy may cause a specific dilated cardiomyopathy—peripartum cardiomyopathy.

Despite its relative rarity, cardiac disease is the leading cause of maternal death in the UK, being responsible for 44 deaths in the three years 2000–2002 inclusive[1,2]. The predominant cardiac causes of maternal death in the UK are pulmonary hypertension, peripartum cardiomyopathy, myocardial infarction, and dissection of the aorta and its branches.

Because of significant physiological changes in pregnancy, symptoms such as palpitations, and signs such as an ejection systolic murmur are very common and innocent findings. The care of the pregnant and parturient woman with heart disease requires a multidisciplinary approach and formulation of an agreed and documented management plan encompassing management of both planned and emergency delivery.

This chapter will cover the most important cardiac conditions relevant to pregnancy.

1 Why Mothers Die 1997–1999. Confidential Enquiry into Maternal Deaths. London: RCOG Press, 2001.
2 Why Mothers Die 2000–2002. Confidential Enquiry into Maternal Deaths. London: RCOG Press, 2004.

Physiological changes in pregnancy

Cardiac output increases early in pregnancy reaching a maximum by the mid second trimester. This is achieved by an increase in both stroke volume and heart rate. There is peripheral vasodilation, and a fall in systemic and pulmonary vascular resistance.

Although there is no increase in pulmonary capillary wedge pressure (PCWP), serum colloid osmotic pressure is reduced. The colloid oncotic pressure–pulmonary capillary wedge pressure gradient is reduced by 28%, making pregnant women particularly susceptible to pulmonary oedema. Pulmonary oedema will be precipitated if there is either an increase in cardiac pre-load (such as infusion of fluids), or increased pulmonary capillary permeability (such as in pre-eclampsia), or both.

In late pregnancy in the supine position, pressure of the gravid uterus on the inferior vena cava causes a reduction in venous return to the heart and a consequent fall in stroke volume and cardiac output. Turning from the lateral to the supine position may result in a 25% reduction in cardiac output. Pregnant women should therefore be nursed in the left or right lateral position wherever possible. If the mother has to be kept on her back, the pelvis should be rotated so that the uterus drops forward and cardiac output as well as uteroplacental blood flow are optimized. Reduced cardiac output is associated with reduction in uterine blood flow and therefore in placental perfusion; this can compromise the fetus.

Labour is associated with further increases in cardiac output (15% in the first stage and 50% in the second stage). Uterine contractions lead to auto transfusion of 300–500 ml of blood back into the circulation and the sympathetic response to pain and anxiety further elevate heart rate and blood pressure. Cardiac output is increased more during contractions but also between contractions.

Following delivery, there is an immediate rise in cardiac output due to the relief of inferior vena cava obstruction and contraction of the uterus that empties blood into the systemic circulation. Cardiac output increases by 60–80% followed by a rapid decline to pre-labour values within about one hour of delivery. Transfer of fluid from the extravascular space increases venous return and stroke volume further. Those women with cardiovascular compromise are therefore most at risk of pulmonary oedema during the second stage of labour and the immediate postpartum period.

Physiological changes in cardiovascular system in pregnancy

Cardiac output	↑	40%
Stroke volume	↑	
Heart rate	↑	10–20 beats per minute
Blood pressure	↓	First and second trimester
	→	Third trimester
Central venous pressure	→	
Pulmonary capillary wedge pressure (PCWP)	→	
Systemic vascular resistance (SVR) and pulmonary vascular resistance (PVR)	↓	25–30%
Serum colloid osmotic pressure	↓	10–15%

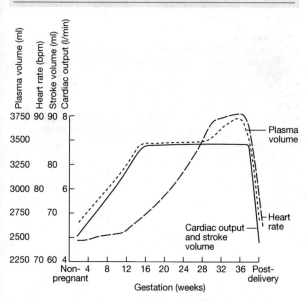

Fig. 14.1 Physiological changes in pregnancy. Systemic and pulmonary vascular resistance fall during pregnancy. Blood pressure may fall in the second trimester, rising slightly in late pregnancy. Note the cardiac output and stroke volume peak by 16 weeks gestation. Reproduced from Throne, SA (2004). Pregnancy in heart disease. *Heart* **90**: 450–456.

Normal findings in pregnancy

On examination
These may include:
- Bounding/collapsing pulse.
- Ejection systolic murmur (present in over 90% pregnant women. May be quite loud, and audible all over the praecordium).
- Third heart sound.
- Relative sinus tachycardia.
- Ectopics.
- Peripheral oedema.

On ECG
These are partly related to changes in the position of the heart:
- Atrial and ventricular ectopics.
- Q wave (small) and inverted T wave in lead III.
- ST segment depression and T wave inversion inferior and lateral leads.
- QRS axis leftward shift.

Investigations
- The amount of radiation received by the fetus during a maternal CXR is negligible and CXRs should never be withheld if clinically indicated in pregnancy.
- Transthoracic and transoesophageal echocardiograms are also safe with the usual precautions to avoid aspiration.
- MRIs are safe in pregnancy.
- Routine investigation with electrophysiological studies and angiography are normally postponed until after pregnancy but should not be withheld in, for example, acute coronary syndromes.

General considerations in pregnancy

The heart has relatively less reserve than the respiratory system. Women with heart disease may not be able to increase their cardiac output adequately to cope with pregnancy and delivery.

The outcome and safety of pregnancy are related to the
- Presence and severity of pulmonary hypertension.
- Presence of cyanosis.
- Haemodynamic significance of the lesion.
- Functional class as determined by the level of activity that leads to dyspnoea (New York Heart Association, NYHA)[1].

Cardiac events such as stroke, arrhythmia, pulmonary oedema and death complicating pregnancies are predicted by[2]:
- A prior cardiac event or arrhythmia.
- NYHA classification >II.
- Cyanosis.
- Left ventricular ejection fraction <40%.
- Left heart obstruction (mitral valve area <2 cm^2, aortic valve area <1.5 cm^2, aortic valve gradient >30 mmHg).

Women with congenital heart disease are at increased risk of having a baby with congenital heart disease, and should therefore be offered detailed scanning for fetal cardiac anomalies.

Women with cyanosis (oxygen saturation <80–85%) have an increased risk of intrauterine growth restriction, fetal loss, and thromboembolism secondary to the reactive polycythaemia. Their chance of a livebirth in one study was less than 20%[3].

Women with the above risk factors for adverse cardiac or obstetric events should be managed and counseled by a multidisciplinary team including cardiologists with expertise in pregnancy, obstetricians, fetal medicine specialists, and paediatricians. Regular antenatal visits and judicious monitoring to avoid or treat expediently any anaemia or infection or cardiac decompensation are essential. There should be early involvement of obstetric anaesthetists and a carefully documented plan for delivery.

1 McCaffrey FM and Sherman FS (1995). Pregnancy and congenital heart disease: The Magee Women's Hospital. *J Mat Fet Med.* **4**: 152–159.
2 Siu SC, Sermer M, Colman et al. (2001). Prospective multicenter study of pregnancy outcomes in women with heart disease. *Circulation* **104**: 515–521.
3 Presbitero P, Somerville J, Stone S et al. (1994). Pregnancy in cyanotic congenital heart disease. Outcome of mother and fetus. *Circulation* **89**: 2673–2676.

Pulmonary hypertension and pregnancy

Pulmonary vascular disease, whether secondary to a reversed large left-to-right shunt such as a VSD, (Eisenmenger's syndrome) or to lung or connective tissue disease (e.g. scleroderma), or due to primary pulmonary hypertension, is extremely dangerous in pregnancy. Women known to have pulmonary vascular disease should be advised from an early age to avoid pregnancy and be given appropriate contraceptive advice. Maternal mortality is 40%[1]. The danger relates to fixed pulmonary vascular resistance and an inability to increase pulmonary blood flow with refractory hypoxaemia. Most deaths can be attributed to thromboembolism, hypovolaemia or pre-eclampsia.

Pulmonary hypertension is defined as a non-pregnant elevation of mean (not systolic) pulmonary artery pressure equal to or greater than 25 mmHg at rest or 30 mmHg on exercise in the absence of a left-to-right shunt. Pulmonary artery systolic (not mean) pressure is usually estimated by using Doppler ultrasound to measure the regurgitant jet velocity across the tricuspid valve. This should be considered a screening test. There is no agreed relation between the mean pulmonary pressure and the estimated systolic pulmonary pressure. If the systolic pulmonary pressure estimated by Doppler is thought to indicate pulmonary hypertension, a specialist cardiac opinion is recommended. If there is pulmonary hypertension in the presence of a left-to-right shunt the diagnosis of pulmonary vascular disease is particularly difficult and further investigation including cardiac catheterization to calculate pulmonary vascular resistance is likely to be necessary. Pulmonary hypertension as defined by Doppler studies may also occur in mitral stenosis and with large left to right shunts that have not reversed and, although such women may not have pulmonary vascular disease and a fixed PVR (or this may not have been established prior to pregnancy), they have the potential to develop it and require very careful monitoring with serial echocardiograms.

Management

- In the event of unplanned pregnancy a therapeutic termination should be offered[1]. Elective termination carries a 7% risk of mortality, hence the importance of avoiding pregnancy if possible.
- If such advice is declined, multidisciplinary care, elective admission for bed rest, oxygen, and thromboprophylaxis are recommended[2].

1 Yentis SM, Steer PJ, Plaat F (1998). Eisenmenger's syndrome in pregnancy: maternal and fetal mortality in the 1990s. *BJOG* **105**: 921–922.

2 Avila, WS, Grinberg, M, Snitcowsky *et al.* (1995). R. Maternal and fetal outcome in pregnant women with Eisenmenger's syndrome. *Eur Heart J* **16**: 460–464.

3 Rosenthal E, Nelson-Piercy C (2000). Value of inhaled nitric oxide in Eisenmenger syndrome during pregnancy (letter). *Am J Obstet Gynecol* **183**: 781–782.

- There is no evidence that monitoring the pulmonary artery pressure pre or intrapartum improves outcome, and indeed insertion of a pulmonary artery catheter increases the risk of thrombosis, which may be fatal in such women[3].
- Vasodilators given to reduce the pulmonary artery pressure will (with the exception of inhaled nitric oxide and prostacyclin), inevitably result in a concomitant lowering of the systemic pressure exacerbating hypoxaemia.
- There is no evidence that abdominal or vaginal delivery nor regional versus general anaesthesia improve outcome in pregnant women with pulmonary hypertension.
- Maternal mortality is extremely high whatever measures are taken and most fatalities occur during delivery or the first week post partum.

Marfan's syndrome and pregnancy

Eighty per cent of Marfan patients have some cardiac involvement, most commonly mitral valve prolapse and regurgitation. Pregnancy increases the risk of aortic rupture or dissection usually in the third trimester or early post-partum. Progressive aortic root dilation and an aortic root dimension >4 cm are associated with increased risk (10%). Those with aortic roots >4.6 cm cm should be advised to delay pregnancy until after aortic root repair[1]. Conversely, in women with minimal cardiac involvement and an aortic root <4 cm pregnancy outcome is usually good[2], although those with a family history of aortic dissection or sudden death are also at increased risk.

Management

- Monthly echocardiograms.
- β-blockers for those with hypertension or aortic root dilation.
- Vaginal delivery for those with stable aortic root measurements but elective caesarean section with regional anaesthesia if there is an enlarged or dilating aortic root[1].

Valvular heart disease in pregnancy

Valvular heart disease affects ~1% of pregnancies and may be associated with an increased risk of adverse maternal, fetal and neonatal outcomes. High risk features include:

- Impaired LV function (EF <40%).
- Left-sided valve stenoses* (AS with valve area <1.5 cm^2 or MS with valve area <2.0 cm^2).
- Previous maternal CVS event (CCF, TIA, CVA), or
- Symptoms* (NYHA class II or higher).

Risk increases with each additive factor, see table opposite.

* Associated with neonatal complications (prematurity, respiratory distress, IUGR, intraventricular haemorrhage, death).

1 Lipscomb KJ, Clayton Smith J, Clarke B et al. (1997). Outcome of pregnancy in women with Marfan's syndrome. *BJOG* **104**: 201–206.

2 Rossiter JP, Repke JT, Morales AJ, et al. (1995). A prospective longitudinal evaluation of pregnancy in the Marfan syndrome. *Am J Obstet Gynecol* **173**: 1599–1606.

Classification of valvular heart disease risk in pregnancy

Low maternal and fetal risk
- Asymptomatic AS with mean gradient <50 mmHg and normal LV function.
- AR, NYHA class I/II and normal LV function.
- MR, NYHA class I/II and normal LV.
- MV prolapse with no MR or with mild-moderate MR and normal LV.
- Mild–moderate MS (MV area >1.5 cm^2, gradient <5mmHg), no severe pulmonary hypertension.
- Mild–moderate PS.

High maternal and fetal risk
- Severe AS with or without symptoms.
- AR and NYHA class III or IV symptoms.
- MS with NYHA class II or higher.
- MR with NYHA class III or IV symptoms.
- AV disease, MV disease, or both, resulting in severe pulmonary hypertension (PA pressure >75% systemic pressure).
- AV disease, MV disease, or both, with LV dysfunction (LVEF <40%).
- Maternal cyanosis.
- Reduced functional status (NYHA class III or IV).

High maternal risk
- Impaired LV systolic function (LVEF <40%).
- Previous heart failure.
- Previous CVA or TIA.

High neonatal risk
- Maternal age <20 or >35 yrs.
- Use of anticoagulant therapy throughout pregnancy.
- Smoking during pregnancy.
- Multiple gestations.

Adapted from Reimold SC, Rutherford JD (2003). Valvular heart disease in pregnancy. *N Engl J Med* **349**: 52–59, with permission.

Mitral stenosis and pregnancy

This is important in pregnancy because although asymptomatic at pregnancy onset, women may deteriorate secondary to tachycardia, arrhythmias, or the increased cardiac output. The commonest complication is pulmonary oedema secondary to increased left atrial pressure, and precipitated by increased heart rate or increased volume (such as occurs during the third stage of labour or following injudicious intravenous fluid therapy)[1]. The risk is increased with severe mitral stenosis (mitral valve area <1 cm^2), moderate or severe symptoms prior to pregnancy, and in those diagnosed late in pregnancy[1].

Management

- Women with severe mitral stenosis should be advised to delay pregnancy until after valvotomy, or, if the valve is not amenable to valvotomy, until after mitral valve replacement.
- β-blockers decrease heart rate, increase diastolic filling time[2], and decrease the risk of pulmonary oedema[2].
- Diuretics should be continued in pregnancy.
- If medical therapy fails, or for those with severe mitral stenosis, balloon mitral valvotomy may be safely and successfully used in pregnancy if the valve is suitable[11]. Percutaneous balloon valvotomy carries a risk of major complications of about 1%, whereas for surgical valvotomy the figures are: closed valvotomy—fetal mortality 5–15%, maternal 3%, open valvotomy—fetal mortality 15–33%, maternal 5%.
- Women with mitral stenosis should avoid the supine and lithotomy positions as much as possible for labour and delivery. Fluid overload must be avoided, and even in the presence of oliguria, without significant blood loss, the temptation to give intravenous colloid must be resisted. Pulmonary oedema if it occurs should be treated in the usual way with oxygen and diuretics and introduction or reintroduction of a β-blocker may be useful to slow the heart rate.

Other valve lesions

Mitral regurgitation Usually due to MV prolapse. Well tolerated as systemic vascular resistance is low in pregnancy. LV function is important in assessing risk (normal function carries a good prognosis).

Aortic stenosis Usually congenital. If severe/symptomatic, advise deferring pregnancy until surgically corrected. If already pregnant and symptomatic early on, consider termination. Surgical replacement/balloon valvuloplasty are both associated with significant risks.

1 Desai DK, Adanlawo M, Naidoo DP et al. (2000). Mitral stenosis in pregnancy: a four-year experience at King Edward VIII Hospital. *BJOG* **107**: 953–958.
2 al Kasab SM, Sabag T, al Zaibag M et al. (1990). Beta-adrenergic receptor blockade in the management of pregnant women with mitral stenosis. *Am J Obstet Gynecol* **163**: 37–40.

Aortic regurgitation Usually wll tolerated as reduced systemic vascular resistance in pregnancy reduces the regurgitant volume. Vasodilators/diuretics usually sufficient treatment (stop ACE-I and replace with nifedipine, hydrallazine, etc).

Mechanical heart valves in pregnancy

The optimal management of women with metal heart valve replacements in pregnancy is controversial, since the interests of the mother and the fetus are in conflict. These women require life-long anticoagulation and this must be continued in pregnancy because of the increased risk of thrombosis. Warfarin is associated with warfarin embryopathy if given between 6 and 12 weeks gestation[1] and increased risks of miscarriage, stillbirth and fetal intracerebral haemorrhage[2]. There is some evidence that the adverse effects of warfarin are related to the dose required to maintain the INR >2, with doses in excess of 5 mg being associated with higher risks of teratogenesis, miscarriage and stillbirth[3]. Heparin and low molecular weight heparin, even in full anticoagulant doses, is associated with increased risks of valve thrombosis and embolic events[1–4].

Management

There are three basic options:
- Continue warfarin throughout pregnancy, stopping only for delivery. This is the safest option for the mother[1,2].
- Replace the warfarin with high dose unfractionated or low-molecular weight heparin from 6 to 12 weeks gestation to avoid warfarin embryopathy.
- Use high dose unfractionated or low-molecular weight heparin throughout pregnancy.

Which option is chosen will depend on several factors.
- The type of mechanical valve. The risk of thrombosis is less with the newer bi-leaflet valves (e.g. CarboMedics) than with the first generation ball and cage (e.g. Starr–Edwards), or second generation single tilting disc (e.g. Bjork–Shiley) valves.
- The position of the valve replacement. Valves in the aortic rather than the mitral position, are associated with a lower risk of thrombosis[5].
- The number of mechanical valves.
- The dose of warfarin required to maintain a therapeutic INR.
- Any previous history of embolic events.

Whichever management option is chosen, warfarin should be discontinued and substituted for heparin for 10 days prior to delivery to allow clearance of warfarin from the fetal circulation. For delivery itself heparin therapy is interrupted. Warfarin is recommended 2–3 days post-partum. In the event of bleeding, or the need for urgent delivery in a fully anticoagulated patient, warfarin may be reversed with fresh frozen plasma

1 Chan WS, Anand S, Ginsberg JS (2000). Anticoagulation of pregnant women with mechanical heart valves. *Arch Intern Med* **160**: 191–196.
2 Sadler L, McCowan L, White H *et al.* (2000). Pregnancy outcomes and cardiac complications in women with mechanical, bioprosthetic and homograft valves. *BJOG* **107**: 245–253.
3 Cotrufo M, De Feo M, De Santo L, *et al.* (2002). Risk of warfarin during pregnancy with mechanical valve prostheses. *Obstet Gynecol* **99**: 35–40.
4 Meschengieser SS, Fondevilla CG, Santarelli MT *et al.* (1999). Anticoagulation in pregnant women with mechanical heart valve prostheses. *Heart* **82**: 23–6.
5 Elkayam U (1999). Pregnancy through a prosthetic heart valve. *J Am Coll Cardiol* **33**: 1642–45.

(FFP) and vitamin K, and heparin with protamine sulphate. Vitamin K should be avoided if possible since it renders the woman extremely difficult to anticoagulate with warfarin after delivery.

Women with metal valve replacements all require antibiotic endocarditis prophylaxis for delivery regardless of the mode of delivery.[6, 7]

Anticoagulation in pregnancy

- **Unfractionated heparin** Often given in early and late pregnancy in patients with mechanical heart valves and valvular heart disease with AF. Used early in pregnancy as not teratogenic. In peri-partum period it is used for rapid control (and reversal) of anticoagulation in case emergency delivery undertaken. Not as effective as other forms of anticoagulation. *Side-effects*: haemorrhage (fetal and maternal), thrombocytopaenia (monitor FBC), osteoporosis, alopecia.
- **Low molecular weight heparin** Effective anticoagulant. Easier to monitor dosage schedule. Less likely to cause thrombocytopaenia (but does still occur). *Side-effects*: maternal and fetal haemorrhage.
- **Warfarin** Effective oral anticoagulant. Studies show it to be more effective than unfractionated heparin at preventing valve thrombosis. *Side-effects*: haemorrhage, teratogenic in first trimester therefore avoid during this period if at all possible (use heparin).
- **Aspirin** Occasionally used in high risk patients (AF, LV dysfunction, previous emboli) or those with previous prosthetic valve thrombosis. *Side-effects*: haemorrhage, prolonged labour, low birth weight (in high doses).

1 Endocarditis Working Party of the British Society for Antimicrobial Chemotherapy (1982). *Lancet* **2**: 1323–26.

2 Dajani AS, Taubert KA, Wilson W *et al.* (1997). Prevention of bacterial endocarditis. Recommendations by the American Heart Association. *JAMA* **277**: 1794–801.

Ischaemic heart disease

The risk factors for myocardial infarction (MI) in pregnancy are the same as for the non-pregnant. The risk is increased in multigravid women and in those who smoke, and women with diabetes, obesity, hypertension, and hypercholesterolaemia. Infarction most commonly occurs in the third trimester and affects the anterior wall of the heart[1]. Maternal death rate is 20%. In pregnancy the underlying aetiology is more likely to be due to non-atherosclerotic conditions (such as coronary artery thrombosis or dissection) than in the non-pregnant[1].

Management
- Management of acute MI is as for the non-pregnant woman.
- Angiography should not be withheld if clinically indicated.
- Intravenous and intracoronary thrombolysis and percutaneous transluminal coronary angioplasty and stenting have all been successfully performed in pregnancy.
- Both aspirin and β-blockers are safe in pregnancy.
- There are less data for clopidogrel and glycoprotein IIb/IIIa inhibitors although there are case reports of their successful use.
- Statins should be discontinued for the duration of pregnancy as they are associated with an increased risk of malformations[2].

Hypertrophic obstructive cardiomyopathy (HOCM)

The danger in pregnancy relates to left ventricular outflow tract obstruction that may be precipitated by hypotension or hypovolaemia. Provided these are avoided, pregnancy is usually well tolerated.

Management
- β–blockers should be continued in pregnancy or initiated for symptomatic women[3].
- Epidural anaesthesia/analgesia carries the risk of vasodilation and hypotension with consequent increased left ventricular outflow tract obstruction. Any hypovolaemia will have the same effect and should be rapidly and adequately corrected.

1 Roth A, Elkayam U (1996). Acute myocardial infarction associated with pregnancy. *Ann. Int. Med* **125**: 751–757.
2 Edison RJ, Muenke M. (2004). Central nervous system and limb anomalies in case reports of first trimester statin exposure. *NEJM* ; **350**: 1579–82.
3 Oakley GD, McGarry K, Limb DG (1979). Management of pregnancy in patients with hypertrophic cardiomyopathy. *BMJ* **1**: 1749–50.

Peripartum cardiomyopathy

This pregnancy-specific condition is defined as the development of cardiac failure between the last month of pregnancy and 5 months post-partum, in the absence of an identifiable cause or recognizable heart disease prior to the last month of pregnancy, and left ventricular systolic dysfunction. The diagnosis should be suspected in the puerperal patient with breathlessness, tachycardia, or signs of heart failure. It is confirmed with echocardiography.

Echocardiographic criteria. for peripartum LV dysfunction[1]:

- Left ventricular ejection fraction <45%.
- Fractional shortening <30%.
- LVEDP (left ventricular end diastolic pressure) >2.7 cm/m^2.
- Often, echocardiography shows the heart is enlarged with global dilation of all four chambers and markedly reduced left ventricular function.

Risk factors include:

- Multiple pregnancy.
- Hypertension (be it pre-existing or related to pregnancy or pre-eclampsia).
- Multiparity.
- Increased age.
- Afro-Caribbean race.

Management

Treatment is as for other causes of heart failure with:

- Oxygen.
- Diuretics.
- Vasodilators.
- ACE inhibitors if post-partum.
- Inotropes if required.
- Heart transplantation

About 50% of women make a spontaneous and full recovery. Most case fatalities occur close to presentation. Recent data show a 5-year survival of 94%[2] Prognosis and recurrence depend on the normalization of left ventricular size within 6 months of delivery[3]. Those women with severe myocardial dysfunction, defined as LV end diastolic dimension ≥ 6cm and fractional shortening ≤ 21% are unlikely to regain normal cardiac function

1 Pearson GD, Veille JC, Rahimtoola S *et al.* (2000). Peripartum Cardiomyopathy. National Heart, Lung and Blood Institute and Office of Rare Diseases (NIH). Workshop Recommendations and Review. *JAMA* **283**: 1183–1188.

2 Felker GM, Thompson RE, Hare JM, *et al.* (2000). Underlying causes and long-term survival in patients with initially unexplained cardiomyopathy. *N Engl J Med*, **342**: 1077–1084.

3 Elkayam U, Tummala PP, Rao K *et al.* (2001). Maternal and fetal outcomes of subsequent pregnancies in women with peripartum cardiomyopathy. *N Engl J Med* **344**: 1567–1571.

on follow-up[4]. Those whose LV function and size do not return to normal within 6 months and prior to a subsequent pregnancy are at significant risk of worsening heart failure (50%) and death (25%) or recurrent peripartum cardiomyopathy in the next pregnancy. They should therefore be advised against pregnancy[5].

4 Witlin AG, Mabie WC, Sibai BM (1997). Peripartum cardiomyopathy: a longitudinal echocardiographic study. *Am J Obstet Gynecol*, **177**:1129–1132.
5 Shotan A, Ostrezega E, Mehra A, *et al.* (1997). Incidence of arrhythmias in normal pregnancy and relation to palpitations, dizziness and syncope. *Am J Cardiol* **79**: 1061–1064.

Arrhythmias in pregnancy

Atrial and ventricular premature complexes (APC, VPC) are common in pregnancy. Many pregnant women are symptomatic from forceful heart beats that occur following a compensatory pause after a VPC. Most women with symptomatic episodes of dizziness, syncope, and palpitations do not have arrhythmias[1].

A sinus tachycardia requires investigation for possible underlying pathology such as:
• Blood loss.
• Infection.
• Heart failure.
• Thyrotoxicosis.
• Pulmonary embolus.

The commonest arrhythmia encountered in pregnancy is supraventricular tachycardia (SVT). First onset of SVT (both accessory pathway-mediated and AV nodal reentrant) is rare in pregnancy but 22% of 63 women with SVT had exacerbation of symptoms in pregnancy[2]. 50% of SVTs do not respond to vagal manoeuvres.

Management
• Propranolol, verapamil, and adenosine have FDA approval for acute termination of SVT. Adenosine has advantages over verapamil including probable lack of placental transfer and may be safely used in pregnancy for SVTs that do not respond to vagal stimulation[3,4].
• Flecanide is safe and is used in the treatment of fetal tachycardias.
• Propafenone and amiodarone should be avoided[5], the latter because of interference with fetal thyroid function.
• Temporary and permanent pacing, cardioversion, and implantable defibrillators are also safe in pregnancy[3].

Cardiac arrest in pregnancy

This should be managed according to the same protocols as used in the non-pregnant with two very important additions:

• Pregnant women (especially those in advanced pregnancy) should be 'wedged' to relieve any obstruction to venous return from pressure of the gravid uterus on the IVC. This can be most rapidly achieved by turning the patient into the left lateral position. If CPR is required then the pelvis can be tilted while keeping the torso flat to allow external chest compressions.
• The most senior member of the obstetric team should be summoned. This is to ensure that obstetric causes of the collapse are considered (e.g. amniotic fluid embolism, massive post-partum haemorrhage) and appropriately treated. In addition emergency caesarean section may be required to aid maternal resuscitation.

1 Lee SH, Chen SA, Wu TJ et al. (1995). Effects of pregnancy on first onset and symptoms of paroxysmal supraventricular tachycardia. Am J Cardiol 76: 675–678.

2 Page RL. (1995). Treatment of arrhythmias during pregnancy Am Heart 130: 871–6.

3 Mason BA, Ricci-Goodman J, Koos BJ. (1992). Adenosine in the treatment of maternal paroxysmal supraventricular tachycardia. Obstetrics & Gynecology 80: 478–480.

4 James PR. Cardiovascular disease. In Nelson-Piercy C. (ed) (2001). Prescribing in pregnancy. Bailliere's Best Practice and Research in Clinical Obstetrics and Gynaecology 15: 903–911.

5 Magee LA, Downar E, Sermer M et al. (1995). Pregnancy outcome after gestational exposure to amiodarone. Am J Obstet Gynecol ; 172: 1307–1311.

Endocarditis prophylaxis

- Antibiotic prophylaxis is mandatory for those with prosthetic valves and for those with a previous episode of endocarditis[1].
- Many cardiologists recommend that women with structural heart defects (eg. VSD) also receive prophylaxis.
- Recommendations of the American Heart Association stratify cardiac conditions into high-, moderate-, and negligible- (not requiring antibiotic prophylaxis) risk[1].
- Fatal cases of endocarditis in pregnancy have occurred antenatally, rather than as a consequence of infection acquired at the time of delivery.

Stratification of cardiac conditions according to risk of bacterial endocarditis[2]

High-risk Endocarditis prophylaxis recommended	• Prosthetic valves (metal, bioprosthetic and homografts) • Previous bacterial endocarditis • Complex cyanotic congenital heart disease (Fallot's, transposition of great arteries) • Surgical systemic/pulmonary shunts.
Moderate-risk Endocarditis prophylaxis recommended	• Other congenital cardiac malformations • Acquired valvular disease • Hypertrophic cardiomyopathy • Mitral valve prolapse with mitral regurgitation.
Negligible-risk Endocarditis prophylaxis not recommended	• Isolated secundum atrial septal defects • Surgically repaired ASD, VSD, PDA • Mitral valve prolapse without regurgitation • Physiological heart murmurs • Cardiac pacemakers.

The current UK recommendations[2] are:
- **Amoxycillin 1 g i.v. plus gentamicin 120 mg i.v.** at the onset of labour or ruptured membranes or prior to caesarean section, followed by amoxycillin 500 mg orally (or i.m/i.v. depending on patient's condition) 6 hours later.
- For women who are allergic to penicillin, vancomycin 1 g i.v. or teicoplanin 400 mg i.v. may be used instead of amoxycillin[1].

1 Dajani AS, Taubert KA, Wilson W et al. (1997). Prevention of bacterial endocarditis. Recommendations by the American Heart Association. *JAMA* **277**: 1794–801.
2 Endocarditis Working Party of the British Society for Antimicrobial Chemotherapy. (1982). *Lancet* **2**: 1323–26.

Major trials in cardiology

ADMIRAL

Abciximab before Direct Angioplasty and stenting in Myocardial Infarction Regarding Acute and Long term follow-up

Purpose: to demonstrate the superiority of abciximab over placebo in primary PTCA with stenting in 300 patients with acute myocardial infarction <12 hours symptom onset. Patients were given unfractionated heparin, aspirin and ticlopidine prior to randomization. Coronary angiography was performed at time of randomization, 24 hours and at 6 months.

Follow-up: 30 days and 6 months.

Results: abciximab in conjunction with primary stenting improved early TIMI 3 flow rate, left ventricular function and 30 day mortality, recurrent MI and rates of any revascularization. There was an excess in minor bleeding in the abciximab group.

Reference: ADMIRAL Investigators. (2001). *N Engl J Med* **344**: 1895–903.

AFCAPS/ TexCAPS

Airforce/Texas Coronary Atherosclerosis Prevention Study

Purpose: To determine if lovastatin 20–40mg/day has a role in the primary prevention of acute coronary events (MI, unstable angina, sudden cardiac death) in 5608 men and 997 women with normal or mildly elevated total or LDL choles-terol, low HDL cholesterol and with no clinically evident atherosclerotic disease in a randomized placebo controlled trial.

Follow-up: 5.2 years.

Results: lovastatin reduced LDL cholesterol by 25% and increased HDL cholesterol by 6%. The incidence of first ma-jor acute coronary events, MI, unstable angina, coronary re-vascularization and cardiovascular events were all significantly reduced. There were too few fatal cardiovascular and fatal coronary heart disease events to perform a survival analysis.

Reference: Downs JR et al. (1998) *JAMA* **279**: 1615–22.

AFFIRM

Atrial Fibrillation Follow-up Investigation of Rhythm Management (AFFIRM) Investigators

Purpose: to evaluate two management strategies in treating AF: 1) cardioversion followed by drugs to maintain sinus rhythm (a choice of amiodarone, disopyramide, flecainide, moroccine, procainamide, propafenone, quinidine, sotalol); 2) rate control drugs, allowing AF to persist (a choice of β-blockers, verapamil, diltiazem, digoxin). Anticoagulation was recommended for both groups. 4060 patients with recent on-set AF and a high risk of stroke or death were randomized. Primary endpoint was overall mortality. 71% had hypertension, 38%

had coronary artery disease. 3311 had echocardiograms, and of these, 65% had enlarged left atria, and 26% had impaired LV function.

Follow-up: 5 years.

Results: mortality at 5 years was 23.8% in the rhythm control group and 21.3% in the rate control group (hazard ratio 1.15, p=0.08). More patients in the rhythm control group were hospitalized and had more adverse drug effects. In both groups, most strokes occurred after warfarin had been stopped or if INR was subtherapeutic, and this occurred more often in the rhythm control group. During the course of the study, 594 patients assigned to the rhythm control group crossed over to the rate control group., mainly due to inability to maintain sinus rhythm and drug intolerance.

Reference: The AFFIRM Investigators. (2002) *NEJM* **347**: 1825–1833.

AFFIRM

Acute Infarction Ramipril Efficacy Study

AIRE

Purpose: to evaluate the effect of ramipril on total mortality of AMI survivors with early clinical evidence of heart failure, and to assess progression to severe/resistant heart failure, non-fatal re-infarction and stroke, compared to placebo. 2006 patients aged ≥ 18yrs with confirmed AMI 3-10 days prior to randomization with clinical evidence of heart failure were given ramipril at a starting dose of 2.5 mg or placebo.

Follow-up: mean 15 months.

Results: all cause mortality was significantly lower at 30 days and was maintained at the end of follow-up in the ramipril group (27% risk reduction), with 30% reduced risk of sudden death. 38% of the reduction in overall mortality was in the sudden death subgroup that had developed severe resistant heart failure. There was no alteration in the risk of stroke or re-infarction in the ramipril group. The study was continued in the AIREX study.

Reference: Cleland JGF et al. (1997). *Eur Heart J* **18**: 41–51.

AIRE Extension study

AIREX

Purpose: to assess the long term (3 years after the end of AIRE) benefit of ramipril in the 603 UK patients from the AIRE study retrospectively, 302 initially on ramipril, 301 on placebo.

Follow-up: 3 years.

Results: all cause mortality occurred in 27% of ramipril treated patients compared to 39% of placebo controls, repre-senting a relative risk reduction of 36%.

Reference: Hall et al. (1997). *Lancet* **349**: 1493–7.

ALLHAT

Antihypertensive and Lipid-Lowering Treatment to Prevent Heart Attack Trial

Purpose: to compare outcomes in high risk hypertensive patients >55 years old in a prospective randomized trial using standard antihypertensive drugs and newer agents as initial monotherapy. Initially, more than 42,000 patients were randomized, but this number dropped to 33,357 after the doxazosin arm was halted due to increased morbidity (mainly stroke and heart failure) in this group compared to the chlorthalidone arm. The remainder was randomized to receive chlorthalidone, amlodipine or lisinopril. 50% were women, and 35% were Black. The primary end point was the combined incidence of fatal CHD or nonfatal MI by intention to treat. Secondary outcomes were all-cause mortality, stroke, combined CHD (fatal CHD, non-fatal MI, coronary re-vascularization, or angina with hospitalization), or combined cardiovascular disease (combined CHD plus stroke, treated angina without hospitalization, heart failure, and peripheral arterial disease).

Follow-up: mean 4.9 years.

Results: all cause mortality was not different between groups. Systolic pressures were higher with both amlodipine and lisinopril compared to chlorthalidone, but diastolic pressures were slightly better with amlodipine. Secondary out-come measures were also better with chlorthalidone compared to lisinopril.

Reference: The ALLHAT Officers and Coordinators for the ALLHAT Collaborative Research Group: Major cardiovascular events in hypertensive patients randomized to doxazosin vs. chlorthalidone: The Antihypertensive and Lipid-Lowering Treatment to Prevent Heart Attack Trial (ALLHAT). (2000). *JAMA*, **283**: 1967–1975.

ASCOT-LLA

Anglo-Scandinavian Cardiac Outcomes Trial—Lipid Lowering Arm

Purpose: to assess benefits of cholesterol lowering in the primary prevention of coronary disease in hypertensive patients not conventionally deemed dyslipidaemic. 19,342 hypertensive patients with at least three other cardiovascular risk factors were randomized to one of two antihypertensive regimens (β blocker plus diuretic, or calcium channel blocker plus ACE inhibitor). Of these, 10,305 had cholesterol of >6.5 mmol/L and were randomized to atorvastatin 10 mg or placebo. Primary endpoint was death from coronary disease and non-fatal MI.

Follow-up: median 3.3 years.

Results: there was a significant reduction in the primary endpoint in the atorvastatin group (hazard ratio 0.64, p = 0.0005), with the benefit being seen by the first year of follow-up. There was a significant reduction in fatal and non-fatal stroke, total cardiovascular events and total coronary events in the atorvastatin group. Atorvastatin lowered cholesterol by 1.1 mmol/L after 3 years follow-up compared to controls. Risk reduction in primary events was unrelated to baseline cholesterol levels.

ASCOT-LLA

Reference: Sever PS *et al.* (2003). *Lancet* **361**: 1149–58.

Assessment of the Safety and Efficacy of a New Thrombolytic-1

ASSENT-1

Purpose: to evaluate the safety of different doses of TNK-tPA (tenecteplase) as a single bolus for AMI patients. 3235 patients with a mean age of 61 years were randomized to receive 30 mg (n=1705), 40 mg (n=1457) and 50 mg (n=73) of TNK-tPA over 5–10 seconds. Aspirin and iv heparin were given concomitantly.

Follow-up: on hospital discharge, and at 30 days.

Results: total stroke incidence at 30 days was 1.5%. Intracranial haemorrhage occurred in 0.77% at 30 days, with most of these occurring in the 30 mg group. The incidence of intracranial haemorrhage was lower in those treated within 6 hours of symptom onset. The incidence of death, nonfatal stroke or severe bleeding were 6.4%, 7.4%, and 1.6% for the 30 mg, 40 mg and 50 mg groups respectively, without significant differences between groups.

Reference: Van de Werf F *et al.* (1999). *Am Heart J* **1737**: 786–91.

Assessment of the Safety and Efficacy of a New Thrombolytic-2

ASSENT-2

Purpose: To compare single bolus tenecteplase (TNK-tPA) and alteplase (t-PA) infusion in treatment of AMI. 16,949 patients with symptom onset within 6 hours and median age 61 years were randomized to receive either drug. Aspirin and iv heparin were given concomitantly.

Follow-up: 30 days.

Results: 30 day mortality, non-fatal stroke and rates of intracranial haemorrhage were similar in the two groups, but fewer bleeding complications and less need for blood transfusion occurred in the TNK-tPA group.

Reference: Assessment of the Safety and Efficacy of a New Thrombolytic (ASSENT-2) Investigators, (1999). *Lancet* **354**: 716–22.

ASSENT-3
and
ASSENT 3
PLUS

Assessment of the Safety and Efficacy of a New Thrombolytic –3 , Assessment of the Safety and Efficacy of a New Thrombolytic –3 PLUS

In ASSENT 3, the aim was to determine the safety and effi-cacy of full doseTNK-tPA in combination with enoxaparin, half dose TNK-tPA plus abciximab plus low dose unfractionated heparin, or full dose TNK-tPA plus weight-adjusted un-fractionated heparin in the treatment of 6095 patients with STEMI presenting within 6 hours of symptom onset. This was the first large-scale trial to investigate the use of low molecular weight heparin in thrombolysis. The combined endpoints of 30 day mortal-ity, recurrent ischaemia, recurrent MI, major bleeding, and intracranial haemorrhage was significantly lower in the enoxaparin and abciximab group. However, if 30 mortality was considered separately, there was no sig-nificant difference between the groups. Major bleeding, mortality, intracranial haemorrhage was higher in the abciximab group, and this effect was more pronounced in patients >75 years and diabetics.

In ASSENT-3 PLUS, TNK-tPA was given to 1639 STEMI pa-tients presenting within 6 hours either with enoxaparin or un-fractionated heparin. Prehospital treatment with enoxaparin plus TNK provided no significant benefit over treatment with unfractionated heparin, although intracranial haemorrhage was greater in the enoxaparin treated patients who were >75 years old, female and weighed <60 kg. 50% of patients were treated within 2 hours compared to just 29% in ASSENT 3. Earlier treatment was associated with better 30 day mortality.

Reference: The ASSENT 3 investigators (2001). *Lancet* **358**: 605–13.

BARI

Bypass Angioplasty Revascularization Investigation

Purpose: to compare percutaneous and surgical revascu-larization strategies in patients with multivessel disease suitable for either procedure, working on the hypothesis that an initial PTCA strategy does not result in a poorer 5 year clinical outcome than CABG. Patients with mul-tivessel disease were randomized to an initial treatment strategy of CABG (n=914) or PTCA (n=915).

Follow-up: mean 5.4 years.

Results: the 5 year survival rates for CABG and PTCA were 89.3% and 86.3% respectively (p=0.19), and the respective rates free from QWMI were 80.4% and 78.7%. 8% of patients in the CABG group vs. 54% in the PTCA group under-went further revascularization procedures. 69% of the PTCA group did not undergo subsequent CABG. In diabetic patients, 5 year survival was 80.6% in the CABG group and 65.5% for the PTCA group. The conclusion was that PTCA initially did not compromise 5 year survival compared to CABG in patients with multivessel disease, except in diabetics. PTCA treated patients underwent more frequent revascularization after initial randomization.

BARI

Reference: Aldermann E *et al.* (1996). *NEJM* **335**: 217–225.

Controlled Abciximab and Device Investigation to Lower Late Angioplasty Complications

CADILLAC

Purpose: to examine the impact of the platelet glycoprotein IIb/IIIa inhibitor abciximab as an adjunct in treating acute myocardial infarction (AMI). 2082 patients with AMI were randomized in an open label 2x2 factorial design trial of primary stenting versus angioplasty, and abciximab treatment (n=1052) versus no abciximab treatment (n=1030). Baseline characteristics were balanced between groups.

Follow-up: 30 days and 1 year.

Results: at 30 days, abciximab treatment vs no abciximab significantly reduced the composite endpoint of death, MI, ischaemia-led target vessel revascularization (TVR) or disabling stroke (4.6% vs 7.0%, p=0.01). However at 12 months, there was no significant difference in composite endpoint. In an angiographic substudy (n=656), restenosis, myocardial salvage and infarct-artery reocclusion were unaffected by abciximab.

Reference: Tcheng *et al.* (2003). *Circulation* **108**:1316–23.

Canadian Amiodarone Myocardial Infarction Trial

CAMIAT

Purpose: to evaluate the impact of amiodarone versus placebo on the risk of VF or death due to arrhythmia in 1202 patients who had MI in the previous 6–45 days having frequent ventricular depolarizations (≥10/hour or ≥1 run of sustained VT). Amiodarone was given initially at 10 mg/kg daily for 2 weeks, then maintenance dose 300-400 mg daily for 3–5 months, 200–300 mg daily for 4 months, and then 200 mg for 5–7 days per week for 16 months. Patients had concomitant therapy with aspirin, β-blockers, calcium antagonist, warfarin, digoxin and ACE inhibitors.

Follow-up: mean 1.79 years.

Results: there was a relative risk reduction in the endpoints of 48.5% in the amiodarone group. Death occurred in 6.0% of the placebo group and 3.3% of the amiodarone group.

Reference: Cairns AJ *et al.* (1997). *Lancet* **349**: 675–82.

CAPRIE

Clopidogrel versus Aspirin in Patients at Risk of Ischaemic Events

Purpose: to evaluate the relative effect of 75–325 mg aspirin and 75 mg clopidogrel in reducing the risk of a composite endpoint of ischaemic stroke, MI or vascular death in 19,185 patients with recent ischaemic stroke, recent MI, or symptomatic peripheral vascular disease.

Follow-up: mean 1.9 years.

Results: compared to aspirin, clopidogrel reduced the combined risk of ischaemic stroke, MI or vascular death by 8.7% (p=0.043). There were no major differences in terms of safety or bleeding risk.

Reference: Harker LA et al. (1999). Drug Safety **4**: 325–35.

CAPTURE

Chimaeric 7E3 Antiplatelet Therapy in Unstable Angina Refractory To Standard Treatment

Purpose: to evaluate the effect of abciximab in mortality, incidence of AMI and urgent intervention for recurrent ischaemia in 1265 patients with refractory unstable angina scheduled for PTCA in a randomized placebo controlled trial. Patients in the abciximab group were given a bolus and infusion beginning 18-24 hours before the PTCA and continuing 1 hour after PTCA. The primary endpoint was death, AMI or urgent intervention within 30 days of enrolment.

Follow-up: 30 days and 6 months.

Results: at 30 days the primary endpoint occurred in 11.3% of the abciximab group and 15.9% of the placebo group (p=0.012). The rate of MI was lower in the abciximab group than placebo both before and during PTCA. Major bleeding occurred more frequently in the abciximab group than placebo. At 6 months, there was no significant difference in the rates of death, MI, or repeat intervention however.

Reference: The CAPTURE Investigators (1997). Lancet **349**: 1429–35.

CARE

Cholesterol and Recurrent Events

Purpose: to evaluate the effect of 40 mg pravastatin on fatal and non-fatal MI in patients with average cholesterol levels. 4159 patients were recruited in a randomized, double blind placebo-controlled trial aged 21–75 years who had MI 3–20 months before randomization. Plasma cholesterol was <240 mg/dL, LDL 115–274 mg/dL, triglycerides <350 mg/dl. If LDL cholesterol increased during the study, dietary counseling was offered as well as cholestyramine.

Follow-up: at least 5 years.

Results: the pravastatin group had 24% lower risk of fatal and non-fatal MI, the risk of CABG was reduced by

26%, risk of PTCA reduced by 23%. There was no reduction in coronary events if baseline total cholesterol was <125 mg/dl.

Reference: Sacks et al. (1996) N Engl J Med **335**: 1001–9.

Carvedilol ACE Inhibitor Remodelling Mild Heart Failure Evaluation Trial

Purpose: to evaluate effects of carvedilol and enalapril, either alone or in combination, upon 572 patients with LVEF<40% in a randomized double-blind parallel group study. Primary outcome was measuring left ventricular end systolic volume index (LVESVI) using echo at baseline and at 6, 12, and 18 months to represent changes in LV remodelling.

Follow-up: 18 months.

Results: Combination therapy significantly reduced LVESVI compared to enalapril alone, and carvedilol significantly improved LVESVI compared to baseline, while enalapril did not.

Reference: Remme et al. (2004). Cardiovasc Drugs Ther. **18(1)**: 57–66.

Candesartan in Heart Failure

Purpose: 7601 patients with symptomatic heart failure were entered into 3 individual component randomized trials in which candesartan was used at 4 or 8 mg a day, titrated to target dose 32 mg vs placebo: 1) CHARM Added- patients with LVEF ≤ 40% and treated with an ACE-inhibitor; 2) CHARM Alternative- patients with LVEF ≤40% and ACE-inhibitor intolerant; 3) CHARM Preserved- patients with LVEF ≤40% with or without ACE-inhibitor. Primary outcome results were all-cause mortality for the trial as a whole, or cardiovascular mortality/CHF hospitalization for component trials.

Follow-up: minimum 2 years.

Results: CHARM Overall: lower cardiovascular mortality compared to placebo (23.3% vs 24.9%, p=0.055), and lower cardiovascular mortality/CHF hospitalizaton (30.2% vs 34.5%, p<0.0001). CHARM Added: lower cardiovascular mortality compared to placebo (23.7% vs 27.3%, p=0.02) and lower heart failure hospitalizations. CHARM Alternative: lower mortality compared to placebo (21.6% vs 24.8%, p=0.072) and lower heart failure hospitalizations. CHARM Preserved: non-significant reduction in death and lower heart failure hospitalizations.

Reference: Pfeffer et al. (2003). Lancet **362**: 759–66.

CIBIS

Cardiac Insufficiency Bisoprolol Study
Purpose: to evaluate effects on mortality 641 of patients with NYHA III and IV heart failure and LVEF <40% using bisoprolol in a randomized double blind placebo-controlled trial.
Follow-up: 2 years.
Results: Significant reduction in hospitalization due to heart failure in the bisoprolol group, and significant improvement in functional class, but no significant difference in mortality, sudden death, or death related to VF or VT.

Reference: CIBIS Investigators and Committees. (1994). Circulation **90**: 1765–73.

CIBIS II

Cardiac Insufficiency Bisoprolol study II
Purpose: to evaluate bisoprolol in reducing mortality in 2647 patients with NYHA III and IV heart failure in a randomized double blind placebo-controlled trial, and also to deter-mine safety and efficacy using cardiovascular death and hospitalization.
Follow-up: mean 1.3 years.
Results: all cause mortality, hospital admission and death were significantly lower in the bisoprolol group. All cause mortality at 2 years was significantly lower in women.

Reference: Simon et al. (1999). Circulation **100** Suppl I: 1–297.

COMET

Carvedilol or Metoprolol European Trial
Purpose: to determine if the beta 2 receptor and alpha 1 blocking effect of carvedilol (target dose 25 mg bd), in addition to its effect of increasing insulin sensitivity, confers a greater benefit in heart failure compared to metoprolol tartrate (target dose 50 mg bd), with which it shares a beta 1 blocking effect, in a randomized double-blind parallel group trial. 3028 Patients had NYHA class II-IV, LVEF <35%, on optimum therapy with ACE-I and diuretics. Primary endpoints was all-cause mortality, composite endpoint was all-cause mortality or all-cause admission.
Follow-up: mean 58 months.
Results: 17% reduction in all cause mortality in carvedilol group.

Reference: Poole-Wilson et al. Comparison of carvedilol and metoprolol on clinical outcomes in patients with chronic heart failure in the Carvedilol Or Metoprolol European Trial (COMET): randomised controlled trial. (2003) Lancet. Jul 5; **362** (9377): 7–13.

Comparison of Medical Therapy, Pacing, and Defibrillation In Heart Failure Trial

Purpose: to compare rates of hospitalization or death of >1600 patients with heart failure and evidence of conduction delay on surface ECG. Patients had NYHA class III or IV, LVEF ≤35%, QRS ≥120 ms, PR>150 ms. They were hospitalized at least once in the previous year. They were treated using optimal drug therapy alone (including β-blockers, ACE-inhibitors, angiotensin receptor blockers, spironolactone), drug therapy plus a biventricular pacemaker (cardiac resynchronization), or drug therapy plus a defibrillator with resynchronization capability.

Follow-up: 12 months.

Results: the combination of all-cause death and all-cause hospitalization was reduced in both resynchronization groups, with a greater being observed for the defibrillator arm com-pared to the pacemaker arm (43.4% and 23.9% mortality reduction respectively). No significant difference in effect was found between patients with ischaemic and non-ischaemic cardiomyopathy.

Reference: Pinski SL. Continuing progress in the treatment of severe congestive heart failure. (2003). *JAMA* Feb 12; **289**(6): 754–6.

Carvedilol Prospective Randomized Cumulative Survival trial

Purpose: to evaluate the impact of carvedilol on mortality in 2289 patients with severe heart failure, LVEF <25% in a randomized double-blind placebo-controlled trial.

Follow-up: mean 10.4 months.

Results: 35% decrease in mortality in the carvedilol group compared to placebo.

Reference: Packer M *et al.* (2001). *N Engl J Med* **344**: 1651–8.

Clopidogrel for Reduction of Events During Observation

Purpose: to evaluate the benefit of long-term clopidogrel after PCI combined with aspirin, and to evaluate the benefit of initiating clopidogrel with loading dose before the procedure. 2116 patients with symptomatic coronary artery disease and objective evidence of ischaemia who were undergoing elective PCI or were deemed highly likely to undergo PCI were enrolled in 99 centres in North America. Patients were randomized to receive a 300 mg clopidogrel loading dose (n=1053) or placebo (n=1063)

CREDO

3 to 24 hours before PCI. After the procedure, all patients received clopidogrel 75 mg/d for 28 days. From day 29 to 12 months, the loading dose group received clopidogrel 75 mg/d, whereas placebo was given to the control group. The 1-year primary end point was a composite of death, myocardial infarction (MI), and stroke in the intent-to-treat population.

Follow-up: 28 days, 6 months, and 1 year.

Results: at 1 year, there was a 26.9% risk reduction in the combined endpoint of the clopidogrel treated group. Pretreatment did not significantly reduce the endpoint, but in a subgroup of patients receiving the loading dose more than 6 hours beforehand there was a significant risk reduction.

Reference: Steinbuhl et al. (2002) JAMA **288**: 2411–2420.

CTOPP

Canadian Trial Of Physiological Pacing

Purpose: to assess potential benefits (measured by risk of cardiovascular death or stroke) of physiological (dual chamber) pacemakers compared non-physiological (single chamber) pacemakers over an extended period. 1474 patients requiring pacemakers for symptomatic bradycardia were randomized to receive one of the two modes of pacemaker.

Follow-up: initially 3 years, extended to a mean 6.4 years

Results: there was no difference between groups in the primary outcome measures of cardiovascular death or stroke, or total mortality. However there was a significant reduction in the risk of developing atrial fibrillation in the physiological pacing group (relative risk reduction 20.1%, p=0.009).

Reference: Kerr CR et al (2004). Circulation **109**: 357–362.

CURE

Clopidogrel in Unstable Angina to Prevent Recurrent Events

Purpose: to evaluate the impact of clopidogrel on 12,562 patients presenting within 24 hours of onset of acute coro-nary syndrome symptoms, either unstable angina (75%) or non ST elevation MI (25%). Patients were randomized to receive 75 mg clopidogrel or placebo, preceded by 75-325 mg aspirin. There were similar rates of use of iv heparin, LMWH, ACE inhibitors, β-blockers and lipid lowering agents in the two groups.

Follow-up: mean 9 months.

Results: The clopidogrel group had a 20% overall reduction in the primary composite endpoint of cardiovascular death, non-fatal MI and non-fatal stroke, and this benefit was seen within 30 days. There was also a reduction in the incidence of refractory ischaemia by 14% and severe ischaemia by 24% in the clopidogrel group. All subgroups benefited from clopidogrel treatment. The incidence of major bleeding was 34% higher in the clopidogrel group (3.6% vs 2.7%, p=0.003), but life-threatening-bleeding did not differ between the groups.

Reference: CURE Study Investigators. (2000). *Eur J Cardiol* **21**: 2033–2041.

CURE

DANish trial in Acute Myocardial Infarction

Purpose: to compare a deferred invasive strategy of PCI or CABG (n=503, within 2-5 week of discharge) with a conservative strategy (n=505) in patients with inducible myocardial ischaemia (on exercise testing) within the first few weeks after receiving thrombolysis for a first AMI. Primary endpoints were death, AMI and admission with unstable angina.

DANAM I

Follow-up: 2.4 years.

Results: in the invasive group, PCI was given to 53% and CABG to 29%. Mortality was not significantly different at 2.4 years between the invasive and conservative groups. However, the invasive group had a lower incidence of AMI, unstable angina, and stable angina. Therefore the recommendation was to refer patients with inducible ischaemia following AMI for a coronary angiogram ± revascularization.

Reference: Madsen *et al* (1997). *Circulation* **96**: 748–755.

DANish trial in Acute Myocardial Infarction 2

Purpose: a comparison of coronary angioplasty with thrombolysis in AMI in patients who require transport from a community hospital to a centre capable of PCI. 1572 patients with AMI were randomized to alteplase or angioplasty; of these, 443 were at invasive-treatment centre. Platelet GpIIb/IIIa inhibitors were given at the discretion of the physician performing PCI; ticlopidine or clopidogrel was given to all patients undergoing PCI for at least 1 month. The primary endpoint was a composite of death, clinical evidence of infarction or disabling stroke at 30 days.

DANAMI II

Results: in those patients randomized from community hospitals, the primary endpoint was reached in 8.5% of the invasive group compared to 14.2 % the thrombolysis group (p=0.002). In invasive centres, the endpoint rates were 6.7% and 12.3% for invasive and thrombolysis groups respectively (attributable mainly due to lower rates of re-infarction). There was no significant difference in death or stroke rates. 96% of patients were transferred from a community hospital to an invasive center within 2 hours. An invasive strategy is better than thrombolysis in patients at community hospitals if the transfer takes less than 2 hours.

Reference: Henning R *et al.* (2003). *NEJM* **349**: 733–742.

DAVID

Dual chamber and VVI Implantable Defibrillator
Purpose: to evaluate efficacy of dual chamber (DDDR) pacing compared with backup ventricular pacing (VVI) in 506 patients with standard indications for ICD implantation but without indications for anti-bradycardia pacing. All had LVEF <40%, no bradycardia indications for pacing, and no persistent atrial arrhythmias. They were randomized to VVI at a backup rate of 40/min or DDDR at a backup rate of 70/min. Optimum medical therapy was continued. Primary composite endpoint was time to death or first hospitalization for CCF.
Follow-up: 1 year.
Results: the VVI group had one year survival free rate of 83.9% vs. 73.3% for the DDDR group. The composite end-point, mortality (6.5% in VVI vs. 10.1% DDDR) as well as hospitalization for heart failure was also better in the VVI group. This suggested that in patients without bradycardia indications for pacing but with indications for ICD and LVEF <40%, DDDR mode may have no advantage and may prove detrimental over VVI.
Reference: Wilkoff BL *et al.* (2002). *JAMA* **288**: 3115–23.

DIAMOND

Danish Investigations of Arrhythmia and Mortality on Dofetilide
Purpose: to evaluate the prophylactic use of dofetilide in 3028 patients at high risk of sudden death. There were two arms; the congestive heart failure (CHF) arm (n=1518), and the AMI arm (n=1510), with patients having had AMI within 7 days. Dofetilide was given at 250 mg once daily initially, titrating to 500 mg twice daily, and was reduced or withdrawn if creatinine clearance fell or QTc was >20% baseline or >550 ms. There were placebo controls. A substudy examined the effect of Dofetilide in the CHF arm upon the rates of cardioversion to sinus rhythm those patients who had AF.
Follow-up: ≥12 months.
Results: one year mortality was 28% in the CHF arm and 22% in the AMI arm. There were fewer hospitalizations for heart failure compared to placebo, but no significant difference in mortality between the dofetilide group as a whole and placebo. In the CHF arm, there was a significantly greater conversion rate of patients to sinus rhythm compared to placebo.
Reference: Torp-Pederson C *et al.* (1999). *NEJM* **341**: 857–65, *Circulation* 2001; **104**: 292–6.

DIG

Digitalis Investigation Group
Purpose: to evaluate the effect of digoxin versus placebo on all-cause mortality in 7788 patients in sinus rhythm with symptoms of heart failure and with LVEF ≤45%.

Follow-up: maximum 5 years.

Results: overall mortality was not reduced by digoxin compared to placebo. However there was a significant reduction in hospitalization for worsening heart failure (p < 0.001).

Reference: The Digitalis Investigation Group. (1997). *NEJM* **336**: 525–33.

Diabetes mellitus Insulin-Glucose infusion in Acute Myocardial infarction

Purpose: to determine if insulin-glucose infusion in diabetic patients with AMI reduces initial high mortality rate, and if strict metabolic control during the early post-infarction period improves prognosis. 620 diabetic patients with suspected AMI and glucose >11 mmol/L were randomized to receive insulin-glucose infusion, and subsequently subcutaneous insulin for ≥ 3months.

Follow-up: 12 months.

Results: at 12 months there was a relative mortality reduction of 29% in the control group. This risk reduction was most pronounced in patients with a low cardiovascular risk profile, who were not previously on insulin, with a relative risk reduction of 52% at 3 months (p=0.046) and 52% at I year (p=0.2).

Reference: Malmberg (1995). *J Am Coll Cardiol* **26**:57–65.

European Myocardial Infarction Amiodarone Trial

Purpose: to evaluate the effect of amiodarone on mortality in 1486 patients enrolled 5–21 days post MI with LVEF <40% in a randomized double blind placebo controlled manner.

Follow-up: median 21 months.

Results: all cause mortality and cardiac mortality did not differ between the groups, but there was a 35% risk reduction in arrhythmic deaths in the amiodarone group (p=0.05).

Reference: Julian DG et al. (1997). *Lancet* **349**: 667–674.

Evaluation in PTCA to Improve Long-Term Outcome with abciximab GPIIb/IIIA blockade

Purpose: to determine the effect of the glycoprotein receptor blocker cF7E3 (abciximab) on mortality and morbidity when used during percutaneous coronary intervention. In a randomized double blind placebo controlled trial 2792 patients were given iv unfractionated heparin as a bolus, and were randomly assigned to receive either placebo, or abciximab. Within the abciximab group, patients could either receive an additional bolus of heparin alone, or an additional bolus plus an infusion of heparin.

Follow-up: 30 days.

DIG

DIGAMI

EMIAT

EPILOG

EPILOG

Results: there was a significant reduction in the composite event rate in the abciximab group, with no significant difference between the high or low dose heparin subgroups within the abciximab group. There was no difference in the risk of major bleeding, although minor bleeding was more frequent in the abciximab group. The trial was stopped after the interim analysis showed a reduction in death and MI that exceeded the predetermined stopping level in the abciximab group.

Reference: The EPILOG investigators. (1997). *N Engl J Med* **336**: 1689–96.

EPISTENT

Evaluation of Platelet IIb/IIIa inhibition in Stenting
Purpose: To evaluate the influence of the platelet glycoprotein inhibitor cF7E3 upon coronary disease treated by PTCA or stenting. Study design was randomized, double blinded, part placebo controlled. 2399 patients who were to undergo elective or urgent intervention, either balloon angioplasty alone or stenting, were randomized to receive abciximab or placebo. Aspirin and heparin were given to all patients, with ticlopidine being given at physician's discretion.
Follow-up: 6 months.
Results: Death, MI, or need for urgent revascularization was lower within 30 days in both the abciximab groups compared to placebo. Within the abciximab group, these rates were lower in the stenting group compared to the PTCA group alone. These trends were also observed at 6 months.

Reference: Lincoff *et al.* (1999). *N Engl J Med* **341**: 319–27.

EUROPA

European trial On reduction of cardiac events with Perindopril in stable coronary Artery disease
Purpose: to evaluate the effect of perindopril on cardiovascular risk in a low risk population and no overt heart failure. 12,218 patients with previous MI, angiographic evidence of coronary disease, coronary revascularization or a positive exercise test were randomized to receive perindopril 8 mg once daily or placebo. Concomitant treatment was with anti-platelet therapy (92%), β-blockers (62%) and lipid lowering agents (58%). Primary endpoint was cardiovascular death, MI or cardiac arrest.
Follow-up: mean 4.2 years.
Results: the primary endpoint was reached by 8% of the perindopril group and 10% of placebo (p=0.0003) representing a 20% risk reduction. Perindopril was well tolerated.

Reference: The EUROPA Investigators (2003). *Lancet* **362**: 782–88.

Fragmin during Instability in Coronary Artery Disease

Purpose: to determine whether the addition of the low molecular weight heparin fragmin (dalteparin) influences the recurrence of cardiac events in patients with unstable angina if added to aspirin and anti-anginal drugs. Study design was randomized, double blind, placebo-controlled, parallel-group. 1506 patients who were in hospital with unstable angina within 72 hours of having chest pain were given either placebo or fragmin 120 U/kg every 12 hours for the first 6 days then 7500 U once a day for 35–45 days thereafter. All patients were on aspirin and β-blockers (unless contra-indicated), with calcium antagonists and nitrates as required.

Follow-up: up to 7 months.

Results: mortality, need for revascularization, re-infarction, and need for iv heparin were lower in the first 6 days in the fragmin group. There was also a significant reduction in the composite endpoint (death, revascularization, iv heparin use, MI) which persisted for up to 40 days for non-smokers (80% of the sample), but this effect was not carried 4 to 5 months after the end of treatment in the group as a whole. If the dose of fragmin were decreased, there was a risk of reinfarction that was more in smokers.

Reference: Fragmin during Instability in Coronary Artery Disease (FRISC) study group. (1996). *Lancet* **347**: 561–8.

Fragmin and Revascularization during Instability in Coronary artery disease

Purpose: To evaluate the impact of 3 months continuous fragmin (dalteparin, a low molecular weight heparin) in patients with unstable angina, and to compare a direct invasive strategy with a stepwise approach, preferably non-invasive. Study design was randomized, double blind, placebo controlled. 2457 patients with anginal symptoms within 48 hours were randomized to have an initial invasive or non-invasive strategy. Within these two groups, patients were randomized to fragmin or placebo for 3 months. All patients received aspirin and β-blockers (unless contra-indicated), as well as nitrates, calcium antagonists, statins, and ACE-inhibitors, although these were optional.

Follow-up: 6 months.

Results: there were significantly fewer deaths and MI in the early revascularization group at 6 months in the invasive group, independent of fragmin treatment. There was a non-significant decrease in deaths when considered separately. At 6 months, 23% of the non-invasive group had an invasive procedure.

Reference: Invasive compared with non-invasive treatment in unstable coronary-artery disease: FRISC II prospective ran-domised multicentre study. (1999). *Lancet* **354**: 708–15.

GISSI-1

Gruppo Italiano per lo Studio della Streptochinasinell'Infarto miocardio

Purpose: to evaluate whether: 1) streptokinase (SK) reduces in-hospital and 1 year mortality after AMI; 2) the effect of reduction, if present, depends on the interval between pain onset and treatment 3) the risks of treatment are acceptable. 11521 patients with AMI were randomized to SK 1.5MU over 1 hour, or control.

Follow-up: 1 year.

Results: at 21 days there was an 18% reduction in mortality in the SK group as a whole (p=0.0002). However in those treated within 3 hours, mortality was reduced by 23% (p=0.0005). At 12 months, total mortality was 17.2% in the SK group vs. 19.0% in controls (relative risk 0.9, p=0.0008).

Reference: GISSI Study Group (1987). *Lancet* **ii**: 871–4.

GISSI-2

Gruppo Italiano per lo Studio della Sopravvivenzanell'Infarto miocardico

Purpose: to compare streptokinase (SK) and alteplase (rt-PA) in 12490 AMI patients, and to evaluate the effects of heparin after thrombolysis with either agent, upon survival and post-ischaemic events in a randomized open label controlled 2x2 factorial design.

Follow-up: 6 months.

Results: there was no significant difference in the combined endpoint of death and severe left ventricular damage, rates of in-hospital complications (15 days post thrombolysis), or rates of reinfarction in all groups, with or without heparin. Major bleeding occurred more frequently in the SK plus heparin group, but stroke rates were similar in all groups (1.14%); rt-PA was associated with a small but excess risk of stroke. Major bleeding was more frequent with SK compared to rt-PA. Hypertensive patients had higher mortality through-out the followup period.

Reference: GISSI 2 Study Group (1996). *J Hypertens* **14**: 743–50.

GISSI-3

Gruppo Italiano per lo Studio della Sopravvivenzanell'Infarto miocardico

Purpose: to evaluate the independent and combined effects of lisinopril and nitrates, on survival and LV function after AMI in 18895 patients presenting within 24 hours of symptoms in a randomized open label controlled factorial trial. Nitrates were given initially as a GTN infusion, then as a patch or oral isosorbide mononitrate after 24 hours. Oral lisinopril was started at a dose of 2.5-5 mg once daily and titrated up to 10 mg after 24 hours. Controls were given neither drug. Trial drugs were continued for 6 weeks.

Follow-up: 6 weeks and 6 months.

Results: overall mortality and LV dysfunction at 6 weeks was significantly reduced by lisinopril, although GTN did not influence outcome. At 6 months, overall mortality was 18.1% in the lisinopril groups compared to 19.3% in those without lisinopril (p=0.015); GTN produced no difference in mortality.

Reference: GISSI 3 Study Group (1996). *J Am Coll Cardiol* **27**: 37–44.

GISSI-3

Gruppo Italiano per lo Studio della Sopravvivenza nell'Infarto miocardico Prevenzione

Purpose: to evaluate the impact of the dietary supplements n-3 polyunsaturated fatty acids (PUFA) and vitamin E within 3 months of MI in 11324 patients in a randomized open parallel group trial. Patients had concomitant therapy with aspirin, β-blockers and ACE-I.

Follow-up: 3.5 years.

Results: vitamin E had no impact, either alone or in combination, upon the risk of death, non-fatal MI or non-fatal stroke, but there was a significant reduction in these endpoints with PUFA (20% reduction in CVS death, non-fatal MI or non-fatal stroke), mainly attributable to decrease in the risk of death and cardiovascular death.

Reference: GISSI-Prevenzione Investigators (1999). *Lancet* **354**: 447–55.

GISSI-Prevenzione

Global Utilization of Streptokinase and t-PA for Occluded coronary arteries

Purpose: to compare in a randomized parallel group the effect of treatment with a) streptokinase (SK) and sc heparin vs. b) streptokinase (SK) and iv heparin vs. c) rt-PA with iv heparin (accelerated regimen) vs. d) rt-PA and streptokinase (SK) and iv heparin simultaneously in the treatment of AMI in 41021 patients <6 hrs after symptom onset. Concomitant therapy included aspirin and atenolol.

Follow-up: 30 days and 1 year.

Results: at both 30 days and 1 year, there was a 14% reduction in mortality in the accelerated t-PA group compared to the two SK only regimens. Combination of SK and t-PA led to no significant difference in 1 year mortality compared to SK only, and a marginal difference when compared to t-PA only. Although the accelerated t-PA group had significantly more haemorrhagic strokes compared to the SK groups and the combination groups, overall there were fewer complications in the accelerated t-PA group, as well as significantly lower endpoint of death and disabling stroke at 1 year. However in patients >75 yrs, those treated by accelerated t-PA had higher mortality at

GUSTO-1

GUSTO-1

30 days compared to younger patients but still had a greater absolute net benefit. Older patients generally had a greater risk of mortality, stroke, bleeding and re-infarction.

Reference: White et al. (1996) Circulation **94**: 1826–33.

GUSTO IV-ACS

Global use of Strategies to Open Occluded Coronary Arteries IV- Acute Coronary Syndrome
Purpose: to investigate long term effects of abciximab in patients with ACS without ST elevation who were not scheduled for coronary intervention. 7800 patients with positive troponin or persistent ST depression were randomized to abciximab bolus and 24 infusion, abciximab bolus and 48 hour infusion, or placebo.
Follow-up: 1 year.
Results: There was no survival benefit in the abciximab group. IN subgroups with low troponin or high CRP, abciximab was associated with a higher mortality.

Reference: Ottervanger et al. (2003) Circulation **107**: 437–442.

HOPE

Heart Outcomes Prevention Evaluation Trial
Purpose: to assess the role of the ACE-inhibitor ramipril and vitamin E in patients at high risk of cardiovascular events who did not have LV dysfunction or heart failure. 9297 patients >55 yrs old with evidence of vascular disease (previous MI, angina, multivessel PTCA or CABG, multivessel coronary artery disease, peripheral vascular disease, cerebrovascular disease) or diabetes plus one other risk factors, not known to have a low LV EF or heart failure were randomly assigned to receive 10 mg ramipril (titrated up from 2.5 mg) or placebo, plus vitamin E 400 U/day or placebo. Primary outcome was composite of MI, stroke or death from cardiovascular events. Secondary endpoints were death from any cause, need for revascularization, hospitalization for unstable angina or heart failure, and complications of diabetes. Patients had approximately similar usage of aspirin, β-blockers, lipid-lowering agents, diuretics and calcium channel blockers in the two groups.
Follow-up: mean 5 years.
Results: more people in the ramipril group stopped treatment due to cough, hypotension or dizziness. However there was a significant reduction in the primary endpoints of MI, stroke, death compared to placebo (14% vs 17%), as well a reduction in total mortality. There was no significant reduction in non-cardiovascular death. In the ramipril group there was also significantly less need for revascularization, complications of diabetes, heart failure, worsening angina, and smaller incidence of

new onset diabetes. The reduction in the primary endpoint and cardiovascular death was even more striking in diabetics (15.3% vs 19.6%). There was a clear benefit in the ramipril group in patients with or without evidence of coronary artery disease, with or without history of MI and EF >40%. Benefits were also seen whether or not patients were taking aspirin, β-blockers, lipid-lowering agents or antihypertensive drugs. In the vitamin E group there were no significant differences in primary or secondary endpoints. The study was stopped 6 months early due to consistent observed benefits in primary endpoints.

HOPE

Reference: The Heart Outcomes Prevention Evaluation (HOPE) Study Investigators. *N Engl J Med*, January 20, 2000.

Heart Protection Study

HPS

Purpose: to evaluate whether the lowering of blood concentrations of low density lipoprotein cholesterol (LDL-C), irrespective of the initial cholesterol measure, is associated with a lower cardiovascular risk. 20,536 patients with coronary disease, other occlusive arterial disease or diabetes were randomized to 40 mg simvastatin once daily or placebo. The average compliance in the statin group was 85%, and in the placebo group the average non-study statin use was 17%. Primary outcome measures were death, and fatal or non-fatal vascular events.

Follow-up: 5 years.

Results: all cause mortality was significantly reduced in the simvastatin group (12.9% vs. 14.7%, p=0.0003) mainly due to an 18% reduction in the coronary death rate. There was a marginal reduction in other vascular deaths, and no significant reduction in non-vascular deaths. There was a significant reduction in the first event rate for non-fatal MI or coronary death, non-fatal or fatal stroke and for coronary revascularization. The proportional reduction in event rate was similar in each subcategory, that is those with diagnosed coronary artery disease, cerebrovascular disease, peripheral vascular disease, diabetes; and separately, in women; in those whose presenting LDL-C was <3.0 mmol/L or total cholesterol <5 mmol/L. The benefits of simvastatin were in addition to existing treatments. There was a 0.01 annual excess risk of myopathy, and no significant adverse effects on cancer incidence or hospitalization for any non-vascular causes.

Reference: Heart Protection Study Collaborative Group (2002). *Lancet* **360**: 7–22.

First International Study of Infarct Survival

ISIS 1

Purpose: to assess the impact on mortality of early use of β-blockers (atenolol 5-10 mg iv over 5 mins followed by 100 mg orally once daily for 7 days) randomized in

ISIS 1

16,027 patients with acute MI (<12 hours), in the first week and after longer follow-up.

Follow-up: mean 20 months.

Results: in first 7 days, 15% reduction (p < 0.02) in vascular deaths in atenolol group, with greatest benefit on day 1, due to reduction of acute myocardial rupture. Further reduction in deaths observed after 1 year.

Reference: Randomized trial of intravenous atenolol among 16027 cases of suspected acute myocardial infarction: ISIS-1 (1986). *Lancet* **ii**: 57–66.

ISIS-2

Second International Study of Infarct Survival

Purpose: to assess effects of iv streptokinase and oral aspirin either alone or in combination in patients with suspected AMI (symptoms <24 hours, median 5 hours). 17,187 patients randomized.

Follow-up: up to 34 months.

Results: reduction on 5 week mortality with streptokinase alone or aspirin alone. There was 25% odds reduction in death with streptokinase and 23% odds reduction with aspirin. There was a 42% odds reduction in death with aspirin and streptokinase combined compared to the placebo group. Streptokinase was associated with more bleeding requiring blood transfusion (0.5% vs. 0.2% in placebo group), but fewer strokes (0.6% vs. 0.8% in placebo group). Aspirin significantly reduced nonfatal re-infarction and nonfatal stroke.

Reference: The ISIS-2 collaborative group (1988). *Lancet* **ii**: 349–60.

ISIS-3

Third International Study of Infarct Survival

Purpose: to compare streptokinase vs. rt-PA vs. anistreplase (APSAC), plus aspirin or aspirin plus heparin in 41299 patients with definite or suspected AMI (symptom onset <24 hrs), in a randomized double-blind parallel group factorial design.

Follow-up: 6 months

Results: the addition of heparin resulted in slightly fewer deaths and more major non-cerebral bleeds, but no significant increase in cerebral haemorrhage; there was no significant difference in mortality after 2 months. The APSAC group had more reports of allergy and cerebral bleeds compared to the streptokinase group, with similar survival rates after 6 months. In the rt-PA group, there were more cerebral bleeds, but fewer re-infarctions compared to the streptokinase group, without any significant difference in mortality between the groups.

Reference: The ISIS-3 (Third International Study of Infarct Survival) collaborative group (1992). *Lancet* **339**:753–70.

Fourth International Study of Infarct Survival

Purpose: to assess the effect on 5 week mortality of oral isosorbide mononitrate, oral captopril or iv magnesium, separately or in combination, on 58,050 patients with definite or suspected AMI (symptom onset <24 hrs) in addition to standard therapy. The study design was randomized, partly placebo controlled, partly open, 2x2x2 factorial.

Follow-up: 5 weeks.

Results: in contrast to magnesium and nitrate, the captopril group had a small but significant survival benefit that was maintained after one year, with greatest benefit in those at highest risk.

Reference: ISIS-4 (Fourth International Study of Infarct Survival) Collaborative Group (1995). *Lancet* **345**: 669–85.

Losartan Intervention For Endpoint Reduction in Hypertension

Purpose: to evaluate the long-term effects of once-daily losartan compared with those of atenolol in patients with diabetes, hypertension and ECG-documented LVH, with respect to the incidence of cardiovascular morbidity and mortality (cardiovascular death, stroke or myocardial infarction). 1195 patients with mean blood pressure 177/96 mmHg after placebo run-in were randomized to losartan or atenolol based treatment.

Follow-up: mean 4.7 years.

Results: all-cause mortality and cardiovascular death were significantly lower in the losartan group. However there was no difference in the risk of stroke or myocardial infarction. Losartan decreased ECG LVH better than atenolol. Losartan seemed to have benefits beyond BP reduction alone.

Reference: Lindholm LH *et al.* (2002). *Lancet* **359**: 1004–1010.

Long-term Intervention with Pravastatin in IHD

Purpose: to evaluate the impact of long term treatment with 40 mg pravastatin upon mortality and morbidity in patients with a history of AMI, and unstable angina within 3–36 months of starting the trial with baseline cholesterol 4–7 mmol/L. 9014 patients aged 31-75 years. The trial was randomized, double blind, placebo controlled.

Follow-up: mean 6.1 years.

Results: in the pravastatin group there was a relative risk reduction of 24% in death from coronary disease, and 22% relative risk reduction in all-cause mortality. There was also a significant reduction in incidence of non-fatal MI, stroke and coronary revascularization.

Reference: The LIPID Study Group (1998). *N Engl J Med* **339**: 1349–57.

MADIT

Multicenter Automatic Defibrillator Implantation Trial
Purpose: to determine if patients at high risk of sudden cardiac death would have reduced mortality if AICD implanted compared to conventional drug therapy. 300 patients with history of ventricular tachycardia or QWMI (>1 month previously) and LVEF <35% randomized to receive either AICD or drug therapy (most commonly amiodarone).
Follow-up: mean 27 months.
Results: 54% reduction in all-cause mortality in AICD group compared to non-device group.

Reference: MADIT Executive Committee. *Pacing Clin Electrophysiol* 1991; **14**: 920–7.

MADIT II

Multicenter Automatic Defibrillator Implantation Trial II
Purpose: to evaluate the impact of prophylactic ICD therapy in patients with MI at lest 30 days prior to enrolment and poor LV EF (≤ 30%). 1232 patients were randomized to receive conventional drug therapy alone (490 patients) or a combination of both ICD and drug therapy (742 patients).
Follow-up: mean 20 months.
Results: mortality rates were 19.8% and 14.2% in the conventional and ICD groups respectively, and there was a 31% reduction in death at any interval in the ICD group.

Reference: Moss A, Zareba W, Hall W, et al, for the Multicenter Automatic Defibrillator Implantation Trial II Investigators. Prophylactic implantation of a defibrillator in patients with myocardial infarction and reduced ejection fraction (2002). *N Engl J Med* **346**:877–883.

MERIT-HF

Metoprolol CR/XL Randomized Intervention Trial I Heart Failure
Purpose: to evaluate the impact of metoprolol succinate when added to standard therapy for chronic heart failure in 3991 patients with LVEF ≤ 40% and NYHA class II-IV, when compared to placebo. Metoprolol was started at 12.5 or 25 mg once daily, aiming to titrated up to 200mg once daily.
Follow-up: 1 year.
Results: at 1 year the trial was terminated early due to the significant reduction in all cause mortality with metoprolol compared to placebo (7.2% vs. 11.0%, p=0.00009), including reductions in cardiovascular death, sudden death and death from worsening heart failure.

Reference: Hjalmarson et al. (2000) *JAMA* **283**:1295–302.

Microalbuminuria, Cardiovascular and Renal Outcomes in the Heart Outcomes Prevention Evaluation

Purpose: to evaluate the impact of Ramipril and vitamin E in the development of diabetic nephropathy in patients with microalbuminuria, or the development of new onset microalbuminuria in the diabetic subset of patients from the HOPE study. Of the HOPE cohort, 3577 were diabetic, 1129 had microalbuminuria.

Follow-up: mean 4 years.

Results: 7% of the ramipril group and 8% of the placebo group (p=0.027) developed proteinuria. There was a trend for reduction in risk of new onset microalbuminuria, although this was not statistically significant (p=0.17). Ramipril reduced the risk of overt nephropathy, dialysis or laser therapy by 16%.

Reference: Heart Outcomes Prevention Evaluation (HOPE) Study Investigators (2000). *Lancet* **355**:253–9.

Myocardial Ischaemia reduction with Aggressive Cholesterol Lowering

Purpose: to determine whether atorvastatin 80 mg once daily initiated 24–96 hours after an acute coronary syndrome (ACS) reduces death, non-fatal MI, cardiac arrest or recurrent symptomatic myocardial ischaemia requiring emergent hospitalization (the primary endpoints) in 3086 patients in a randomized placebo controlled trial.

Follow-up: 16 weeks.

Results: the primary endpoint occurred in 14.8% of the atorvastatin group and 17.4% of the placebo group (p=0.48). There were no significant differences in risk of death, non-fatal MI or cardiac arrest between the two groups. However the atorvastatin group had a lower risk of recurrent ischaemic events requiring hospitalization.

Reference: Schwartz GG *et al.* (2001). *JAMA* **285**:1711–18.

MultiCentre InSycnh Randomized Clinical Evaluation Trial

Purpose: to evaluate whether cardiac resynchronization therapy (CRT) through atrial-synchronized biventricular pacing produces clinical benefit in patients with heart failure and IV conduction delay. 453 patients with NYHA class III and IV heart failure, LVEF ≤35% and QRS >130 ms were randomized to a CRT group (n=228) or a control group (n=225), while continuing optimal medical therapy. Primary endpoints were 6 minute walk distance and NYHA functional class.

Follow-up: 6 months.

Results: patients in the resynchronization group had significantly improved walking distance, quality of life score, NYHA class after 1 month which was maintained throughout the study, compared to non-paced controls. Significant

MIRACLE

improvements were also seen in secondary endpoints of LVEF, peak oxygen consumption, total exercise time, duration of the QRS interval. The risk of major clinical events (death and hospitalization for heart failure) were also significantly lower.

Reference: Abraham WT et al. (2002) N Engl J Med **346**:1845–1853, Jun 13, 2002.

MIRACLE ICD

Multicentre InSync ICD Randomized Clinical Evaluation

Purpose: To evaluate the safety and efficacy of combined cardiac resynchronization therapy (CRT) through biventricular pacing and implantable cardiac defibrillator (ICD) in 369 patients with NYHA III (n=328) or IV (n=41) despite appropriate medical management. LVEF was ≤35%, and QRS 130 ms. Of these 369 patients, 182 were controls (ICD on, CRT off), while 187 were in the CRT group (ICD on, CRT on). Primary endpoints were quality of life, 6 minute walk distance, and functional class compared to baseline.

Follow-up: 6 months.

Results: The CRT group had greater improvement in quality of life score and functional class compared to controls. There was no difference in 6 minute walk distance, but peak exercise oxygen consumption and treadmill exercise duration increased in the CRT group. There was no difference in survival (15 deaths in control arm, 14 deaths in CRT arm), LV size or function, overall heart failure status, and rates of hospitalization.

Reference: Young JB et al. (2003). JAMA **289**: 2719–21.

MOST

Mode Selection Trial in Sinus-Node Dysfunction

Purpose: To evaluate whether dual chamber pacing would provide better event free survival and quality of life than single chamber pacing for sinus node dysfunction. 2010 patients were randomized to dual chamber or ventricular pacing. Primary endpoint was all-cause mortality or non-fatal stroke. Secondary endpoints included the composite of death, stroke or heart failure related hospitalization, AF, heart failure score, pacemaker syndrome and quality of life.

Follow-up: mean 33.1 months.

Results: incidence of the primary endpoint did not differ between groups. The risk of AF was lower in the dual chamber group (hazard ratio 0.79, p=0.0008, heart failure scores were better, as were quality of life scores. Rates of hospitalization for heart failure, death and stroke were not different. 16.5% of the ventricular pacing group experienced pacemaker syndrome and were crossed over to dual chamber pacing.

Reference: Gervasio et al. (2002). NEJM **346**:1854–62.

Multisite Stimulation in Cardiomyopathies Trial

Purpose: to evaluate the impact of biventricular pacing upon 67 patients with severe heart failure (NYHA III) and QRS >150 ms in a single-blind controlled randomized cross-over study. The primary endpoint was distance walked in 6 minutes, with secondary endpoints of quality of life measures, peak oxygen consumption, patients' treatment preference, (active vs. inactive pacing), hospitalizations due to heart failure, and mortality.

Follow-up: 6 months.

Results: mean distance walked in 6 minutes was 23% longer in the active pacing group. 85% preferred the active pacing period. Quality of life score and peak oxygen uptake were both significantly improved, and hospitalizations were 66% less when paced. Longer follow-up was required to determine impact on mortality.

Reference: Cazeau et al. (2001). Effects of multisite biventricular pacing in patients with heart failure and intraventricular conduction delay. N E J Med **344**:873–880.

Multicenter UnSustained Tachycardia Trial

Purpose: To identify individuals at greatest risk of sudden cardiac death using signal averaged ECG and electrophysiological studies, and then optimizing anti-arrhythmic therapy on the basis of the data to reduce sudden death and mortality. 2139 patients ≤80 yrs old were enrolled with coronary heart disease, or MI more than 4 days previously, with LVEF ≤40% and asymptomatic non-sustained VT. 704 patients had inducible sustained VT after electrophysiological testing and were entered into the randomized trial (184 drug therapy, 167 ICD, 353 no therapy). β-blockers were recommended for all patients, but drug therapy varied included sotalol, amiodarone, procainamide, dispyramide, prpafenone, quinindine, and mexiletine. The remaining 1435 patients were entered into a registry.

Follow-up: 5 years.

Results: β-blockers reduced all-cause mortality in the whole cohort, but did not influence death from arrhythmia or cardiac arrest. Patients with inducible sustained VT, the incidence of death from cardiac arrest or arrhythmia was significantly lower in the EP-guided treatment group compared to the no treatment group, but the benefit only occurred in those receiving ICDs. Similarly, the ICD group had significantly reduced risk of arrhythmic death, cardiac arrest, and overall mortality compared to the other groups.

Reference: Buxton AE et al. (1999) N Engl J Med **341**: 1882–90.

OPTIMAAL

Optimal Therapy in Myocardial Infarction with the Angiotensin II Antagonist Losartan
Purpose: to compare the effects on all-cause mortality of losartan 50 mg once daily and captopril 50 mg twice daily in 5477 patients with confirmed acute MI acute anterior QWMI or re-infarction, and heart failure during the acute phase, were randomized in a double-blind parallel method. Primary end-point was all cause mortality.
Follow-up: 2.7 years.
Results: there was a non-significant difference in total mortality in favour of captopril, but losartan was better tolerated.

Reference: Dickstein et al. (2002). Lancet **360**:752–60.

PASE

Pacemaker Selection in the Elderly
Purpose: to assess the effect of the pacing mode (DDDR or VVIR) on the long-term health-related quality of life of 407 elderly patients (65–96 years, mean age 76 years) with pacemakers, randomized to one of these two modes. All patients were in sinus rhythm requiring pacing for bradycardia. Primary endpoint was quality of life. Secondary endpoints included all cause mortality, hospitalization due to heart failure, nonfatal stroke, new AF or the pacemaker syndrome.
Follow-up: 30 months.
Results: quality of life improved significantly for both groups after implantation, but there was no significant difference between groups in this endpoint, or in cardiovascular events or death. 26% of the VVIR group crossed over due to the pacemaker syndrome. Patients with sinus node disease however had an improved quality of life with dual chamber compared to single chamber pacing (explored more fully in MOST trial).

Reference: Gervasio et al. (1998). NEJM **338**:1097–1104.

PCI-CURE

Percutaneous Coronary Intervention and Clopidogrel in Unstable Angina to Prevent Recurrent Events
Purpose: to evaluate the effect of pretreatment of patients undergoing PCI with clopidogrel followed by long term therapy, in addition to concomitant use of aspirin. 2658 patients with NSTEMI undergoing PCI in the CURE study were randomly assigned double-blind treatment with clopidogrel or placebo. Patients were pretreated with aspirin and clopidogrel for a median of 10 days overall. After PCI, >80% of patients in both groups received open-label clopidogrel for 4 weeks. After this, clopidogrel was restarted in the randomized individuals for a mean of 8 months (up to 1 year). The primary composite endpoint was cardiovascular death,

MI or urgent target vessel revascularization within 30 days of PCI.

Follow-up: up to 1 year.

Results: there was a 30% reduction in cardiovascular death or MI in the clopidogrel group, as well as a lower rate of re-vascularization, without any significant difference in major bleeding.

Reference: Mehta SR *et al.* (2001). *Lancet* **358**: 527–533.

PCI-CURE

PRimary angioplasty in AMI patients from General community hospitals transported to PCI Units versus Emergency thrombolysis

PRAGUE Trials

PRAGUE 1: a comparison of long-term outcomes of 3 reperfusion strategies in 300 patients with acute STEMIs presenting to community hospitals: 1) thrombolysis alone in a community hospital; 2) thrombolysis during immediate transportation for angioplasty; 3) immediate transportation for angioplasty without thrombolysis. After one year, there were no significant differences in total mortality in the group as a whole, but in a subset of patients randomized within 2 hours of symptoms, total mortality was lower in the angioplasty group. Primary angioplasty patients however had a lower combined endpoint of total mortality and nonfatal reinfarction rate. Combining thrombolysis and PCI was not superior to PCI alone.

PRAGUE 2: 850 patients with STEMI <12 hours were randomized to thrombolysis in a community hospital without PCI, or immediate transport for PCI. PCI strategy decreased mortality in patients presenting >3 hours after symptom on-set, but in those presenting within 3 hours, thrombolysis had similar results to PCI (primary endpoint was 30 day death, secondary endpoints were death, reinfarction or stroke at 30 days).

PRAGUE 4: 400 patients scheduled for CABG were randomized to off-pump and on-pump surgery by a cardiologist. The surgeon was allowed to change technique after randomization. Primary endpoint at 30 days was death, MI, stroke or new renal failure needing dialysis. There was no significant difference in the primary endpoint. The of pump group had lower post-op CKMB levels, lower total hospital costs, less blood loss and fewer distal anastamoses, suggesting that the off-pump technique was at least as clinically safe and effective as on-pump surgery.

Reference: Bednar *et al.* (2003). *Can J Cardiol.* Sep; **19(10):**1133–7. Widimsky *et al.* (2003). *Eur Heart J* **24**: 21–3. Straza *et al.* (2004). *Ann Thorac Surg* **77**:789–93.

PRISM

Platelet Receptor Inhibition Ischaemic Syndrome Management

Purpose: to compare tirofiban with unfractionated heparin in 3232 patients with unstable angina (last chest pain <24 hours, documented coronary artery disease) on aspirin in a double blind randomized control trial.

Follow-up: 48 hours and 30 days.

Results: at 48 hours, the incidence of death, MI and refractory ischaemia was lower in the tirofiban group, but at 30 days theses rates were not significantly different. In 2240 patients who were troponin T positive at 24 hours, mortality and the incidence of MI was lower at 30 days for the tirofiban group. This benefit was not seen in troponin negative patients.

Reference: Hamm CW et al. (1999). Circulation 100 Suppl I: 1–775.

PRISM PLUS

Platelet Receptor Inhibition in Ischaemic Syndrome Management in patients limited by Unstable Signs and Symptoms

Purpose: to evaluate the effect of tirofiban in the treatment of unstable angina and NQWMI. 1915 were randomized to tirofiban, heparin, or tirofiban and heparin. The study drugs were infused for a mean of 71.3 hours, during which coronary angiography and intervention were performed when indicated after 48 hours. The drug infusion was maintained for 12–24 hours after an intervention. The composite primary endpoint was death, MI , or refractory ischaemia within 7 days randomization. All patients were given aspirin unless here were any contraindications.

Follow-up: 6 months.

Results: the study was stopped prematurely for the group who received tirofiban alone due to excess mortality at 7 days. The composite endpoint was reached by fewer people in the tirofiban plus heparin group compared to those who had heparin alone (12.9% vs. 17.9%, p=0.004). The composite endpoint rates, as well as rates of death and MI, were lower in the tirofiban plus heparin group compared to the heparin alone group at 30 days and at 6 months. There was no significant difference in rates of bleeding between the tirofiban plus heparin group and the heparin alone group.

Reference: The PRISM-PLUS Study Investigators (1998). *NEJM* **338**: 1488–1497.

Perindopril Protection against Recurrent Stroke Study

Purpose: to evaluate the effects of BP reduction on risk of stroke in 6105 patients, normotensive or hypertensive, with a proven TIA or stroke in the previous 5 years. They were randomized to perindopril 4 mg/day plus 2.5 mg indapamide if required, or placebos.

Follow-up: 3.9 years.

Results: BP was reduced by 9/4 mmHg in the treatment group compared to placebo. There was a relative risk reduction in stroke of 28% in the treatment group (p<0.0001), and the risk of total vascular events was also lower in the treatment group. Risk of stroke was reduced in both normotensive and hypertensive patients. The combination of perindopril and indapamide reduced BP by 12/5 mmHg and stroke risk by 43%, but in the perindopril alone group BP was reduced by 5/3 mmHg and did not lead to a reduced stroke risk.

Reference: PROGRESS Collaborative Group (2001). *Lancet* **358**:1033–41.

Platelet IIb/IIIa Underpinning the Receptor for Suppression of Unstable Ischaemia Trial

Purpose: to evaluate the effects of integrelin on the frequency and duration of ischaemia in 227 patients with unstable angina in a randomized double blind, placebo controlled trial. PCI was performed in 11.2% of patients during a period of medical therapy with integrelin that lasted for 72 hours in total and for 24 hours after the intervention. All patients received iv heparin.

Follow-up: 72 hours.

Results: Holter monitoring measured ischaemic episodes, and their frequency and duration were lower in the integrelin group, as well as refractory ischaemia and MI. There was no excess bleeding risk in the integrelin group.

Reference: Schulman SP et al. (1996). *Circulation* **94**:2083–9.

Rate Control versus Electrical Cardioversion for Persistent Atrial Fibrillation

Purpose: to evaluate whether ventricular rate control in AF is inferior to maintenance of sinus rhythm. 522 patients with persistent AF after electrical cardioversion rate control or rhythm control group. The endpoint was a composite of death from cardiovascular disease, heart failure, thromboembolism, bleeding, permanent pacemaker implantation, and adverse drug effects. Rate control was achieved by digoxin, calcium channel blockers (non-dihydropyridine), and β-blockers, either alone or in combination, to achieve a target heart rate

RACE

<100/minute. All patients were orally anticoagulated unless contraindicated. The rhythm control group underwent DCCV without prior treatment with anti-arrhythmics. Then they were placed on sotalol. If AF recurred within 6 months, DCCV was repeated and sotalol was replaced by flecainide or propafenone. If further AF recurred, a loading dose of amiodarone was given at 600 mg daily for 4 weeks then DCCV was repeated, and the anti-arrhythmic drug continued. Patients were orally anticoagulated until one month of sinus rhythm was maintained, after which the anticoagulant was stopped or changed to aspirin. Aspirin was allowed in the rate control group if they were <65 years old without under-lying cardiac disease.

Follow-up: mean 2.3 years.

Results: 39% of the rhythm control vs. 10% of the rate control group were in sinus rhythm, The primary end-point occurred in 17.2% of the rate control vs. 22.6% of the rhythm control group, indicating that rate control was not inferior to rhythm control for preventing death and morbidity from cardiovascular causes in patients with recurrent AF after DCCV.

Reference: Van Gelder et al. (2002). NEJM **347**:1834–40.

RALES

Randomized Aldactone Evaluation Study Mortality Trial
Purpose: To evaluate the effect of adding 25 mg spironolactone in 1663 patients with LVEF <35%, already on ace inhibitors and loop diuretic, and most also on digoxin. The primary endpoint was all-cause mortality.

Follow-up: mean 24 months.

Results: There was a 30% risk reduction in the spironolactone group, p <0.001, due to lower deaths from both sudden cardiac death and also progressive heart failure. There was also 35% less frequent hospitalization in the spironolactone group, this group had a significant improvement in NYHA functional class. There was a 10% incidence of gynaecomastia and breast pain in men treated with spironolactone. There was minimal risk of serious hyperkalaemia in either group. The trial was discontinued early after an interim analysis showed spironolactone to be efficacious,

Reference: Pitt B. (1999). NEJM **341**:709–717.

RAVEL

A Randomized (double blind) study with the Sirolimus coated BX Velocity balloon expandable stent (CYPHER) in the treatment of patients with de novo native coronary Lesions
Purpose: 237 patients with single de novo lesions <18 mm in length and 2.5-3.5 mm in diameter received clopidogrel for a 2 month period and randomized to

receive either a Cypher or bare-metal stent. All patients underwent angiography at the end of the study.

Follow-up: 6 months.

Results: Event free survival was 97% at 6 months compared to 72% in the bare metal stent group. There was no restenosis in the Cypher group compared to 26% in the control. There were no reported cases of subacute thrombosis in the Cypher group.

Reference: Regar et al. (2002). *Circulation* **106**:1949–56.

Reversal of Atherosclerosis with Aggressive Lipid Lowering

Purpose: to evaluate the effect of two different lipid lowering drugs on coronary atheroma burden and progression. Patients were enrolled who required coronary angiography for a clinical indication and demonstrated at least 1 obstruction with angiographic luminal narrowing of ≥20%. Lipid criteria required a low density cholesterol level (LDL-C) of 3.24–5.44 mmol/L after a 4–10 week washout period. 654 patients were initially randomized in a double-blinded manner to receive the study drug, either 40mg pravastatin or 80 mg atorvastatin. 502 patients had intravascular ultrasound (IVUS) examinations that could be evaluated both at baseline and after 18 months treatment. The target vessel for IVUS must not have undergone angioplasty or have a luminal narrowing of more than 50% throughout a target segment with a minimum length of 30 mm, The main outcome measure was the percentage change in atheroma volume. A secondary outcome measure was change in percentage atheroma volume, a measure of an absolute change in atheroma volume as opposed to a relative change.

Follow-up: 18 months.

Results: The baseline LDL-C value (mean 3.89 mmol/L in both groups) was reduced to 2.85 mmol/L in the pravastatin group and 2.05 mmol/L in the atorvastatin group (p <0.001). C-reactive protein (CRP) decreased 5.2% in the pravastatin group and 36.4% with atorvastatin. There was a significantly lower reduction in progression of the percentage change in atheroma volume (the primary endpoint) in the atorvastatin group compared with pravastatin. There was no significant progression of atheroma burden in the atorvastatin group, but here was in the pravastatin group compared to baseline. These changes may be related to reduction in LDL-C and CRP. There were no significant numbers of adverse drug reactions in either group.

Reference: Nissen SE et al. (2004). *JAMA* **291**:1071–1080.

RITA-2

Second Randomized Intervention Treatment of Angina
Purpose: to compare the long-term consequences in 1018 patients with unstable angina randomized to PTCA vs conservative therapy.
Follow-up: median 7 years.
Results: death or MI occurred in 14.5% PTCA patients, and in 12.3% medical patients which was not significantly different. CABG and repeat arteriography were more common in the PTCA group. The PTCA group had improved exercise tolerance and anginal symptoms however.

Reference: Lancet 1997 Aug 16;**350**(9076):461-8, (2003). *J Am Coll Cardiol* **42**:1161–70.

SAVE

Survival and Ventricular Enlargement Study
Purpose: to evaluate the effect of captopril starting 3–16 days after MI in improving mortality and left ventricular function in 2231 patients with LVEF <40% but no overt heart failure.
Follow-up: mean 42 months.
Results: all-cause mortality risk was reduced in the captopril arm by 19%. Recurrent MI risk was reduced by 25% and death after recurrent MI by 32%. The captopril arm patients were less likely to require coronary revascularization but there was no difference in hospitalization rates compared to placebo. Symptoms of cough, dizziness, diarrhoea, and taste alteration were more common on the captopril group.

Reference: Rutherford JD *et al.* (1994). *Circulation* **90**:1731–8.

SIRIUS

A Randomized Trial of a Sirolimus-Eluting Stent versus a Standard Stent in patients at High risk of coronary restenosis
Purpose: to evaluate the effect of sirolimus drug eluting stents vs a bare metal stents upon 1058 patients with de novo coronary artery stenosis.
Follow-up: 12 months.
Results: at 9 months, clinical restenosis (target lesion revascularization) was 4.1% in the sirolimus limb and 16.6% in the control (p <0.001). At 12 months these values were 4.9% and 20% respectively (p <0.001). There were no differences in death or MI rates. In high risk subsets and in presence of diabetes, there was a reduction of 70–80% clinical restenosis at 1 year. At 9 months, clinical restenosis (target lesion revascularization) was 4.1% in the sirolimus limb and 16.6% in the control (p <0.001). At 12 months these values were 4.9% and 20% respectively (p <0.001). There were no differences in death or MI rates.

Reference: Holmes *et al* (2004) *Circulation* **105**:634–640.

Scandinavian Simvastatin Survival Study

Purpose: To evaluate the impact of 20mg simvastatin in patients with total serum cholesterol 5.5–8 mmol/L (after 8 weeks of dietary therapy) upon mortality and the incidence of major coronary artery disease. 4444 patients aged 35–69 years.

Follow-up: median 5.4 years.

Results: there was a 30% relative risk reduction in all-cause mortality, 42% reduction in coronary mortality, 34% reduction in coronary events, 32% reduction in cost of hospitalization and 37% reduction in revascularization procedures in the simvastatin group. Simvastatin significantly reduced the risk of major coronary events in all quartiles of baseline total, LDL and HDL cholesterol to a comparable degree in each quartile. There was on case of reversible myopathy that was the most serious drug-related adverse event.

Reference: Jönsson B et al. (1996) Eur Heart J **17**:1001–7.

Studies of Left Ventricular Dysfunction

Purpose: to evaluate the impact of enalapril on long-term survival in patients with LVEF ≤0.35 with or without a history of cardiac failure, and on LV function and volume, arrhythmias and quality of life. Study design was randomized, double blind placebo controlled. 4228 patients aged 21–80 years had no overt congestive cardiac failure, and 2568 patients had overt cardiac failure. Both groups were randomized to receive enalapril (starting at 2.5 mg twice daily, titrating to 10 mg twice daily) or placebo.

Follow-up: 3 years.

Results: In the group without heart failure there was no statistically significant decrease in mortality, either all-cause or related to cardiovascular disease. There was however a 29% risk reduction in the combined incidence of death and development of overt cardiac failure. In the group with symptoms of heart failure, there was a 16% risk reduction in all-cause mortality. There was no change in the quality of life in either group compared to placebo after 1 year, or in the incidence of ventricular arrhythmias. However left ventricular end diastolic volumes and left ventricular mass increased in the placebo group but did not in the enalapril treated groups. Enalapril treated patients lived 0.16 years longer than the placebo group, translating into a lifetime increase of 0.4 years over placebo. The enalapril groups had significantly fewer hospitalizations than the placebo group.

Reference: Glick H et al. (1995). J Card Fail **1**:371–80.

SPORTIF III

Stroke Prevention Using Oral Thrombin Inhibitor in Atrial Fibrillation

Purpose: to determine if the oral direct thrombin inhibitor ximelagatran is a potential alternative to warfarin in the management of non-valvular atrial fibrillation, in preventing stroke or systemic embolization (primary endpoints). 3410 patients with AF and at least 1 stroke risk factor were randomized to open-label warfarin (to maintain INR 2–3) or fixed dose ximelagatran (36 mg twice daily).

Follow-up: 17.4 months.

Results: there was no significant difference between the groups in primary event rates on an intention-to-treat analysis, or in rates of mortality, fatal stroke and major bleeding. Raised serum ALT levels were commonly found in the ximelagatran group. Hence ximelagatran was at least as effective as warfarin this patient population in preventing stroke and systemic embolization.

Reference: Olsen *et al.* (2003). **362**:1691–8.

SPORTIF IV

This trial protocol was identical to SPORTIF III except SPORTIF III had open label design with blinded event assessment, and SPORTIF V had double blinded assessment. SPORTIF V enrolled 3922 patients who were randomized to ximelagatran and warfarin. Combining the results of SPORTIF III and SPORTIF V demonstrated a relative risk reduction of combined rates of death, primary events and major bleeding of 16% in the ximelagatran group.

Reference: Halperin JL. AHA Scientific Sessions (2003). Nov 9–12.

TAXUS

Trials evaluating a Slow-Release Paclitaxel-Eluting Stent (TAXUS) for Coronary Lesions

TAXUS 1: This trial was to evaluate the safety and feasibility of a TAXUS stent delivering paclitaxel locally to coronary plaques via a slow-release polymer coating, compared to a bare-metal control stent. 61 patients with de novo or restenotic lesions (≤12 mm) were randomized to receive a TAXUS stent or control stent that was non-drug eluting (diameters 3.0 or 3.5 mm). The primary endpoint, 30 day major adverse clinical event (MACE), rate was 0% in both groups. At 12 months, the MACE rate was 3% in the TAXUS group and 10% in the control. The restenosis rate measured by QCA was 0% in the TAXUS group vs 10% in controls at 6 months. IVUS showed significant improvements in normalized neointimal hyperplasia in TAXUS group compared to controls.

TAXUS 2: A comparison of slow release (SR) and moderate release (MR) paclitaxel eluting stents with control bare metal stents (BMS). All 536 patients had post-procedure and 6 month follow-up with IVUS. There was significant reduction in MACE rates, in-stent restenosis (ISR) and in-stent volume reduction with SR or MR stents compared to controls. There was no significant difference between the TAXUS groups.

TAXUS

TAXUS 3: 28 patients with ISR with lesions <30 mm length and 50-99% diameter stenosis in 3.0–3.5 mm vessels were treated with one or more TAXUS stents. 25 people completed the angiographic follow-up at 6 months. The MACE rate was 29% (8 patients). IVUS was recommended to ensure good stent deployment and complete coverage of target lesion.

TAXUS 4: A trial to evaluate the safety and efficacy of slow release polymer based paclitaxel stents after implantation in de novo coronary lesions after 1 year. 1314 patients with de novo coronary lesions 10–28 mm length, diameter 2.5–3.75 mm, coverable by a single stent, were randomized to a TAXUS or bare metal (EXPRESS) stent. At 1 year, MACE rates and target vessel revascularization rates were lower in the TAXUS group. However, rates of cardiac death, MI and subacute thrombosis were not significantly different.

Reference: Grube E et al. (2003). *Circulation* **107**:38–32. Columbo et al. (2003) *Circulation* **108**:788–94. Tanabe et al. (2003). *Circulation* **107**:559–564. Stone et al. (2004) *Circulation* **109**:1942–47.

Comparing efficacy of tPA (with iv heparin) to streptokinase in achieving reperfusion in 290 patients presenting with acute STEMI <6 hrs after symptom onset. All patients underwent baseline coronary angiography after randomization. There were significantly higher rates of perfusion in the TPA arm. Patients with a patent artery at 90 minutes after starting reperfusing therapy had lower 6 month and 1 year mortality regardless of treatment group.

TIMI 1

Patients with acute MI were given tPA within 4 hours of symptom onset and randomized to an immediate invasive strategy (angiogram within 2 hours), delayed invasive (within 18–48 hours) and conservative (angiogram if ETT positive at 6 weeks or further ischaemia). They were then given a pre-discharge angiogram, 6 week ETT and followed up at one year. At 6 weeks, there was no difference between the three groups in death or re-infarction. Infarct related artery patency at time of discharge was similar in all groups with more complications in the invasive arms.

TIMI 2A

TIMI 2B   3339 patients with AMI were given tPA within 4 hours of symptom onset and randomized to an invasive strategy (angiogram within 18–48 hrs) or a conservative strategy (angiogram if ETT positive at 6 weeks or further ischaemia). Patients were also randomized to immediate iv followed by oral β-blockade, or deferred β-blockade. There was no difference in the composite endpoint of death or recurrent MI at 42 days between the invasive and conservative groups. However, those in the invasive arm were twice as likely to need PTCA or CABG at 1 year. In the early β-blockade group, there was significantly lower reinfarction and recurrent ischaemia at 6 weeks.

TIMI 3A   391 patients with unstable angina or NQWMI were given aspirin, iv heparin, beta-blockers, nitrates and calcium antagonists, and then randomized to receive tPA or placebo after baseline angiography had excluded patients with left main stem disease or no coronary disease. They then underwent repeat angiography at 18–36 hrs and were followed up at 6 weeks with an ETT. Baseline angiography showed 35% had apparent thrombus, and 30% had possible thrombus, with no difference in the degree of lesion improvement at angiography after randomization (25% tPA vs 19% placebo).

TIMI 3B   1473 patients with unstable angina or NQWMI were treated with maximal medical therapy and randomized in a 2x2 factorial design to receive tPA or placebo, and to follow invasive or conservative strategies. There was no difference in composite endpoints of death, infarction, or ischaemia in tPA and placebo groups, although the risk of MI, death, or cerebral bleeding was higher in the tPA group. Similarly, there was no difference between the conservative and invasive groups in the primary endpoints, although the invasive group required more re-admission to hospital for angina. The TIMI 3 registry showed that ST deviation was a prognostic indicator in unstable angina, whereas new T wave inversion was not.

TIMI 4   382 patients with AMI <6 hrs were randomized to tPA, APSAC or a combination of the two (at reduced dosage). Each underwent angiograms at 90 mins, and at 18-36 hrs. tPA was shown to have higher patency than APSAC or the combination, fewer unsatisfactory outcomes prior to discharge and lower mortality at 1 year.

TIMI 5   Patients with AMI <6 hrs were randomized to hirudin (a direct thrombin inhibitor) or unfractionated heparin, combined with aspirin and tPA, followed by angiography at 90 mins and 18–36 hrs. The hirudin arm had higher TIMI 3 flow rates and fewer re-occlusions.

TIMI 5

This compared different doses of hirudin and unfractionated heparin in AMI pts in combination with streptokinase and aspirin. There was a lower incidence of death, recurrent MI or new onset CHF in the hirudin groups compared to the heparin groups.

TIMI 6

Hirulog was used to treat 250 patients with unstable angina at a high and low dose, and the incidence of death and MI was lower using higher doses of hirulog.

TIMI 7

This was a follow-on trial comparing hirulog and heparin in a multicentre, double blind randomized study, but was stopped by the sponsor after enrolment for business reasons.

TIMI 8

A trial evaluating the safety and efficacy of hirudin compared to heparin as an adjunct to thrombolysis with tPA or streptokinase. As there were higher rates of bleeding than expected with hirudin, TIMI 9B was designed using lower hirudin doses.

TIMI 9A

Similar to TIMI 9A but using lower doses of hirudin. No significant difference in death or reinfarction was seen between the hirudin and heparin groups.

TIMI 9B

A dose ranging trial of TNK-tPA with aspirin and unfractionated heparin for treating acute STEMI.

TIMI 10A

Using TIMI 10A data, bolus doses of 30, 40, and 50 mg of TNK-tPA were chosen for comparison with accelerated tPA in conjunction with aspirin and iv heparin. A single bolus of TNK 40 mg achieved similar TIMI 3 flow to tPA at 90 minutes.

TIMI 10B

A dose ranging trial for iv enoxaparin treating patients with unstable angina/NQWMI. Due to higher than expected bleeding rate, the trial was reconfigured to look at a 1 mg/kg of enoxaparin to give bleeding rates similar to the heparin plus placebo arm of TIMI 3B.

TIMI 11A

A comparison of enoxaparin and unfractionated heparin to treat unstable angina/NQWMI looking at the benefit of an extended courses of enoxaparin compared to a shorter course (8 vs 43 days). Those randomized to unfractionated heparin continued on placebo. The enoxaparin group had reduced death, MI and revascularization at both timepoints.

TIMI 11B

TIMI 12   A dose ranging study for the GP IIb/IIIa inhibitor sibrafiban in patients 1–7 days after presenting with acute coronary syndrome. Results showed a dose-dependent rise in platelet inhibition

TIMI 14   Evaluating abciximab for the treatment of STEMI, in combination with tPA, streptokinase, reteplase, or with no thrombolytic drug, compared to a group receiving tPA and heparin only. The combination of abciximab and half dose tPA achieved the highest rates of reperfusion.

TIMI 15A   A dose ranging study of the GP IIb/IIIa inhibitor Klerval (avail-able both orally and iv) for acute coronary syndrome, that showed a dose dependent increase in platelet inhibition. The data was used in selecting the dose for the TIMI 15B trial.

TIMI 15B   A dose ranging trial examining iv Klerval for 24–96 hrs then oral Klerval for 4 weeks in the management of acute coronary syndromes (unstable angina, NSTEMI, STEMI), versus placebo. Results showed potent predictable dose dose-related platelet inhibition with intravenous use, but moderate inhibition only with oral use.

TIMI 16   **(OPUS TIMI 16)** Patients with acute coronary syndrome were randomized to two dosing strategies of oral orbofiban, versus placebo to evaluate the benefit of orbofiban in addition to standard therapy. No significant benefit was observed.

TIMI 17   **(InTIME II)** A multicentre trial of bolus lanoteplase vs accelerated tPA for 15087 patients with STEMI. No significant difference was observed in mortality at 30 days between the two groups.

TIMI 18   **(TACTICS TIMI-18) Treat Angina with Aggrastat and determine Cost of Therapy with an Invasive or Conservative Strategy TIMI 18**
2220 patients with an unstable angina or NQWMI had base-line troponin measured and were given aspirin, heparin and tirofiban. They were then randomized to an early invasive (angiogram in 4–48 hrs) or early conservative strategy, and would proceed to PCI or CABG depending on their symptoms, treadmill testing or other evidence of ischaemia. They were followed up for 6 months. The combined primary end-point of death, MI, and rehospitalization at 6 months was 19.4% in the conservative arm and 15.9% in the invasive arm. The reduction in patients who reached the primary endpoint was most marked in the 54% who were troponin positive

(>0.01 ng/ml), and in patients who had an intermediate and high-risk TIMI score. There was no significant difference in stroke, although major bleeding rate was higher in the invasive group. Hence there was benefit for 'upstream' use of tirofiban in early intervention, using troponin levels and TIMI scores to guide potential usefulness of an early interventional approach.

TIMI 18

PRavastatin Or atorVastatin Evaluation and Infection Therapy (PROVE IT)

TIMI 22

A study to evaluate whether statins are effective in reducing events in patients with an acute coronary syndrome (ACS), and to see whether intensive lipid lowering of LDL-C (to an average 65 mg/dL) achieves greater reduction in clinical events than standard lowering (to an average 95 mg/dL). 4162 patients with an ACS within 10 days were given standard therapy and randomized to pravastatin 40 mg (standard therapy) or atorvastatin 80 mg (intensive therapy), as well as gatifloxacin vs. placebo in a 2x2 factorial manner. There was a mean 2 year follow-up after which the following primary endpoints were measured: death, MI, documented unstable angina requiring hospitalization, revascularization (>30 days after randomization), and stroke. The findings were that the atorvastatin group the risk of all-cause mortality or major cardiac events were reduced by 16% (p=0.005). The benefits emerged at 30 days post ACS and were maintained throughout follow-up, and were consistent across all cardiovascular endpoints except stroke, and most clinical subgroups.

Veterans Affairs Non-Q Wave Infarction Strategies in Hospital

VANQUISH

Purpose: to compare the role of early invasive versus conservative management strategies in patients with NQWMI with or without prior MI. The background of this study was that patients with a first NQWMI have a better prognosis than those with prior myocardial infarction who suffer another NQWMI. 920 patients were enrolled; 396 had prior MI, 524 did not. These two groups were randomly assigned to an invasive strategy or conservative strategy, with subsequent invasive management if there was spontaneous or inducible ischaemia within 72 hrs of the NQWMI. The combined primary endpoint was death or non-fatal MI.
Follow-up: mean 23 months.
Results: Mortality did not differ significantly between the invasive and conservative strategy groups. Those with previous MI were identified as a high risk subset of NQWMI patients who have similar outcomes

VANQUISH

regardless of the strategy used. But patients with a first infarct had better prognosis if managed conservatively, or with an ischaemia-guided approach.

Reference: VANQWISH trial Investigators (1998). *NEJM* **338**:1785–92.

V-HEFT II

Vasodilator Heart Failure Trial II
Purpose: to compare the impact of enalapril with the combination of hydralazine plus isosorbide dinitrate in treating 804 patients with chronic congestive cardiac failure.
Follow-up: mean 2.5 years.
Results: The enalapril group had significantly lower mortality attributable mainly to a reduction in sudden cardiac death. Blood pressure reduction was greater in the enalapril group in the first 13 weeks. There was increased incidence of symptomatic hypotension and cough in the enalapril group, and increased headache in the hydralazine plus isosorbide dinitrate group.

Reference: Cohn JN *et al.* (1991) *NEJM* **325**:303–310.

WOSCOPS

West Of Scotland Coronary Prevention Study
Purpose: A primary prevention study to evaluate the effect of 5 years of once daily 40 mg pravastatin on the risk of MI, in 6595 men aged 45-64 years with LDL cholesterol 4-6 mmol/L and no history of MI, in a randomized double blind placebo controlled trial.
Follow-up: mean 4.9 years.
Results: total cholesterol and LDL cholesterol were lowered by 20% and 26% respectively in the pravastatin group. There was a 31% relative risk reduction in the number of definite coronary events in the pravastatin group, and a 31% reduction in non-fatal MI, 33% reduction in death from coronary heart disease and 32% reduction in death from all cardiovascular causes. All-cause mortality was reduced by 22% in the pravastatin group (p=0.051).

Reference: The WOSCOPS study Group.(1996). *Eur Heart J* **17**:163–4.

Eponymous syndromes

Syndromes listed in alphabetical order

Aase syndrome A clinical triad of congenital anaemia, triphalangeal thumbs, and VSD. The aetiology is unknown.

Adams–Stokes syncope See Stokes–Adams syndrome (p597).

Alfidi's syndrome Hypertension resulting from occlusion of the celiac axis, leading to diversion of collateral blood flow from the right renal artery. Originally described as renal-splanchnic steal syndrome[1].

Andersen syndrome A triad of periodic paralysis, ventricular tachyarrythmias, and dysmorphic features (hypertelorism, micrognathia, low-set ears, and high arched or cleft palate, short stature, scoliosis, syndactyly, and clinodactyly). The periodic paralysis can be associated with hyper-, hypo- or normokalaemia. It is an autosomal dominant condition associated with mutations in the KCNJ2 gene encoding the inward-rectifying K^+ channel Kir2.1[2].

Barlow's syndrome A familial form of mitral valve prolapse which is sometimes inherited as an autosomal dominant trait. It is a genetically heterogenous syndrome, characterized by 'billowing' of one or both of the mitral valve leaflets into the left atrium during systole. On auscultation there is a midsystolic click and a late or pansystolic murmur. 20% are asymptomatic. Females are twice as commonly affected[3].

Barth syndrome An X-linked mutation of the TAZ gene, leading to dilated cardiomyopathy, skeletal myopathy, short stature and neutropenia. 3-methylglutaconic acid excretion in the urine has been observed in almost all reported cases.

Beemer lethal malformation syndrome A lethal syndrome of double outlet right ventricle, hydrocephalus, dense bones, thrombocytopenia, and abnormal nasal development.

Bouillaud's syndrome An eponym for rheumatic fever. Bouillaud was the first to emphasize the importance of cardiac involvement in the acute articular phase of rheumatic fever[4].

1 Alfidi RJ, et al. (1967) Renal-splanchnic steal. Report of a case. *Cleveland Clinic Quarterly* **34**: 43–54.
2 Donaldson MR, Jensen JL, Tristani-Firouzi, M, et al. (2003) PIP2 binding residues of Kir2.1 are common targets of mutations causing Andersen syndrome. *Neurology* **60**(11): 1811–1816.
3 Barlow J, Marchand BP, Pocock WA, Denny D (1963) The significance of late systolic murmurs. *American Heart Journal* **66**: 443.
4 Bouillaud B (1832) *Traité clinique du rheumatisme articulaire.* Paris.

Bourneville–Pringle disease Hamartomas of the heart and kidney associated with epilepsy, learning difficulties, cerebral cortical hamartomas (tuberose sclerosis) and adenoma sebaceum. It is inherited in an autosomal dominant manner. Renal cysts or carcinomas may occur[1].

Bradbury–Egglseton syndrome An idiopathic disorder of autonomic failure characterized by orthostatic hypotension, with more widespread manifestations of thermoregulatory, bowel, bladder, and sexual function disturbance.

Brugada's syndrome One of the principal causes of sudden cardiac death in young adults in the absence of structural heart disease, secondary to mutation of the SCN5A gene on chromosome inherited in an autosomal dominant fashion. This results in malfunction of a sodium channel leading to initiation and perpetuation of ventricular arrhythmias. Clinically there is RBBB, ST elevation in V1 to V3, and sudden death/syncope. The clinical phenotype may be unmasked by the administration of ajmaline or procainamide. The only effective treatment is with an ICD[2].

Carney syndrome Also known as the Carney complex. There is association of atrial myxomas with myxomas in other locations, e.g. breast or skin, spotty pigmentation, and endocrine overactivity, e.g. pituitary or testicular tumours. The inheritance is autosomal dominant, the mutation being in the PRKAR1A gene on chromosome 17. It tends to affect individuals in their third decade. They are more likely to have bilateral myxomas and develop recurrences of the myxoma after removal, in contrast to sporadic cases.

DiGeorge syndrome A disorder resulting from deletion of the TBX1 gene on chromosome 22q11.2 leading to parathyroid hypoplasia (and hypocalcaemia), thymic hypoplasia (and low T cell counts), and outflow tract defects of the heart including tetralogy of Fallot, truncus ateriosus, interrupted aortic arch, right-sided aortic arch, and aberrant right subclavian artery. Affected individuals typically have micrognathia, low set ears, short philtrum and small mouth. The Shprintzen syndrome is also caused by a disorder in the same gene.

1 Bourneville DM (1880) Sclérose tubéreuse des circonvolution cérébrales: Idiotie et épilepsie hemiplégique. *Archives de neurologie, Paris,* **1**: 81–91.
2 Brugada P, Brugada J (1992) Right bundle branch block, persistent ST segment elevation and sudden cardiac death: a distinct clinical and electrocardiographic syndrome. A multicenter report. *J Am Coll Cardiol.* 20(6): 1391–6.

Dressler syndrome A myocardial infarction-associated pericarditis, usually occurring one week after the onset of infarction, but may occur several months afterwards. An autoimmune aetiology is suspected due to the delay in development of the syndrome, the presence of antibodies against the heart, evidence of altered lymphocyte subsets and complement activation, frequent recurrences, associated pleuritis and pleural effusions, and response to non-steriodal drugs and steroids. There may be a pericardial rub, fever, pericardial and pleural effusions, with PR abnormalities, as well as ST and T wave changes suggestive of pericarditis.

Duchenne muscular dystrophy An X-linked disorder of the dystrophin gene. There is severe skeletal muscle weakness, which may mask dilated cardiomyopathy. There is a tendency for fibrosis to affect the posterolateral and posterobasal left ventricular wall. Supraventricular arrhythmias are more common than ventricular arrhythmias and heart block, which occur as the fibrosis becomes more widespread.

Ebstein's anomaly A malformation in which there is an abnormal attachment of the tricuspid valve leaflets leading to a downward displacement of the tricuspid valve. A portion of the right ventricle therefore lies between the AV ring and the origin of the valve, so that the proximal part of the right ventricle is 'atrialized', and a small RV chamber exists. Tricuspid valve tissue is dysplastic. There is spectrum of severity in this condition, and it is associated with pulmonary stenosis or atresia, as well as VSD and ostium primum ASD.

Eisenmenger syndrome Any systemic to pulmonary circulation shunt that eventually leads to reversal or bi-directional flow of the shunt, with subsequent pulmonary hypertension and cyanosis. It was first described in a 32 year old man with a ventricular septal defect in 1897[1].

Ellis–Van Creveld syndrome An autosomal recessive condition characterized by short stature caused by metaphyseal dysplasia, polydactyly, dysplastic nails and teeth, and, most commonly, primum ASD. Coarctation of the aorta, hypoplastic left heart and PDA occur in 20% of cases.

1 Eisenmenger, V (1897). Die angeborenen Defekte der Kammerscheidewände des Herzens. *Zeitschrift für klinische Medizin* **32** (Supplement): 1–28.

Emery–Dreifuss muscular dystrophy A clinical triad of early contractures of the elbow, Achilles tendon and posterior cervical muscles, progressive skeletal myopathy, and cardiac manifestations. These include sinus bradycardia, atrial fibrillation and atrial flutter initially, progressing to higher levels of AV block, sustained ventricular tachycardia and ventricular fibrillation. Heart failure may also be present. Sudden death before the age of 50 is common. It is X-linked in its transmission, with the gene responsible encoding a nuclear membrane protein called emerin[1].

Fallot's tetralogy The association of pulmonary stenosis, ventricular septal defect, over-riding aorta and right ventricular hypertrophy, causing cyanosis in the newborn. This forms 10% of all congential heart disease, and is slightly more common in males. Fallot's trilogy comprises pulmonary stenosis, strial septal defect and intact ventricular septum, Fallot's pentalogy is the addition of an atrial septum defect or patent foramen ovale to the tetralogy[2].

Friedreich's ataxia A spinocerebellar degenerative disease characterized by limb and trunk ataxia, skeletal deformities, dysarthria, and cardiomyopathy. Concentric left ventricular hypertrophy frequently occurs, as well as asymmetrical septal hypertrophy. Rarer is dilated cardiomyopathy. There may be associated atrial arrhythmias. The condition is inherited in an autosomal dominant manner, with the mutation identified as an amplified, unstable GAA trinucleotide repeat found in the first intron of the frataxin gene on chromosome 9q13.

Friedreich's disease Sudden collapse of the cervical veins that were previously distended at each diastole, caused by an adherent pericardium. Also known as mediostinopericarditis adhesiva, or Friedreich's sign.

Holt–Oram syndrome An autosomal dominant condition, sometimes known as heart–hand syndrome, in which there is dysplasia of the upper limbs associated most commonly with secundum ASD, but also with VSD, MVP, and PDA. The arm deformities may be subtle, from having distally placed or triphalangeal thumbs, to more severe forms including hypolplastic clavicles and phocomelia.

1 Muntoni, F (2003) Cardiomyopathy in muscular dystrophies. *Current Opinion in Neurology.* 16(5): 577–583.
2 Fallot: ELA (1888) Contribution à l'anatomie pathologique de la maladie bleue (cyanose cardiaque). Marseille médical.

Heyde's syndrome The association of gastrointestinal bleeding and calcific aortic stenosis. Since Heyde's original description in 1958, the bleeding has been shown to be due to an acquired von Willebrands disease type 2a caused by high shear stress around the aortic valve, leading to haemorrhage from arteriovenous malformations in the gut. The bleeding abnormality ceases after replacement of the valve[1].

Hurler's syndrome An autosomal recessive mucopolysaccharide storage disorder resulting from deficiency of the lysosomal enzyme alpha-L-iduronate. It is also designated mucopolysaccharidosis type IH (MPSIH). Clinical features include coarse facial characteristics, corneal clouding, hepatosplenomegaly, thickened skin, mental retardation, and cardiac problems. These consist of restrictive cardiomyopathy due to endomyocardial fibroelastosis, coronary artery stenosis, and valvular thickening (left side more than right side) and regurgitation. Most die in the first decade. Hunter's syndrome is MPS II, and pursues a slower course. Scheie syndrome is MPS IS and has the most benign course of the mucopolysaccharidoses[2].

Jervell–Lange–Nielsen syndrome An autosomal recessive condition associated with deafness caused by mutation in the KVLQT1 gene, or the KCNE1 gene, both encoding components of the delayed rectifier potassium channel involved in the action potential. As a result, the QT interval is prolonged and affected individuals have a variable risk of developing torsade de pointes and sudden cardiac death (SCD).

Kartagener's syndrome A clinical triad of situs inversus, abnormal frontal sinuses and immotile cilia. The patient has recurrent respiratory infections, sinusitis, bronchiectasis and infertility. Some may have anosmia, or low levels of IgA. Inheritance is autosomal recessive. The defect lies in the genes encoding the dynein protein that contributes to the structure of cilia. Also known as the Siewert Syndrome[3].

Kawasaki disease An acute vasculitis that affects children, which manifests with fever, cervical lymphadenopathy, bilateral conjunctivitis, erythema or desquamation of the palms and soles, and coronary artery aneurysms or ectasia. These may lead to myocardial infarction and sudden death. The aetiology is unknown[4].

1 Heyde EC (1958) Gastrointestinal bleeding in aortic stenosis. NEJM, 259: 196; Pelin Batur (2000) Increased Prevalence of Aortic Stenosis in Patients with Arteriovenous Malformations of the Gastrointestinal Tract in Heyde Syndrome. *Arch Int Med*, 163: 1821–1824.
2 Hurler G (1919) Über einen Typ multipler Abartungen, vorwiegend am Skelettsystem. *Zeitschrift für Kinderheilkunde*, Berlin, 24: 220–234.
3 Kartagener M (1933) *Zur Pathogenese der Bronchiektasien: Bronchiektasien bei Situs viscerum inversus.Beiträge zum Klinik der Tuberkulose*, 83: 489–501.
4 Kawasaki T (1967) Acute febrile mucocutaneous syndrome with mucoid involvement with specific desquamation of the fingers and toes in children. *Jpn J Allergy* 116: 178.

Kearns–Sayre syndrome A clinical triad of AV block, pigmentary retinopathy and progressive external ophthalmoplegia. It is caused by the deletion of several mitochondrial genes. In most cases it occurs sporadically and is not inheritable[1].

Leber hereditary optic neuropathy A mitochondrial encephalomyopathy characterized by painless loss of vision in a young man. There may be an associated short PR interval and pre-excitation[2].

Lenegre–Lev disease Also known as progressive familial heart block type I (PFHBI). An autosomal dominant disorder mapped to chromosome 19, defined by evidence of bundle branch block wide QRS complexes that may progress to complete heart block. This is distinct from progressive familial heart block type II (PFHBII) which has narrow QRS complexes. There is an accelerated degenerative process that affects primarily the conduction tissue.

Løffler's syndrome A rare form of endocarditis associated with high levels of circulating eosinophils. The underlying cause may be helminthic infection or leukaemia, but in most is unknown. Typically the lungs are involved with diffuse reticular nodular shadowing on the chest X-ray. The acute form is characterized by an eosinophilic vasculitis that leads to dilated cardiac chambers, whereas the chronic form leads to fibrosis of myocardium leading to a clinical syndrome of restrictive cardiomyopathy, resulting in reduced effort tolerance, wheezing, hepatomegaly, heart block, mitral and tricuspid regurgitation, and systemic embolization.

Lown–Ganong–Levine syndrome A ventricular pre-excitation phenomenon characterized by a short PR interval (<120 ms) and normal QRS duration, in association with paroxysms of supraventricular tachycardia but not atrial flutter or fibrillation. Patients without a history of tachycardia may be described as having accelerated AV nodal conduction. Although first described by Clerc in 1938, the eponymous individuals reported this syndrome in 1952. No single structural abnormality has been found to be the cause of LGL. It may be due to intranodal or paranodal fibres that bypass the AV node. Most patients at electrophysiological study have been found to have a reason other than a bypass tract for their paroxysmal tachycardia, such as AVNRT. Therefore LGL is a syndrome of a pre-electrophysiological study era that describes a clinical phenomenon of paroxysmal tachycardia with a short PR interval that may be at one end of the normal range (2–4% of adults have PR <120 ms)[3].

1 Schmitz K, Lins H, Behrens-Baumann W (2003) Bilateral spontaneous corneal perforation associated with complete external ophthalmoplegia in mitochondrial myopathy (Kearns-Sayre syndrome). *Cornea* 22(3): 267–270.
2 Leber (1868) Beiträge zur Kenntniss der atrophischen Veränderungen des Sehnerven nebst Bemerkungen über normale Structur des Nerven. *Archiv für Ophthalmologie, Berlin,* 14: 164–176.
3 Lown B, Ganong WF, Levine SA (1952) The syndrome of short PR interval, normal QRS complex, and paroxysmal rapid heart action. *Circulation* 5: 693–706.

Libman–Sacks syndrome A cardiac manifestation of systemic lupus erythematosus which occurs late in the disease process, and is found in 50% of patients with fatal lupus at post mortem. It characterized by sterile, verrucous lesions on valve leaflets and chordae comprised of fibrin, neutrophils, lymphocytes, and histiocytes. The mitral and aortic valves are most commonly affected, although most cases are clinically silent. Valvular regurgitation is more common than stenosis. Similar lesions may occur in association with the antiphospholipid syndrome. Women are more commonly affected[1].

Lutembacher's syndrome The combination of mitral stenosis (congenital or acquired) and atrial septal defect (congenital or iatrogenic), with left to right shunt. If the ASD is large, pulmonary hypertension is avoided, but with the consequence of progressive right heart dilatation[2].

Marfan's syndrome A disorder resulting from mutations in the FBN1 gene on chromosome 15q21.1 encoding fibrillin-1 which constitutes the microfibrils that make up the extracellular matrix. Some features include tall stature, kyphosis, scoliosis, pectus excavatum, upwards lens dislocation, dural ectasia, retinal detachment, and a variety of cardiac abnormalities. These include mitral valve prolapse and regurgitation, dilated sinuses of Valsalva, aortic root dilatation with aortic regurgitation and increased risk of dissection, and arrhythmias. Patients may be at increased risk of endocarditis secondary to the valve abnormalities. 75% are inherited as autosomal dominant; the remainder occurs sporadically[3].

Morquio's syndrome One of the mucopolysaccharide storage disorders, designated mucopolysaccaridosis IVB (MPSIVB), inherited in an autosomal recessive manner. Two types are recognized. Type A is caused by deficiency of galactosamine-6-sulfatase, whereas type B is caused by deficiency in beta galactosidase. Clinical features include short stature, skeletal and joint abnormalities, cloudy corneas, hepatomegaly, aortic and mitral regurgitation. Heart failure may result from either an infiltrative cardiomyopahthy or from valvular regurgitation[4].

Noonan's syndrome A dysmorphic syndrome characterized by cardiac anomalies, short stature, low set ears, hypertelorism, deafness, and bleeding diathesis. It is inherited in an autosomal dominant manner. Cardiac problems include valvular pulmonary stenosis. This syndrome has sometimes been called 'male Turner's syndrome' although it affects both sexes, and in contrast has no chromosomal abnormalities[5].

1 Libman E, Sacks B (1924) A hitherto undescribed form of valvular and mural endocarditis. *Archives of Internal Medicine, Chicago*, 33: 701–737.
2 Lutembacher R (1916) De la sténose mitrale avec communication interauriculaire. Archives des maladies du coeur et des vaisseaux, Paris, 9: 237–260.
3 Marfan AB (1896) Un cas de déformation congénitale des quatre membres, plus prononcée aux extrémités, caractérisée par l'allongement des os avec un certain degré d'aminicissement. Bulletins et memoires de la Société medicale des hôpitaux de Paris, 13: 220–226.
4 Morquio L (1929) Sur une forme de dystrophie osseuse familiale. *Archives de médecine des enfants, Paris*, 32: 129–135.
5 Noonan A. Ehmke DA (1963) Associated noncardiac malformations in children with congenital heart disease. *Journal of Pediatrics, St. Louis*, 63: 468–470.

Ortner's syndrome First described as compression of the recurrent laryngeal nerve by a dilated left atrium in mitral valve stenosis, giving rise to a hoarse voice from vocal cord paresis. Sometimes used to describe any non-malignant cardiac or intrathoracic process that damages the recurrent laryngeal nerve. The left nerve is more commonly affected than the right due to its longer course around the aortic arch.

Prinzmetal's (variant) angina Angina resulting from spasm of a coronary artery, which may lead to heart block and myocardial infarction. It may be prevented by long-acting calcium antagonists[1].

Romano–Ward syndrome An autosomal dominant condition caused by mutation in genes on chromosomes 3, 4, 7, 11, and 21 encoding different components of both sodium and potassium channels. The QT interval is prolonged and there is a high risk of developing torsades de pointes and sudden cardiac death (SCD). It not associated with deafness and is therefore distinct from Jervell–Lange–Nielson syndrome.

Shprintzen syndrome A disorder caused by mutation in the TBX1 gene, which is also responsible for the Di-George syndrome. The characteristic features are cardiac anomalies (most commonly VSD), cleft palate, learning difficulties, and typical facies including prominent nose, narrow palpebral fissures, and micrognathia. Also known as the velocardiofacial syndrome.

Stokes–Adams syndrome Syncope caused by cardiac arrhythmia. Also known as Spens syndrome and Morgagni's syndrome[2].

Sydenham's chorea A delayed manifestation of rheumatic fever, due to an inflammatory reaction caused by autoantibodies in the basal ganglia and caudate nuclei following group A streptococcal infection. It usually occurs three months after the initial infection and symptoms may last for up to two weeks. It is characterized by involuntary movements, muscle incoordination and emotional lability.

Taussig–Bing syndrome A congenital anomaly in which the aorta arises from the right ventricle, the pulmonary artery arises from both ventricles, and there is an associated VSD[3].

1 Prinzmetal M Massumi RA (1955) The anterior chest wall syndrome-chest pain resembling pain or cardiac origin. *JAMA*, 159: 177–184.
2 Adams R, (1827) Cases of Diseases of the Heart, Accompanied with Pathological Observations. *Dublin Hospital Reports*, 4: 353–453. Stokes W (1846) Observations on some cases of permanently slow pulse. *Dublin Quarterly Journal of Medical Science*, 2: 73–85.
3 Taussig HB, Bing RJ (1949) Complete transposition of the aorta and levoposition `of the pulmonary artery: clinical, physiological, and pathological findings. *American Heart Journal*, St. Louis, 37: 551–559.

Tietze's syndrome Inflammation of the costochondral cartilages of unknown aetiology. There is characteristic swelling of the cartilages, which distinguishes the syndrome from other types of costochondritis, and the swelling may persist after the pain has resolved. Mostly men in their third decade are affected[1].

Townes–Brocks syndrome An autosomal dominant condition describing the association of imperforate anus, abnormalities of the kidneys, hand, foot, and ear, sporadically associated with cardiac malformations including VSD and ASD.

Turner's syndrome A disorder resulting from the absence of one of the X chromosomes, XO. Features include coarctation of the aorta, short stature, absence of secondary sexual characteristics, webbing of the neck, cubitus valgus, and lymphoedema. It is one of the most common chromosomal abnormalities[2].

Twiddler's syndrome Not strictly an eponym. The phenomenon of permanent malfunction of a pacemaker due to the patient's manipulation of the pulse generator[3].

Wenkebach's heart A description of a heart located in the midline which is smaller than normal. Also known as mesocardia, or the 'hanging heart'.

Wenkebach's phenomenon A form of second degree atrioventricular heart block characterized by progressive lengthening of the PR interval on the ECG until a P wave is not conducted to the ventricles[4].

Williams syndrome A congenital supravalvular aortic stenosis associated with peripheral pulmonary artery stenosis, hypercalcaemia, elfin facies, outgoing personality, learning difficulties, strabismus, and dental anomalies. The left ventricle may be hypertrophied, and the sinuses of Valsalva may be dilated. In addition, the coronary arteries may be dilated or tortuous, and demonstrate accelerated atherosclerosis. The patient is at higher risk of endocarditis and sudden death than unaffected individuals. Autosomal dominant transmission is observed if this syndrome is inherited.

1 Tietze A (1921) Über eine eigenartige Häufung von Fällen mit Dystrophie der Rippenknorpel. Berliner klinische Wochenschrift, 58: 829–831.

2 Turner HH, (1938) A syndrome of infantilism, congenital webbed neck, and cubitus valgus. Endocrinology, 23: 566–574.

3 Bayliss CE, Turner H H. The pacemaker-twiddler's syndrome: a new complication of implantable transvenous pacemakers. Can Med Assoc J. 1968 Aug 24–31; 99(8): 371–3.

4 Wenckeback KF (1898) De Analyse van den onregelmatigen Pols. III. Over eenige Vormen van Allorythmie en Bradykardie. Nederlandsch Tijdschrift voor Geneeskunde, Amsterdam, 2: 1132.

Wolff–Parkinson–White syndrome Tachyarrhythmias that occur as a result of an accessory atrioventricular pathway, typified by the ECG features in sinus rhythm of a PR interval less than 120 ms and QRS duration greater than 120 ms caused by a delta wave, representing antegrade conduction through the accessory pathway. Patients can have intermittent conduction via this pathway, leading to variable ECG patterns[1].

1 Wolff, Parkinson J, White PD (1930) Bundle-branch block with short P-R interval in healthy young people prone to paroxysmal tachyardia. *Am Heart J St. Louis*, 5: 685.

Cardiovascular emergencies

Adult basic life support

Basic life support is the backbone of effective resuscitation following a cardiorespiratory arrest. The aim is to maintain adequate ventilation and circulation until the underlying cause for the arrest can be reversed. 3–4 minutes without adequate perfusion (less if the patient is hypoxic) will lead to irreversible cerebral damage. The usual scenario is an unresponsive patient found by staff who alert the cardiac arrest team. The initial assessment described below should have already been performed by the person finding the patient. The same person should have also started cardiopulmonary resuscitation (CPR). Occasionally you will be the first to discover the patient and it is important to rapidly assess the patient and begin CPR. The various stages in basic life support are described here and summarized on p603.

1. **Assessment of the patient**
* Ensure safety of rescuer and victim
* **Check whether the patient is responsive.** Gently shake victim and ask loudly *'are you all right?'*
   a) If victim responds place him/her in the recovery position and get help
   b) If victim is unresponsive shout for help and move on to assess airway (see below).

2. **Airway assessment**
* **Open the airway.** With two fingertips under the point of the chin, tilt the head up. If this fails place your fingers behind the angles of the lower jaw and apply steady pressure upwards and forwards. Remove ill-fitting dentures and any obvious obstruction. If the patient starts breathing, roll the patient over into the recovery position and try to keep the airway open until an orophyrangeal airway can be inserted.
* **Keep airway open, look, listen and feel for breathing.** Look for chest movements, listen at the victim's mouth for breathing sounds and feel for air on your cheek (for no more than 10 seconds).
   a) If patient is breathing turn patient into the recovery position, check for continued breathing and get help
   b) If patient is not breathing, making occasional gasps, or weak attempts at breathing send someone (or go for help if alone). (On return) start rescue breaths by giving two slow effective breaths each resulting in a visible rise and fall in the chest wall.

3. **Assessment of circulation**
* Assess signs of circulation by feeling the carotid pulse for no more than ten seconds.
   a) If there are signs of circulation but no breathing continue rescue breaths and check for signs of breathing every 10 breaths (approximately one breath a minute).
   b) If there are no signs of circulation start chest compression at a rate of 100 times per minute. Combine rescue breaths and compression at the rate of 15 compressions to two effective breaths.
* The ratio of compressions to lung inflation remains the same for resuscitation with two persons.

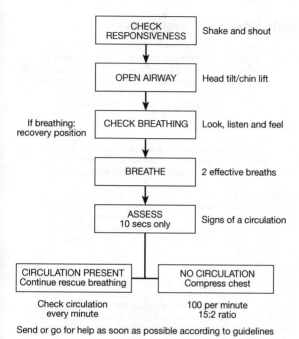

Fig. 17.1 For further information see The Resuscitation Council (UK) website (http://www.resus.org.uk/pages/bls.htm).

Adult advanced life support

- It is unlikely that an effective spontaneous cardiac activity will be restored by basic life support without more advanced techniques (intubation for effective ventilation, drugs, defibrillation, etc.). Do not waste time. As soon as help arrives, delegate CPR to someone less experienced in ACLS, so that you are able to continue.
- Attach the patient to a cardiac monitor as soon as possible to determine the cardiac rhythm and treat appropriately **(see p608 for universal treatment algorithm).**
- Orophyrangeal (Guedel) or nasopharyngeal airways help maintain the patency of the airway by keeping the tongue out of the way. They can cause vomiting if the patient is not comatose. ET intubation is the best method of securing the airway. *Do not attempt this if you are inexperienced.*
- Establish venous access. Central vein cannulation (internal jugular or subclavian) is ideal but requires more training, practise, and is not for the inexperienced. If venous access fails, drugs may be given via an ET-tube into the lungs (except for bicarbonate and calcium salts). Double the dose of drug if using this route as absorption is less efficient than iv.

Post resuscitation care

- Try to establish the events that precipitated the arrest from the history, staff, witnesses and the hospital notes of the patient. Is there an obvious cause (MI, hypoxia, hypoglycaemia, stroke, drug overdose or interaction, electrolyte abnormality, etc.)? Record the duration of the arrest in the notes with the interventions, drugs (and doses) in chronological order.
- Examine the patient to check both lung fields are being ventilated; check for ribs that may have broken during CPR. Listen for any cardiac murmurs. Check the neck veins. Examine the abdomen for an aneurysm or signs of peritonism. Insert urinary catheter. Consider an NG-tube if patient remains unconscious. Record the Glasgow Coma Score and perform a brief neurological assessment.
- Investigations: **ECG** [looking for MI, ischaemia, tall T-waves ($\uparrow K^+$)]; **ABG** [mixed metabolic and respiratory acidosis is common and usually responds to adequate oxygenation and ventilation once the circulation is restored. If severe, consider bicarbonate]; **CXR** (check position of ET-tube, look for pneumothorax); **U&Es, and glucose.**
- After early and successful resuscitation from a primary cardiac arrest, the patient may rapidly recover completely. Patient must be transferred to HDU or CCU to monitor for 12–24h. Commonly the patient is unconscious post-arrest and should be transferred to ITU for mechanical ventilation and haemodynamic monitoring and support for ≥ 24 hours
- Change any venous lines that were inserted at the time of arrest for central lines inserted with sterile technique. Insert an arterial line and consider PA catheter (Swan–Ganz) if requiring inotropes.

- Remember to talk to the relatives. Keep them informed of events and give a realistic (if bleak) picture of the arrest and possible outcomes.
- When appropriate consider the possibility of organ donation and do not be frightened to discuss this with the relatives. Even if discussion with the relatives is delayed, remember corneas and heart valves may be used up to 24 hours after death.

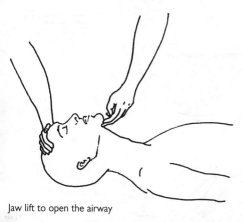

Jaw lift to open the airway

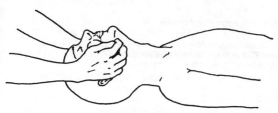

Jaw thrust (thrust the angle of th mandible upwards)

Fig. 17.2 Opening airways. Reproduced with permission from Ramrakha PS, Moore KPK (2004). Oxford Handbook of Acute Medicine. Oxford: Oxford University Press, pp.5–6.

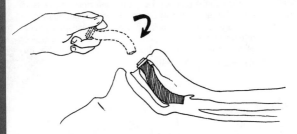

Insertion of oropharyngeal airway

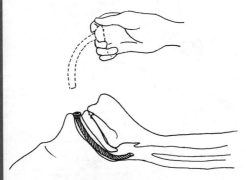

Inertion of nasopharyngeal airway

Fig. 17.3 Insertion of nasopharyngeal airway. Reproduced with permission from Ramrakha PS, Moore KPK (2004). *Oxford Handbook of Acute Medicine.* Oxford: Oxford University Press, pp.5–6.

Universal treatment algorithm

- Cardiac rhythms of cardiac arrest can be divided into two groups:
    1. **Ventricular fibrillation/pulseless ventricular tachycardia (VF/VT).**
    2. **Other cardiac rhythms,** which include **asystole** and **PEA**.
- The principle difference in treatment of the two groups of arrhythmias is the need for attempted defibrillation in the VF/VT group of patients.
- The figure opposite summarizes the algorithm for management of both groups of patients.

VF/VT

- VF/VT are the most common rhythms at the time of cardiac arrest.
- Success in treatment of VF/VT is dependent on the delivery of prompt defibrillation. With each minute the chances of successful defibrillation declines by 7–10%.
- **Precordial thump:** if arrest is witnessed or monitored a sharp blow with a closed fist on the patient's sternum may convert VF/VT back to a perfusing rhythm. It is particularly effective if delivered within thirty seconds after cardiac arrest.
- Shock cycles are generally in groups of three. Initially 200J, 200J and 360J, with subsequent cycles at 360J.
- After each shock (or sequences) the carotid pulse should be palpated only if the waveform changes to one usually capable of providing a cardiac output.
- Shock cycle is repeated every minute if VF/VT persist.
- Myocardial and cerebral viability must be maintained after each shock cycle with chest compressions and ventilation.
- In between cycles of defibrillation reversible factors must be identified and corrected, patient intubated (if possible) and obtain venous access.
- Adrenaline should be given every 3 minutes (1 mg IV and 2–3 mg via endotracheal route).

Non-VF/VT rhythms

- The outcome from these rhythms is generally worse than VF/VT unless a reversible cause can be identified and treated promptly.
- Chest compressions and ventilation should be undertaken for three minutes with each loop of the algorithm (1 min if directly after a shock).
- With each cycle attempts must be made to intubate the patient, gain IV access and give adrenaline.

Asystole

- Atropine 3 mg IV should be given to block all vagal output.
- In the presence of p waves on the ECG strip/monitor, pacing (external or transvenous) must be considered.

Pulseless electrical activity (PEA)

- Identification of the underlying cause and its correction are both vital for successful resuscitation. Resuscitation must be continued whilst reversible causes are being sought.

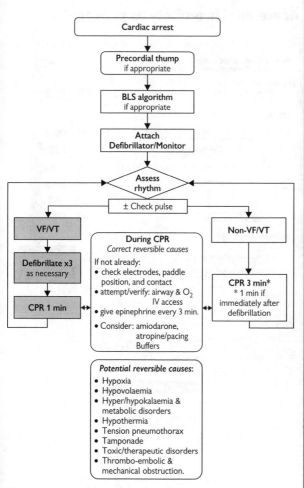

Fig. 17.4 The Advanced Life Support universal algorithm for the management of cardiac arrest in adults. (For further details see The Resuscitation Council (UK) website http://www.resus.org.uk/pages/als.htm)

Acute MI: thrombolysis protocol

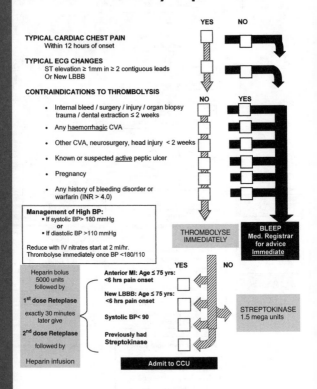

TYPICAL CARDIAC CHEST PAIN
Within 12 hours of onset

TYPICAL ECG CHANGES
ST elevation ≥ 1mm in ≥ 2 contiguous leads
Or New LBBB

CONTRAINDICATIONS TO THROMBOLYSIS

- Internal bleed / surgery / injury / organ biopsy
  trauma / dental extraction ≤ 2 weeks

- Any haemorrhagic CVA

- Other CVA, neurosurgery, head injury < 2 weeks

- Known or suspected active peptic ulcer

- Pregnancy

- Any history of bleeding disorder or
  warfarin (INR > 4.0)

Management of High BP:
■ If systolic BP> 180 mmHg
  or
■ If diastolic BP >110 mmHg

Reduce with IV nitrates start at 2 ml/hr.
Thrombolyse immediately once BP <180/110

THROMBOLYSE
IMMEDIATELY

BLEEP
Med. Registrar
for advice
Immediate

Heparin bolus
5000 units
followed by

1st dose Reteplase

exactly 30 minutes
later give

2nd dose Reteplase

followed by

Heparin infusion

Anterior MI: Age ≤ 75 yrs:
<6 hrs pain onset

New LBBB: Age ≤ 75 yrs:
<6 hrs pain onset

Systolic BP< 90

Previously had
Streptokinase

STREPTOKINASE
1.5 mega units

Admit to CCU

Acute myocardial infarction

Treatment options in tachyarrhythmias

Sinus tachycardia	Look for cause. β-blockade if anxious		
Atrial fibrillation **Atrial flutter** **SVT** (p378)	*Rate control* *(AV node)* • Digoxin • β-blockade • calcium blocker (e.g. veraoamil)	*Version to SR* • Flecainide • Amiodarone • Sotalol • Disopyramide • Synchronised DC shock	*Prevention* • Amiodarone • Sotalol • Quinidine • Procainamide
Junctional **tachycardia (AVNRT)** (p382)	• Adenosine • β-blockade • Verapamil • (Vagal stimulation)	• Digoxin • Flecainide • Synchronised DC shock	
Accessory pathway **tachycardias** **(i.e. AVRT)** (p382)	*At AV Node* • Adenosine • β-blockade	*At accessory* *pathway* • Sotalol • Flecainide • Disopyramide • Quinidine • Amiodarone	*Termination only* Synchronised DC shock
Ventricular **tachycardia** (p390)	*Termination and* *prevention* • Lignocaine • Procainamide • Amiodarone • Magnesium	• Flecainide • Disopyramide • Propafenone • β-blockade	*Termination only* DC Shock

Ventricular tachycardia: drugs

Dosages of selected anti-arrhythmics for the acute treatment of VT

Drug	Dosage
Magnesium sulphate	*Loading dose* 8mmol (2g) iv over 2–15 min (repeat once if necessary) *Maintenance dose* 60 mmol/48 ml saline at 2–3 ml/hr
Lignocaine	*Loading dose* 100 mg iv over 2 min (repeat once if necessary) *Maintenance dose* 4 mg/min for 30 min 2 mg/min for 2 hours 1–2 mg/min for 12–24 hours
Procainamide	*Loading dose* 100 mg iv over 2 min Repeat every 5 min to max 1 g *Maintenance dose* 2–4 mg/min iv infusion 250 mg q6h po
Amiodarone	*Loading dose* 300 mg iv over 60 min via central line followed by 900 mg iv over 23 hours OR 200 mg po tds x 1 week then 200 mg po bd x 1 week *Maintenance dose* 200–400 mg od iv or po
Disopyramide	*Loading dose* 50 mg iv over 5 min repeated up to maximum 150 mg iv 200 mg po *Maintenance dose* 2–5 mg/min iv infusion 100–200 mg q6h po
Flecainide	*Loading dose* 2 mg/kg iv over 10 min (max 150 mg) *Maintenance dose* 1.5 mg/kg iv over 1 hour then 100–250 µg/kg/hour iv for 24 hours or 100–200 mg po bd

Supraventricular tachyarrhythmias

Dosages of selected antiarrhythmics for SVT

Drug	Dosage
Digoxin	*Loading dose:* iv 0.75–1 mg in 50 ml saline over 1–2 hrs. po 0.5 mg q12h for 2 doses then 0.25 mg q12h for 2 days *Maintenance dose:* 0.0625–0.25 mg daily (iv or po)
Propranolol	iv 1 mg over 1 min, repeated every 2 min up to maximum 10 mg po 10–40 mg 3–4 times a day
Atenolol	iv 5–10 mg by slow injection po 25–100 mg daily
Sotalol	iv 20–60 mg by slow injection po 80–160 mg bd
Verapamil	iv 5 mg over 2 min; repeated every 5 min up to maximum 20 mg po 40–120 mg tds
Procainamide	iv 100 mg over 2 min; repeated every 5 min up to maximum 1 g po 250 mg q6h
Amiodarone	*Loading dose:* iv 300 mg over 60 min via central line followed by 900 mg iv over 23 hours OR po 200 mg tds x 1 week then 200 mg po bd x 1 week *Maintenance dose:* 200–400 mg od iv or po
Disopyramide	iv 50 mg over 5 min; repeated every 5 min up to maximum 150 mg iv 100–200 mg q6h po
Flecainide	2 mg/kg iv over 10 min (max 150 mg) or 100–200 mg po bd

Acute pulmonary oedema: assessment

Presentation

- Acute breathlessness, cough, frothy blood-stained (pink) sputum.
- Collapse, cardiac arrest, or shock.
- Associated features may reflect underlying cause:
  - Chest pain or palpitations—? IHD/MI, arrhythmia.
  - Preceding history of dyspnoea on exertion—? IHD, poor LV.
  - Oliguria, haematuria—? acute renal failure.
  - Seizures, signs of intracranial bleed.

Causes

A diagnosis of pulmonary ooedema or 'heart failure' is not adequate. An underlying cause must be sought in order to direct treatment appropriately. These may be divided into:

- Increased pulmonary capillary pressure (hydrostatic).
- Increased pulmonary capillary permeability.
- Decreased intravascular oncotic pressure.

Often a combination of factors are involved (e.g. pneumonia, hypoxia, cardiac ischaemia) See table p652.

The main differential diagnosis is acute (infective) exacerbation of COPD (previous history, quiet breath sounds ± wheeze, fewer crackles). It may be difficult to differentiate the two clinically.

The principles of management are:

1 Stabilize the patient—relieve distress and be.g.in definitive treatment.
2 Look for an underlying cause.
3 Address haemodynamic and respiratory issues.
4 Optimise and introduce long-term therapy.

Initial rapid assessment

- If the patient is very unwell (e.g. unable to speak, hypoxic, systolic BP <100 mmHg) introduce stabilizing measures and begin treatment immediately before detailed examination and investigations (p624).
- If the patient is stable and/or if there is doubt as to the diagnosis, give oxygen and diuretic, but await the outcome of clinical examination and CXR before deciding on definitive treatment.

Urgent investigations for all patients

- ECG   Sinus tachycardia most common.
           ? any cardiac arrhythmia (AF, SVT, VT).
           ? evidence of acute ST change (STEMI, NSTEMI, UA).
           ? evidence of underlying heart disease (LVH, p mitrale).
- CXR   To confirm the diagnosis, looking for interstitial shadowing, enlarged hila, prominent upper lobe vessels, pleural effusion and Kerley B lines. Cardiomegaly may or may not be present. Also exclude pneumothorax, pulmonary embolus (oligaemic lung fields) and consolidation.
- ABG   Typically $\downarrow P_aO_2$. P_aCO_2 levels may be $\downarrow$ (hyperventilation) or $\uparrow$ depending on severity of pulmonary oedema. Pulse oximetry may be inaccurate if peripherally shut down.

- U&Es   ? pre-existing renal impairment. Regular K^+ measurements (once on iv diuretics).
- FBC   ? anaemia or leukocytosis indicating the precipitant.
- ECHO   As soon as practical to assess LV function, valve abnormalities, VSD or pericardial effusion.

Investigations for patients with pulmonary oedema

All patients should have:

- FBC, U&Es, CRP
- Serial biochemical markers of myocardial injury (CK, CK-MB, troponins)
- LFTs, albumin, total protein
- ECG
- CXR
- ECHO (± TOE)
- Arterial blood gases.

Where appropriate consider:-

- Septic screen (sputum, urine, blood cultures)
- Holter monitor (?arrhythmias)
- Coronary angiography (?IHD)
- Right and left heart catheter (if ECHO unable to provide adequate information on pressures, shunts, valve disease)
- Endomyocardial biopsy (myocarditis, infiltration)
- MUGA scan
- Cardiopulmonary exercise test with an assessment of peak oxygen consumption.

Pulmonary oedema: causes

Look for an underlying cause for pulmonary oedema

Increased pulmonary capillary pressure (hydrostatic)

↑ Left atrial pressure	• Mitral valve disease • Arrhythmia (e.g. AF) with pre-existing mitral valve disease • Left atrial myxoma.
↑ LVEDP	• Ischaemia • Arrhythmia • Aortic valve disease • Cardiomyopathy • Uncontrolled hypertension • Pericardial constriction • Fluid overload • High output states (anaemia, thyrotoxicosis, Paget's, AV fistula, beri-beri) • Reno vascular disease.
↑ Pulmonary venous pressure	• L → R shunt (e.g. VSD) • Veno-occlusive disease.
Neurogenic	• Intracranial haemorrhage • Cerebral oedema • Post-ictal.
High altitude pulmonary oedema	

Increased pulmonary capillary permeability

Acute lung injury	• ARDS

Decreased intravascular oncotic pressure

Hypoalbuminaemia	• ↑ losses (e.g. nephrotic syndrome, liver failure) • ↓ production (e.g. sepsis) • Dilution (e.g. crystalloid transfusion).

(Note: the critical LA pressure for hydrostatic ooedema = serum albumin (g/L) x 0.57)

Pulmonary oedema: management

Stabilize the patient

- Patients with acute pulmonary oedema should initially be continuously monitored and managed where full resuscitation facilities are available.
- Sit the patient up in bed.
- Give 60–100% oxygen by facemask (unless contraindicated, COPD)
- If the patient is severely distressed, summon the 'on-call' anaesthetist and inform ITU. If dyspnoea cannot be significantly improved by acute measures (below) the patient may require CPAP or mechanical ventilation.
- Treat any haemodynamically unstable arrhythmia (urgent synchronized DC shock may be required (p702).
- Give:
  - Diamorphine 2.5–5 mg IV (caution abnormal ABGs)
  - Metoclopramide 10 mg IV
  - Frusemide 40–120 mg slow IV injection.
- Secure venous access and send blood for urgent U&Es, FBC, and cardiac enzymes (including troponin).
- Unless thrombolysis is indicated take ABG.
- If the systolic blood pressure is ≥90 mmHg and the patient does not have aortic stenosis:
  - Give sublingual GTN spray (2 puffs)
  - Start IV GTN infusion 1–10 mg/hr, increase the infusion rate every 15–20 minutes, titrating against blood pressure (aiming to keep systolic BP ~100 mmHg).
- If the systolic blood pressure is < 90 mmHg treat patient as cardiogenic shock (see p204).
- Insert a urinary catheter to monitor urine output.
- Repeat ABG and K^+ if the clinical condition deteriorates/fails to improve, or after 2 hrs if there is improvement and the original sample was abnormal.
- Monitor pulse, BP, respiratory rate, O_2 saturation with a pulse oximeter (if an accurate reading can be obtained) and urine output.

If the patient responds arrange appropriate investigations as listed on p621 to help with further management. However, if there is further deterioration specific measures should be taken to address problems.

Further management

The subsequent management of the patient is aimed at ensuring adequate ventilation/gas exchange, ensuring haemodynamic stability and correcting any reversible precipitins of acute pulmonary ooedema.

- **Assess the patient's respiratory function**
  - Does the patient require respiratory support?
- **Assess the patient's haemodynamic status**
  - Is the patient in shock?   p190
- **Look for an underlying cause**   p622
- **Conditions that require specific treatment**
  - Acute aortic and mitral regurgitation.
  - Diastolic left ventricular dysfunction.

- Fluid overload.
- Renal failure.
- Severe anaemia.
- Hypoproteinaemia.

If the patient remains unstable and/or deteriorates:

Assess the patient's respiratory function

- Wheeze may be caused by interstitial pulmonary oedema. If there is a history of asthma, give nebulized salbutamol (2.5–5 mg), nebulized ipratropium bromide (500 µg) and hydrocortisone (200 mg) IV. Consider commencing aminophylline infusion. This will relieve bronchospasm, as well as 'off-load' by systemic vasodilatation. However, it may worsen tachycardia, can be arrhythmogenic and lower K^+ (supplement to ensure K^+ 4–5 mmol/L).
- *Indications for further respiratory support include:*
  - Patient exhaustion or continuing severe breathlessness.
  - Persistent P_aO_2 <8 kPa.
  - Rising P_aCO_2.
  - Persistent or worsening acidosis (pH < 7.2).
- **Continuous positive airways pressure (CPAP):** This may be tried for co-operative patients, who can protect their airway, and have adequate respiratory muscle strength and who are not hypotensive. The positive pressure reduces venous return to the heart and may compromise BP.
- **Endotracheal intubation and mechanical ventilation** may be required, and some positive end expiratory pressure (PEEP) should be used.
- Discuss the patient with the on-call anaesthetist or ITU team early.

Assess the patient's haemodynamic status

It is important to distinguish between cardiogenic and non-cardiogenic pulmonary oedema, as further treatment is different between the two groups. This may be difficult clinically. A PA (Swan–Ganz) catheter must be inserted if the patient's condition will allow.

- **Non-cardiogenic pulmonary oedema** occurs when the hydrostatic pressure within the capillary system overcomes the plasma oncotic pressure. In patients with hypoalbuminaemia this will occur at PCWP less than 15 mmHg. The critical PCWP may be estimated by *serum albumin (g/L) x 0.57*. Thus a patient with a serum albumin of 15 g/L will develop hydrostatic pulmonary oedema at a LA pressure of 8 mmHg; a serum albumin of 30 g/L will require an LA pressure of >17 mmHg and so on…
- **Cardiogenic pulmonary oedema** is often associated with significant systemic hypotension or low output states. Contributing factors include conditions where there is 'mechanical' impairment to forward flow (e.g. valvular heart disease (especially if acute), VSD), or severe myocardial disease (large MI, ongoing ischaemia, acute myocarditis, cardiomyopathy).
- The gradient between PA diastolic pressure and PCWP (PAD–PCWP) is generally <5 mmHg in cardiogenic and >5 mmHg in non-cardiogenic pulmonary oedema (e.g. ARDS).

- The pulse and BP are most commonly elevated due to circulating catecholamines and over activity of the renin-angiotensin system. Examination reveals sweating, cool 'shut-down' peripheries, high pulse volume (assess carotid or femoral pulses).

Management

The general approach involves combination of diuretics, vasodilators ± inotropes. Patients may be divided into two groups:
- Patients in shock (with systolic BP <100 mmHg)—p627
- Haemodynamically stable patients with systolic BP >100 mmHg— see p628.

Patients with systolic BP <100 mmHg

- The patient is in incipient (or overt) shock. The most common aetiology is cardiogenic shock but remember non-cardiogenic causes (e.g. ARDS, septic shock).
- **Optimal monitoring and access:** central line ± PA catheter (Swan–Ganz), urinary catheter, arterial line (monitoring BP and ABGs). Internal jugular lines are preferable as the risk of pneumothorax is lower.
- Ensure patient is not under filled using PCWP as a guide (<10 mmHg) (mistaken diagnosis e.g. septic shock from bilateral pneumonia).
- **Is there a mechanical cause that may require emergency surgery?**
  - Arrange an urgent ECHO to rule out:
    —VSD and acute MR in all patients with recent MI with/without new murmur (pp178–180)
    —Prosthetic heart valve dysfunction (e.g. dehiscence, infection) or pre-existing native aortic or mitral disease that may require surgery.
  - Discuss patient early on with cardiologist/cardiac surgeon.

The **choice of inotropic agent** depends on the clinical condition of the patient and to some extent, the underlying diagnosis:
- **Systolic BP 80–100 mmHg** and cool peripheries: start **dobutamine** infusion at 5 µg/kg/min, increasing by 2.5 µg/kg/min every 10–15 minutes to a maximum of 20 µg/kg/min until BP >100 mmHg. This may be combined with dopamine (2.5–5 µg/kg/min). However, tachycardia and/or hypotension secondary to peripheral vasodilation my limit its effectiveness. **Phosphodiesterase inhibitors** (enoximone or milrinone) should be considered where dobutamine fails.
- **Systolic BP <80 mmHg** give a slow IV bolus of **epinephrine** (2–5 ml of 1 in 1000 solution Min-I-Jet®) and repeated if necessary.
  - **Dopamine** at doses of >2.5 µg/kg/min has a pressor action in addition to direct and indirect inotropic effects and may be used at higher doses (10–20 µg/kg/min) if the blood pressure remains low. However it tends to raise the pulmonary capillary filling pressure further and should be combined with vasodilators (e.g. nitroprusside or hydralazine) once the blood pressure is restored (see below). Beware of arrhythmias at these doses.

- **Epinephrine** infusion may be preferred to high-dose dopamine as an alternative inotrope. Once the blood pressure is restored (>100 mmHg), vasodilators such as nitroprusside/hydralazine or GTN infusion should be added to counteract the pressor effects. Epinephrine can be combined with dobutamine and/or a phosphodiesterase inhibitor, especially in the context of a poor ventricle.
- **Intra-aortic balloon counter pulsation** should also be used with/without inotropes in the context of a potentially reversible cause for the pulmonary oedema and shock (e.g. ongoing myocardial ischaemia, VSD, acute MR).
- Further doses of diuretic may be given.

Patients with systolic BP ≥100 mmHg
- Further doses of diuretic may be given (frusemide 40–80 mg iv q3–4h or as a continuous infusion (20–80 mg/hr)).
- Continue the GTN infusion, increasing the infusion rate every 15–20 minutes up to 10 mg/hr, titrating against blood pressure (aiming to keep systolic BP ~100 mmHg).
- ACE inhibitors can be used if BP is adequate and there are no other known contraindications (e.g. RAS, renal failure). Arteriolar vasodilators (nitroprusside or hydralazine) may also be added in or used instead of GTN (± ACE inhibitor) in patients with adequate BP (pXX for dose). Arterial pressure should be monitored continuously via an arterial line to prevent inadvertent hypotension.

Long-term management
- Unless a contraindication exists, start an ACE inhibitor increasing the dose to as near the recommended maximal dose as possible. In the context of LV impairment, ACE inhibitors have significant prognostic benefit.
- If ACE inhibitors are contraindicated or not tolerated, consider the use of hydralazine and long-acting oral nitrate in combination.
- If the patient is already on high doses of diuretics and ACE inhibitors consider the addition spironolactone (25–50 mg) (NB monitor renal function and serum potassium).
- In the context of stable patients (no clinical features of failure) and poor LV function β–blockers have significant mortality and some symptomatic benefit (NB start very small dose and increase gradually every 2 weeks with re.g.ular monitoring). Bisoprolol, carvedilol and metoprolol can all be used.
- Ensure all arrhythmias are treated.
- Digoxin can be used for symptomatic improvement.
- Consider multisite pacing (biventricular) in the context of severe LV dysfunction, broad QRS complex ± MR on ECHO.
- Patients in AF, or poor LV function should be considered for long term anticoagulation.
- Patients <60 years with severe irreversible LV dysfunction and debilitating symptoms must be considered for cardiac transplantation.

Pulmonary oedema: specific conditions

Diastolic LV dysfunction

- This typically occurs in elderly hypertensive patients with LV hypertrophy, where there is impaired relaxation of the ventricle in diastole. There is marked hypertension, pulmonary oedema, and normal, or only mild, systolic LV impairment.
- With tachycardia, diastolic filling time shortens. As the ventricle is 'stiff' in diastole, LA pressure is increased and pulmonary ooedema occurs (exacerbated by AF as filling by atrial systole is lost).
- Treatment involves control of hypertension with IV nitrates (and/or nitroprusside), calcium blockers (verapamil or nifedipine) and even certain β-blockers (e.g. carvedilol, bisoprolol).

Fluid overload

- Standard measures are usually effective.
- In extreme circumstances venesection may be necessary.
- Check the patient is not anaemic (Hb ≥ 10 g/dL). Remove 500 ml blood via a cannula in a large vein and repeat if necessary.
- If anaemic (e.g. renal failure) and acutely unwell, consider dialysis.

Known (or unknown) renal failure

- Unless the patient is permanently anuric, large doses of IV frusemide may be required (up to 1 g given at 4 mg/min) in addition to standard treatment.
- If this fails, or patient is known to be anuric, dialysis will be required.
- In patients not known to have renal failure an underlying cause should be sought.

Anaemia

- Cardiac failure may be worsened or precipitated by the presence of significant anaemia. Symptoms may be improved in the long term by correcting this anaemia.
- Generally transfusion is unnecessary with Hb >9 g/dL unless there is a risk of an acute bleed. Treatment of pulmonary ooedema will result in haemoconcentration and a 'rise' in the Hb.
- If the anaemia is thought to be exacerbating pulmonary ooedema, ensure that an adequate diuresis is obtained prior to transfusion. Give slow transfusion (3–4 hrs per unit) of packed cells, with IV frusemide 20–40 mg before each unit.

Hypoproteinaemia

- The critical LA pressure at which hydrostatic pulmonary ooedema occurs is influenced by the serum albumin and approximates to serum albumin concentration (g/L) x 0.57.
- Treatment involves diuretics, cautious albumin replacement, spironolactone (if there is secondary hyperaldosteronism), and treatment of the underlying cause for hypoproteinaemia.

Acute aortic regurgitation

Presentation

- Sudden, severe aortic regurgitation presents as cardiogenic shock and acute pulmonary ooedema.
- The haemodynamic changes are markedly different from those seen in chronic AR. The previous normal sized LV results in a smaller effective forward flow and higher LVEDP for the same de.g.ree of AR.
- Patients are often extremely unwell, tachycardic, peripherally shut down and often have pulmonary oedema. Unlike chronic AR, pulse pressure may be near normal.
- If available, ask for a history of previous valvular heart disease, hypertension, features of Marfan's syndrome, and risk factors for infective endocarditis.
- Physical signs of severe AR include a quiet aortic closure sound (S2); an ejection systolic murmur over aortic valve (turbulent flow); high pitched and short, early diastolic murmur (AR); quiet S1 (premature closure of the mitral valve).
- Examine specifically for signs of an underlying cause (see table p76).
- Where there is no obvious underlying cause (e.g. acute MI), assume infective endocarditis until proven otherwise.

Causes

- Infective endocarditis.
- Ascending aortic dissection.
- Collagen vascular disorders (e.g. Marfan's).
- Connective tissue diseases (large and medium vessel arteritis).
- Trauma.
- Dehiscence of a prosthetic valve.

Diagnosis

Is based on a combination of clinical features and transthoracic and/or transoesophageal ECHO.

Management

Acute AR is a surgical emergency and all other management measures are only aimed at stabilizing patient until urgent AVR can take place. Patient's clinical condition will determine the urgency of surgery (and mortality). Liaise immediately with local cardiologists.

General measures (see p624)

- Admit the patient to intensive care or medical HDU.
- Give oxygen, begin treating any pulmonary ooedema with diuretics.
- Monitor blood gases; mechanical ventilation may be necessary.
- Blood cultures x 3 are essential.
- Serial ECG: watch for developing AV block or conduction defects.

Specific measures

- Every patient must be discussed with your regional cardiothoracic centre.
- In the context of good systemic BP, vasodilators such as sodium nitroprusside or hydralazine may temporarily improve forward flow and relieve pulmonary oedema.
- Inotropic support may be necessary if hypotensive. However, inotropes are best avoided as any increase in systemic pressures may worsen AR.
- All patients with haemodynamic compromise should have immediate or urgent aortic valve replacement.
- Infective endocarditis: indications for surgery are given on p106.
- IABP must be avoided as it will worsen AR.

Acute mitral regurgitation

Presentation

- Patients most commonly present with acute breathlessness and severe pulmonary ooedema. Symptoms may be less severe, or spontaneously improve as left atrial compliance increases. There may be a history of previous murmur, angina, or myocardial infarction.
- The signs are different to those seen in chronic MR because of the presence of a non-dilated, and relatively non-compliant LA. Acute MR results in a large LA systolic pressure wave ('v' wave), and hence pulmonary oedema.
- Patients may be acutely unwell with tachycardia, hypotension, peripheral vasoconstriction and pulmonary oedema, and a pan-systolic murmur of MR.
- Later in the illness, probably because of sustained high left atrial and pulmonary venous pressures, right heart failure develops.
- Examine for signs of any underlying conditions (see p633).
- The important differential diagnosis is a VSD. Transthoracic ECHO and Doppler studies can readily differentiate between the two conditions. Alternatively, if ECHO not available, pulmonary artery catheterization in acute MR will exclude the presence of a left to right shunt and the PCWP trace will demonstrate a large 'v' wave.
- Where there is no obvious underlying cause (e.g. acute MI), assume the patient has infective endocarditis until proven otherwise.

Diagnosis

Is based on a combination of clinical features and ECHO. Transthoracic ECHO can readily diagnose and quantify MR. It also provides information on LV status (in particular regional wall motion abnormalities which can give rise to MR). TOE can provide specific information about aetiology of valve dysfunction including papillary muscle rupture and MV leaflet (anterior and posterior) structural abnormalities. This information will be vital for a decision regarding definitive management.

General measures (see p624)

- Admit the patient to intensive care or medical HDU.
- Give oxygen, begin treating any pulmonary oedema with diuretics.
- Monitor blood gases; mechanical ventilation may be necessary.
- Blood cultures x 3 are essential.
- If present, MI should be treated in the standard manner.

Specific measures

- Pulmonary ooedema may be very resistant to treatment.
- In the presence of good BP, reduction in preload (GTN infusion and afterload especially with ACE inhibitors important. Systemic vasodilators such as hydralazine (12.5–100 mg tds) can also be added in.
- An IABP will help decrease LVEDP and increase coronary blood flow.
- *Patients may require inotropic support.* There are multiple combinations and aetiology of MR, haemodynamic status, and local policy/expertise should dictate choice of agent.

- CPAP and intubation and positive pressure ventilation are extremely useful and must be considered in all severe and/or resistant cases.
- Haemodynamic disturbance and severe pulmonary oedema in the context of acute MR is a surgical emergency.
- *Infective endocarditis:* indications for surgery are given on p106.
- *Post-infarct MR:* management depends upon the patient's condition following resuscitation. Patients who are stabilized may have MVR deferred because of the risks of surgery in the post infarct patient. Their pre-operative management should consist of diuretics and vasodilators, including ACE inhibitors if tolerated. Advise patients regarding endocarditis prophylaxis.

Causes of acute mitral regurgitation

- Infective endocarditis
- Papillary muscle dysfunction or rupture (post MI, p178).
- Rupture of chordae tendinae (e.g. infection, myxomatous degeneration, SLE)
- Trauma (to leaflets, papillary muscle, or chordae)
- Prosthetic valve malfunction (e.g. secondary to infection)
- Left atrial myxoma
- Acute rheumatic fever
- Collagen vascular disorders (e.g. Marfan's)
- Connective tissue diseases (large and medium vessel arteritis).

Deep vein thrombosis: assessment

Presentation

- Most commonly asymptomatic. Minor leg discomfort or isolated swelling (>65%) in the affected limb are the most common clinical features. Breathlessness or chest pain may be secondary to PE.
- Signs include erythema and swelling of the leg, dilated superficial veins, and calf discomfort on dorsiflexion of the foot (Homan's sign). The thrombus may be palpable as a fibrous cord in the popliteal fossa. Confirm the presence of swelling (>2 cm) by measuring the limb circumference 15 cm above and 10 cm below the tibial tuberosity.
- In all case of leg swelling abdominal and rectal (and pelvic in women) examination must be carried out to exclude an abdominal cause.

Risk factors for DVT

Procoagulant states

Congenital	Acquired
Factor V$_{Leiden}$	Malignant disease (~5%)
Antithrombin III deficiency	Antiphospholipid syndrome
Protein C deficiency	Myeloproliferative disorders
Protein S deficiency	Oral contraceptive pill (especially with Factor V$_{Leiden}$ mutation)
	Nephrotic syndrome (via renal AT III losses)
	Homocystinuria
	Paroxysmal nocturnal haemoglobinuria

Venous stasis

Immobility (e.g. long journeys)	Recent surgery
Pelvic mass	Pregnancy or recent childbirth
	Severe obesity

Miscellaneous

Hyperviscosity syndromes
Previous DVT or PE
Family history of DVT/PE

Investigations

- **Real time B-mode venous compression ultrasonography** of leg veins is largely replacing venography as the initial investigation of choice. It is quick, non-invasive, with sensitivity and specificity of over 90% and does not carry the risk of contrast allergy or phlebitis. It can simultaneously assess extent of proximal progression of the thrombus in particular extension into pelvic vessels.
- **D-Dimers** have a high negative predictive value for DVT. A low clinical probability of DVT and a negative D-Dimer does not require

further investigation. A positive D-Dimer result should be followed by ultrasonography.
- **Venography:** use if results uncertain and clinical suspicion is high.
- Consider baseline investigations (FBC, U&Es, ECG, CXR, urinalysis and pulse oximetry [± ABG]) on all patients.
- If appropriate, look for an underlying cause.
- Coagulation screen.
- Pro-coagulant screen: refer to local screening policy and get haematology advice (e.g. CRP, ESR, Protein C and S, Antithrombin III levels, Factor V$_{Leiden}$ mutation, auto-Ab screen, immunoglobulins and immunoelectrophoretic strip, anticardiolipin antibody, Ham test, etc.).
- Screen for malignancy: Ultrasound ± CT (abdomen and pelvis), CXR, LFTs, PSA, CEA, CA-125, CA-19.9, β-HCG etc.

Deep vein thrombosis: management

- If there is a high clinical suspicion of DVT (the presence of risk factors and absence of an alternative diagnosis), start empiric anticoagulation with LMWH. This may be stopped if subsequent investigations are negative.
- **Below knee DVT:** thrombi limited to the calf have a lower risk of embolization and may be treated with compression stockings and subcutaneous prophylactic doses of LMWH until mobile to deter proximal propagation of thrombus. A brief period of systemic anticoagulation with LMWH may lessen the pain from below-knee DVT.
- **Above knee DVT:** thrombi within the thigh veins warrant full anticoagulation with LMWH/UFH and subsequently warfarin.

Anticoagulation

Heparin

- LMWHs have now superceded UFH for management of both DVT and PE. They require no monitoring on a daily basis and also allow outpatient treatment.
- There must be a period of overlap between LMWH/UFH therapy and anticoagulation with warfarin until INR is within therapeutic range and stable.
- LMWH are administered primarily as once daily sc injection and dosage is determined by patient weight.

Warfarin

- Always anticoagulate with LMWH/UFH before starting warfarin. Protein C (a vitamin K dependent anticoagulant) has a shorter half-life than the other coagulation factors and levels fall sooner resulting in a transient pro-coagulant tendency.
- If DVT is confirmed commence warfarin and maintain on LMWH/UFH until INR >2.
- Anticoagulate (INR 2–2.5) for 3 months.
- If recurrent DVT, or patient at high-risk of recurrence consider lifelong anti-coagulation.

Thrombolysis

- This should be considered for recurrent, extensive, proximal venous thrombosis (e.g. femoral or iliac veins), as it is more effective than anticoagulation alone in promoting clot dissolution and produces a better clinical outcome.
- Catheter-directed thrombolytic therapy (rt-PA or SK) is superior to systemic thrombolysis.
- One approach is streptokinase 250,000 U over 30 min then 100,000 U every hour for 24–72 hours (see data sheet). See p166 for contraindications to thrombolysis.

Further management
- Women taking the combined OCP should be advised to stop this.
- If there are contraindications to anti-coagulation, consider the insertion of a caval filter to prevent PE.
- All patients should be treated with thigh-high compression stockings to try to reduce symptomatic venous distension when mobilizing.

Pulmonary embolism (PE): assessment

Symptoms

- Classically presents with sudden onset, pleuritic chest pain, associated with breathlessness and haemoptysis. Additional symptoms include postural dizziness or syncope.
- Massive PE may present as cardiac arrest (particularly with electromechanical dissociation) or shock.
- Presentation may be atypical i.e. unexplained breathlessness or unexplained hypotension or syncope only.
- Pulmonary emboli should be suspected in all breathless patients with risk factors for deep vein thrombosis (DVT) or with clinically proven DVT (p634).
- Recurrent PEs may present with chronic pulmonary hypertension and progressive right heart failure.

Signs

- Examination may reveal tachycardia and tachypnoea only. Look for postural hypotension (in the presence of raised JVP).
- Look for signs of raised right heart pressures and cor pulmonale (raised JVP with prominent 'a' wave, tricuspid regurgitation, parasternal heave, right ventricular S3, loud pulmonary closure sound with wide splitting of S2, pulmonary regurgitation).
- Cyanosis suggests a large pulmonary embolism.
- Examine for a pleural rub (may be transient) or effusion.
- Examine lower limbs for obvious thrombophlebitis.
- Mild fever (>37.5°C) may be present. There may be signs of co-existing COPD.

Causes

Most frequently secondary to DVT (leg >> arm; see p634).

Other causes:

- Rarely secondary to right ventricular thrombus (post MI).
- Septic emboli (e.g. tricuspid endocarditis).
- Fat embolism (post fracture).
- Air embolism (venous lines, diving).
- Amniotic fluid.
- Parasites.
- Neoplastic cells.
- Foreign materials (e.g. venous catheters).

Prognostic features

The prognosis in patients with pulmonary emboli varies greatly associated in part with any underlying condition. Generally worse prognosis is associated with larger PE, poor prognostic indicators include:

- Hypotension.
- Hypoxia.
- ECG changes (other than non-specific T-wave changes).

Pulmonary embolism: investigations

General investigations

- ABG: Normal ABG **does not** exclude a PE.
  $\downarrow P_aO_2$ is invariable with larger PEs. Other changes include mild respiratory alkalosis and $\downarrow P_aCO_2$ (due to tachypnoea) and metabolic acidosis ($2°$ to shock).

- ECG: Commonly shows sinus tachycardia $\pm$ non-specific ST and T wave changes in the anterior chest leads. The classical changes of acute cor pulmonale such as $S_1Q_3T_3$, right axis deviation, or RBBB are only seen with massive PE. Less common findings include AF.

- CXR: May be normal and a near normal chest film in the context of severe respiratory compromise if highly suggestive of a PE. Less commonly may show focal pulmonary oligaemia (*Westermark's sign*), a raised hemidiaphragm, small pleural effusion, wedge shaped shadows based on the pleura, subsegmental atelectasis, or dilated proximal pulmonary arteries.

- Blood tests: There is no specific test. FBC may show neutrophil leukocytosis; mildly elevated CK, Troponin and bilirubin may be seen.

- ECHO/TOE are insensitive for diagnosis but can exclude other causes of hypotension and raised right sided pressures (e.g. tamponade, RV infarction). In PE it will show RV dilatation and global hypokinesia (with sparing of apex (*McConnell's sign*)), pulmonary artery dilation and Doppler may show tricuspid/pulmonary regurgitation allowing estimation of RV systolic pressure. Rarely, the thrombus in the pulmonary artery may be visible.

Specific investigations

D-dimer

- A highly sensitive, but non-specific test.
- Useful in ruling out PE in patients with low or intermediate probability.
- Results can be effected by advancing age, pregnancy, trauma, surgery, malignancy, and inflammatory states.

Ventilation/perfusion (V/Q) lung scanning

A perfusion lung scan (with iv Technetium-99 labeled albumin) should be performed in all suspected cases of PE. A ventilation scan (inhaled Xenon-133) in conjunction increases the specificity by assessing whether the defects in the ventilation and perfusion scans 'match' or 'mismatch'. Pre-existing lung disease makes interpretation difficult.

- A normal perfusion scan rules out significant sized PE.
- Abnormal scans are reported as low, medium or high probability:
  - A high probability scan is strongly associated with a PE, but there is a significant minority of false positives.
  - A low probability scan with a low clinical suspicion of PE should prompt a search for another cause for the patient's symptoms.

- If the clinical suspicion of PE is high and the scan is of low or medium probability, alternative investigations are required.

Investigations for an underlying cause for PEs

- Ultrasound deep veins of legs
- USS abdomen and pelvis (?Occult malignancy/pelvic mass)
- CT abdomen/pelvis
- Screen for inherited pro-coagulant tendency (e.g. Protein C, S, Anti thrombin III, Factor V$_{Leiden}$ etc.)
- Autoimmune screen (anticardiolipin antibody, ANA)
- Biopsy of suspicious lymph nodes/masses.

CT pulmonary angiography (CTPA)

- **This is the recommended initial lung imaging modality in patients with non-massive PE.**
- Allows direct visualization of emboli as well as other potential parenchymal disease, which may explain alternative explanation for symptoms.
- Sensitivity and specificity are high (>90%) for lobar pulmonary arteries but not so high for segmental and subsegmental pulmonary arteries.
- A patient with a positive CTPA does not require further investigation.
- A patient with a negative CTPA in the context of a high/intermediate probability of a PE should undergo further investigation.

Evaluation of leg veins with ultrasound

- Not very reliable. Almost half of patients with PE do not have evidence of a DVT and therefore a negative result can not rule out a PE.
- Useful second line investigation as an adjunct to CTPA/VQ scan.
- Outcome studies have demonstrated that it would be safe not to anticoagulate patients with a negative CTPA and lower limb US who have an intermediate/low probability of a PE.

Pulmonary angiography

- Is the 'gold standard' investigation.
- It is indicated in patients in whom diagnosis of embolism can not be established by non-invasive means. Look for sharp cut-off of vessels or obvious filling defects.
- Invasive investigation and can be associated with 0.5% mortality.
- If there is an obvious filling defect, the catheter or a guide wire passed through the catheter, may be used to disobliterate the thrombus.
- After angiography, the catheter may be used to give thrombolysis directly into the affected pulmonary artery (see below).
- The contrast can cause systemic vasodilatation and haemodynamic collapse in hypotensive patients.

MR pulmonary angiography

- Results are comparable to pulmonary angiography in preliminary studies.
- It can simultaneously assess ventricular function.

Pulmonary embolism: management

1. Stabilize the patient

- Unless an alternative diagnosis is made the patient should be treated as for a pulmonary embolus until this can be excluded.
- Monitor cardiac rhythm, pulse, BP, respiration rate every 15 minutes with continuous pulse oximetry and cardiac monitor. Ensure full resuscitation facilities are available.
- Obtain venous access and start IV fluids (crystalloid or colloid).
- Give maximal inspired oxygen via facemask to correct hypoxia. Mechanical ventilation may be necessary if the patient is tiring (beware of cardiovascular collapse when sedation is given for endotracheal intubation).
- **Give LMWH or UFH to all patients with high or intermediate risk of PE until diagnosis is confirmed.** Meta analysis of multiple trials has shown LMWH to be superior to UFH with a reduction in mortality and bleeding complications. For doses consult local formulary.
- If there is evidence of haemodynamic instability (systemic hypotension, features of right heart failure) or cardiac arrest patients may benefit from thrombolysis with rtPA or streptokinase (same doses used for treatment of STEMI (see p167)).

2. Analgesia

- Patients may respond to oral NSAIDs.
- Opiate analgesia to be used with caution. The vasodilatation caused by these drugs may precipitate or worsen hypotension. Give small doses (1–2 mg diamorphine IV) slowly. Hypotension should respond to IV colloid.
- Avoid im injections (anticoagulation and possible thrombolysis).

3. Investigations with view to a definite diagnosis

(see previous section)

4. Anticoagulate

- Patients with a positive diagnosis must undergo anticoagulation with warfarin. There should be period of overlap with LMWH/UFH until INR values are therapeutic. Target INR is 2–3 for most cases.
- Standard duration of anticoagulation is:
  - 4–6 weeks for temporary risk factor.
  - 3 months first idiopathic cases.
  - At least 6 months for other cases
  - With recurrent events and underlying predisposition to thromboembolic events (e.g. antiphospholipid antibody syndrome) lifelong anticoagulation may be needed (as well as higher target INR > 3).

Dosage of thrombolytic agents for pulmonary embolus

rtPA	100 mg over 2 hours or 0.6 mg/kg over 15 min (maximum of 50 mg) followed by heparin.
Streptokinase	250,000 U over 30 minutes followed by 100,000 U/hr infusion for 24 hours

NB contraindications for thrombolysis identical to ones for STEMI (p166).

Cardiac arrest (also see p604)

- Massive PE may present as cardiac arrest with electromechanical dissociation (EMD). Exclude the other causes of EMD (see p608).
- Chest compressions may help break up the thrombus and allow it to progress more distally, thereby restoring some cardiac output.
- If clinical suspicion of PE is high and there is no absolute contraindication to thrombolysis, give rt-PA (similar in dose to STEMI with a maximum of 50 mg (see p167) followed by heparin).
- If cardiac output returns, consider pulmonary angiography or inserting a PA catheter to try to mechanically disrupt the embolus.

Hypotension

The acute increase in pulmonary vascular resistance results in right ventricular dilatation and pressure overload, which mechanically impairs LV filling and function. Patients require a higher than normal right-sided filling pressure, but may be worsened by fluid overload.

- Insert an internal jugular sheath prior to anticoagulation. This can be used for access, later if necessary.
- If hypotensive give colloid (e.g. 500 ml *Haemacell*® stat).
- If hypotension persists invasive monitoring and/or inotropic support is required. The JVP is a poor indicator of the left-sided filling pressures in such cases. Adrenaline is the inotrope of choice.
- Femoro-femoral cardiopulmonary bypass may be used to support the circulation until thrombolysis or surgical embolectomy can be performed.
- Pulmonary angiography in a hypotensive patient is hazardous as the contrast may cause systemic vasodilatation and cardiovascular collapse.

Pulmonary embolectomy

- In patients who have contraindications to thrombolysis and are in shock requiring inotropic support, there may be a role for embolectomy if appropriate skills are on site.
- This can be performed percutaneously in the catheterization laboratory using a number of devices or surgically on cardiopulmonary bypass.
- Percutaneous procedures may be combined with peripheral or central thrombolysis.
- Seek specialist advice early. Best results are obtained before onset of cardiogenic shock.

- Radiological confirmation of extent and site of embolism is preferable before thoracotomy.
- Mortality is ~25–30%.

Inferior vena cava (IVC) filter
- Infrequently used as little to suggest improved short or long-term mortality.
- Filters are positioned percutaneously and if possible patients must remain anticoagulated to prevent further thrombus formation.
- Most are positioned infra-renally (bird's nest filter), but can also be supra-renal (Greenfield filter).
- Indications for IVC filter use include:
  - Anticoagulation contraindicated: e.g. active bleeding, heparin induced thrombocytopenia, planned intensive chemotherapy.
  - Anticoagulation failure despite adequate therapy.
  - Prophylaxis in high-risk patients: e.g. progressive venous thrombosis, severe pulmonary hypertension.

Fat embolism

Commonly seen in patients with major trauma. There is embolization of fat and micro-aggregates of platelets, RBCs, and fibrin in systemic and pulmonary circulation. Pulmonary damage may result directly from the emboli (infarction) or by a chemical pneumonitis and ARDS.

Clinical features

- There may be a history of fractures followed (24–48 hrs later) by breathlessness, cough, haemoptysis, confusion, and rash.
- Examination reveals fever (38–39°C), widespread petechial rash (25–50%), cyanosis and tachypnoea. There may be scattered crepitations in the chest, though examination may be normal. Changes in mental state may be the first sign with confusion, drowsiness, seizures, and coma. Examine the eyes for conjunctival and retinal haemorrhages; occasionally fat globules may be seen in the retinal vessels. Severe fat embolism may present as shock.

Investigations

- ABG   Hypoxia and a respiratory alkalosis (with low P_aCO_2) as for thromboembolic PE.
- FBC   Thrombocytopenia, acute intravascular haemolysis.
- Coagulation Disseminated intravascular coagulation.
- U&Es & glucose   Renal failure, hypoglycaemia.
- Ca^{2+} May be low.
- Urine   Microscopy for fat and dipstick for haemoglobin.
- ECG   Usually non-specific (sinus tachycardia; occasionally signs of right heart strain).
- CXR   Usually lags behind the clinical course. There may be patchy, bilateral, air space opacification. Effusions rare.
- CT head   Consider if there is a possibility of head injury with expanding subdural or epidural bleed.

Differential diagnosis

- Pulmonary thromboembolism, other causes of ARDS, septic shock, hypovolaemia, cardiac or pulmonary contusion, head injury, aspiration pneumonia, transfusion reaction.

Management

- Treat respiratory failure. Give oxygen (maximal via face mask; CPAP and mechanical ventilation if necessary).
- Ensure adequate circulating volume and cardiac output. CVP is not a good guide to left sided filling pressures and a PA catheter (Swan–Ganz) should be used to guide fluid replacement. Try to keep PCWP 12–15 mmHg and give diuretics if necessary. Use inotropes to support circulation as required.

- Aspirin, heparin and Dextran 40 (500 ml over 4–6 h) are of some benefit in the acute stages, but may exacerbate bleeding from sites of trauma.
- High dose steroids (methylprednisolone 30 mg/kg q8h for 3 doses) has been shown to improve hypoxaemia[1] but steroids are probably most effective if given prophylactically.

1 Lindeque BG et al (1987) J Bone Joint Surg, 69: 128–131.

Hypertensive emergencies

Hypertensive crisis

Hypertensive crisis is defined as a severe elevation in blood pressure (SBP > 200 mmHg, DBP > 120 mmHg). Rate of change in BP is important. A rapid rise is poorly tolerated and leads to end-organ damage, whereas a gradual rise in a patient with existent poor BP control is tolerated better. Hypertensive crisis are classified as:

1. **Hypertensive emergency** where a high BP is complicated by acute target organ dysfunction (see p649) and includes:
   - *Hypertensive emergency with retinopathy* where there is marked elevation in BP (classically DBP >140 mmHg) with retinal haemorrhages and exudates (previously called accelerated hypertension) and
   - *Hypertensive emergency with papilloedema* with a similarly high BP and papilloedema (previously called malignant hypertension).
2. **Hypertensive urgency** where there is a similar rise in BP, but without target organ damage.

Conditions which present as hypertensive emergency

- Essential hypertension.
- Renovascular hypertension: atheroma, fibromuscular dysplasia, acute renal occlusion.
- Renal parenchymal disease: acute glomerulonephritis, vasculitis, scleroderma.
- Endocrine disorders: phechromocytoma, Cushing's syndrome, primary hyperaldosteronism, thyrotoxicosis, heperparathyroidism, acromegaly, adrenal carcinoma.
- Eclampsia and pre-eclampsia.
- Vasculitis.
- Drugs: cocaine, amphetamines, MAOI interactions, cyclosporine, β-blocker, and clonidine withdrawal.
- Autonomic hyperactivity in presence of spinal cord injury.
- Coarctation of the aorta.

Presentation

- Occasionally minimal non-specific symptoms such as mild headache and nose bleed.
- A small group of patients present with symptoms resulting from BP-induced microvascular damage:
  - Neurological symptoms: severe headache, nausea, vomiting, visual loss, focal neurological deficits, fits, confusion, intracerebral haemorrhage, coma (see below).
  - Chest pain (hypertensive heart disease, MI, or aortic dissection) and congestive cardiac failure.
  - Symptoms of renal failure: renal impairment may be chronic (secondary to long-standing hypertension) or acute (from the necrotising vasculitis of malignant hypertension).

- Patients may present with hypertension as one manifestation of an underlying 'disease' (renovascular hypertension, chronic renal failure, CREST syndrome, phaeochromocytoma, pregnancy).
- Examination should be directed at looking for evidence of end-organ damage even if the patient is asymptomatic (heart failure, retinopathy, papillooedema, focal neurology).

Hypertensive emergencies

- Hypertensive emergency with retinopathy/papillooedema
- Hypertensive encephalopathy
- Hypertension induced intracranial haemorrhage/stroke
- Hypertension with cardiovascular complications:
  - Aortic dissection (p660)
  - MI
  - Pulmonary ooedema (p620)
- Pheochromocytoma
- Pregnancy associated hypertensive complications
  - Eclampsia and pre-eclampsia
- Acute renal insufficiency
- Hypertensive emergency secondary to acute withdrawal syndromes (e.g. β-blockers, centrally acting anti-hypertensives).

Hypertensive emergencies: management

Priorities in management are:
1   Confirm the diagnosis and assess the severity.
2   Identify those patients needing specific emergency treatment.
3   Plan long-term treatment.

Diagnosis and severity

- **Ask about** previous BP recordings, previous and current treatment, sympathomimetics, antidepressants, non-prescription drugs, recreational drugs.
- **Check the blood pressure** yourself, in both arms, after a period of rest and if possible on standing. Monitor the patient's blood pressure regularly while they are in A&E.
- **Examine** carefully for clinical evidence of cardiac enlargement or heart failure, peripheral pulses, renal masses or focal neurological deficit. Always examine the fundi—dilate if necessary.

Investigations

All patients should have:

- **FBC**   Microangiopathic haemolytic anaemia with malignant HT.

- **U&E**   Renal impairment and/or $\downarrow K^+$ (diffuse intra-renal ischaemia and $2°$ hyperaldosteronism).

- **Coag screen**   DIC with malignant HT.

- **CXR**   Cardiac enlargement.
                       Aortic contour (dissection?).
                       Pulmonary oedema.

- **Urinalysis**   Protein and red cells ± casts.

Other investigations depending on clinical picture and possible aetiology include:

- **24 hr urine collection**   Creatinine clearance.
                               Free catecholamines, metanephrines or vanilmandellic acid (VMA).

- **ECHO**   LVH, aortic dissection.
- **Renal USS & Doppler**   Size of kidneys and renal artery stenosis.
- **MR renal angiogram**   Renal artery stenosis.
- **CT/MR brain**   Intracranial bleed.
- **Drug screen**   Cocaine, amphetamine, others.

Indications for admission

- Diastolic blood pressure persistently ≥120 mmHg.
- Retinal haemorrhages, exudates or papillooedema.
- Renal impairment.

Voltage criteria for LVH

- Tallest R (V4–V6) + deepest S (V1–V3) >40 mm
- Tallest R (V4–V6) >27 mm
- Deepest S (V1–V3) >30 mm
- R in aVL >13 mm
- R in aVF >20 mm
- QRS complex >0.08 secs (2 small sq.)
- Abnormal ST depression or T inversion in V4–V6

Treatment principles

- **Rapid reduction in BP is unnecessary, must be avoided and can be very dangerous.** This can result in cerebral and cardiac hypoperfusion (an abrupt change of >25% in BP will exceed cerebral BP autoregulation).
- Initial BP reduction of (25%) to be achieved over 1–4 hours with a less rapid reduction over 24 hours to a DBP 100 mmHg.
- The only two situations where BP must be lowered rapidly are in the context of aortic dissection and MI.

Treatment

- The majority of patients who are alert and otherwise well may be treated with oral therapy to lower BP gradually.
- First line treatment should be with a β-blocker (unless contraindicated) with a thiazide diuretic, or a low dose calcium antagonist.
- Urgent invasive monitoring (arterial line) prior to drug therapy is indicated for patients with:
  - Evidence of hypertensive encephalopathy.
  - Complications of hypertension
    (e.g. aortic dissection, acute pulmonary ooedema or renal failure).
  - Treatment of underlying condition
    (e.g. glomerulonephritis, phaeochromocytoma, CREST crisis).
  - Patients with persistent diastolic BP ≥140 mmHg.
  - Eclampsia
- Sublingual nifedipine must be avoided.

Conditions requiring specific treatment
(see p652)

Long term management

- Investigate as appropriate for an underlying causes.
- Select a treatment regime, which is tolerated and effective. Tell the patient why long-term therapy is important.
- Try to reduce all cardiovascular risk factors by advising the patient to stop smoking, appropriate dietary advice (cholesterol), and aim for optimal diabetic control.
- Monitor long-term control and look for end-organ damage (regular fundoscopy, ECG, U&Es). Even poor control is better than no control.

Conditions requiring specific treatment

- Accelerated and malignant hypertension (p656)
- Hypertensive encephalopathy (p658)
- Eclampsia
- Phaeochromocytoma
- Hypertensive patients undergoing anaesthesia

Drugs for hypertensive emergencies

Drugs for the treatment of hypertensive emergencies: IV therapy

Drug	Dosage	Onset of action	Comments
Labetalol	20–80 mg iv bolus q10min 20–200 mg/min by iv infusion increasing every 15 min.	2–5 minutes	Drug of choice in suspected phaeochromocytoma (p598) or aortic dissection (p170). Avoid if there is LVF May be continued orally (see below)
Nitroprusside	0.25–10 µg/kg/min iv infusion (p698)	Seconds	Drug of choice in LVF and/or encephalopathy.
GTN	1–10 mg/hr iv infusion	2–5 minutes	Mainly venodilatation. Useful in patients with LVF or angina.
Hydralazine	5–10 mg iv over 20 min 50–300 µg/kg/min iv infusion	10–15 minutes	May provoke angina
Esmolol HCl	500 µg/kg/min iv loading dose 50–200 µg/kg/min iv infusion	Seconds	Short acting β-blocker also used for SVTs
Phentolamine	2–5 mg iv over 2–5 minutes prn	Seconds	

NB: It is dangerous to reduce the blood pressure quickly. Aim to reduce the diatolic BP to 100–110 mmHg within 2–4 hours. Unless there are good reasons to commence iv therapy, always use oral medicines

Drugs for the treatment of hypertensive emergencies: Oral therapy

Drug	Dosage	Onset of action	Comment
Atendol	50–100 mg po od	30–60 minutes	There are numerous alternative β-blockers—see BNF
Nifedipine	10–20 mg po q8h (q12h if slow release)	15–20 minutes	Avoid sublingual as the fall in bp is very rapid.
Labetalol	100–400 mg po q12h	30–60 minutes	Use if phaeochromocytoma suspected. Safe in pregnancy
Hydralazine	25–50 mg po q8h	20–40 minutes	Safe in pregnancy
Minoxidil	5–10 mg po od	30–60 minutes	May cause marked salt and water retention Combine with a loop diuretic (e.g. frusemide 40–240 mg daily)
Clonidine	0.2 mg po followed by 0.1 mg hourly max.30–60 minutes 0.8 mg total for urgent therapy, or 0.05–0.1mg po q8 h increasing every 2 days	30–60 minutes	Sedation common. Do not stop abruptly as here is a high incidence of rebound hypertensive crisis

NB: Aim to reduce diastolic bp to 100–110mmHg in 2–4 hours and normalize bp in 2–3 days.

Hypertensive emergency with retinopathy (accelerated and malignant hypertension)

This is part of a continuum of disorders characterized by hypertension (diastolic BP often >120 mmHg) and acute microvascular damage (seen best in the retina but present in all organs). It may be difficult to decide whether the damage in some vascular beds is the cause or effect of hypertension (e.g. an acute glomerulonephritis).

- Accelerated hypertension (Grade 3 retinopathy) may progress to malignant hypertension, with widespread necrotizing vasculitis of the arterioles (and papillooedema).
- Presentation is commonly with headache or visual loss and varying degrees of confusion. More severe cases present with renal failure, heart failure, microangiopathic haemolytic anaemia and DIC.

Management

- Transfer the patient to medical HDU/ITU.
- Insert an arterial line and consider central venous line if there is evidence of necrotizing vasculitis and DIC. Catheterize the bladder.
- Monitor neurological state, ECG, fluid balance.
- Aim to lower the DBP to 100 mmHg or by 15–20 mmHg, whichever is higher, over the first 24 hours.
- Those with early features may be treated successfully with oral therapy (β-blockers, calcium channel blockers—see table p655)
- Patients with late symptoms or who deteriorate should be given parenteral therapy aiming for more rapid lowering of BP.
  - If there is evidence of pulmonary oedema or encephalopathy give frusemide 40–80 mg IV.
  - If there is no LVF, give a bolus of labetalol followed by an infusion. For patients with LVF, nitroprusside or hydralazine are preferable.
- Consult renal team for patients with acute renal failure or evidence of acute glomerulonephritis (>2+ proteinuria, red cell casts). Dopamine should be avoided as it may worsen hypertension.
- Consider giving an ACE inhibitor. High circulating renin levels may not allow control of hypertension, which in turn causes progressive renal failure. ACE inhibitors will block this vicious circle. There may be marked first dose hypotension so start cautiously.
- Haemolysis and DIC should recover with control of BP.

Hypertension in the context of acute stroke/intracranial bleed

- Stroke/bleed may be the result of hypertension or vice-versa.
- In the acute setting there is impaired autoregulation of cerebral blood flow and autonomic function. Small changes in systemic BP may result in catastrophic falls in cerebral blood flow.
- Systemic BP should not be treated unless DBP >130 mmHg and/or presence severe cerebral oedema (with clinical manifestations).
- In most cases BP tends to settle over 24–36 hours. If treatment is indicated above BP reduction principles must be adhered to and a combination of nitroprusside, labetalol and calcium channel blockers can be used.
- Centrally acting agents must be avoided as they cause sedation.
- In patients with SAH, a cerebroselective calcium channel blocker, such as nimodipine, is used to decrease cerebral vasospasm.
- Systemic BP must also be treated if qualifies above principles and/or if it remains elevated after 24 hours. There is no evidence that this reduces further events in the acute phase.

Hypertensive retinopathy

Grade 1	Tortuous retinal arteries, silver wiring
Grade 2	AV nipping
Grade 3	Flame shaped haemorrhages and cotton wool exudates
Grade 4	Papilloedema

Hypertensive encephalopathy

- Is caused by cerebral ooedema secondary to loss of cerebral autoregulatory function.
- Usually gradual onset and may occur in previously normotensive patients at blood pressures as low as 150/100. It is rare in patients with chronic hypertension and pressures are also much higher.

Symptoms

- Headache, nausea and vomiting, confusion, grade III and IV hypertensive retinopathy.
- Late features consist of focal neurological signs, fits, and coma.

Diagnosis

- Is a diagnosis of exclusion and other differential diagnosis must be ruled out (e.g. stroke, encephalitis, tumours, bleeding, vasculitis).
- History is helpful; particularly of previous seizures, SAH usually being sudden in onset and strokes being associated with focal neurological deficit.
- Always exclude hypoglycaemia.
- Starting hypotensive treatment for hypertension associated with a stroke can cause extension of the stroke.
- **An urgent MRI or CT brain must be obtained** to rule out some of the differential diagnosis.

Management

- The primary principle of blood pressure control is to reduce DBP by 25% or reduce DBP to 100 mmHg, whichever is higher, over a period of 1–2 hours.
- Transfer the patient to ITU for invasive monitoring (see previous section).
- Monitor neurological state, ECG, fluid balance.
- Correct electrolyte abnormalities (K^+, Mg^{2+}, Ca^{2+}).
- Give frusemide 40–80 mg IV.
- Nitroprusside is the first line agent as it is easy to control of BP changes, despite its tendency to increase cerebral blood flow.
- Labetolol and calcium channel blockers are second line agents and should be added in if necessary.
- It is vital to avoid agents with potential sedative action such as β–blockers, clonidine and methyldopa.
- In selected patients who are stable and present at the very early stages oral therapy with a combination of β–blockers and calcium blockers may be sufficient.

Aortic dissection: assessment

Aortic dissection is a surgical/medical emergency and untreated has a >90% one year mortality. Dissection begins with formation of a tear in the intima and the force of the blood cleaves the media longitudinally to various lengths. Predisposing factors are summarized on p661.

Classification

There are three classifications as illustrated in Fig. 17.5 p663—DeBakey, Stanford, and Descriptive. Dissections involving the ascending and/or aortic arch are surgical emergencies and ones exclusive to the descending aorta are treated medically.

Presentation

- **Chest pain:** classically abrupt onset, very severe in nature and most commonly anterior chest pain radiating to the interscapular region. Usually tearing in nature and unlike the pain of myocardial infarction most severe at its onset. Pain felt maximally in the anterior chest is associated with ascending aortic dissection, whereas interscapular pain suggests dissection of the descending aorta. Patients often use adjectives such as 'tearing', 'ripping', 'sharp' and 'stabbing' to describe the pain.
- **Sudden death** or **shock:** usually due to aortic rupture or cardiac tamponade.
- **Congestive cardiac failure:** due to acute aortic incompetence and/or myocardial infarction.
- Patients may also present with symptoms and signs of occlusion of one of the branches of the aorta. Examples include:
  - Stroke or acute limb ischaemia—due to compression or dissection.
  - Paraplegia with sensory deficits—spinal artery occlusion.
  - Myocardial infarction—usually the right coronary artery.
  - Renal failure and renovascular hypertension.
  - Abdominal pain—coeliac axis or mesenteric artery occlusion.
- Aortic dissection may be painless.
- Ask specifically about history of hypertension, previous heart murmurs or aortic valve disease and previous chest X-rays that may be useful for comparison.

Examination

- This may be normal.
- Most patients are hypertensive on presentation. Hypotension is more common in dissections of the ascending aorta (20–25%) and may be due to blood loss, acute aortic incompetence (which may be accompanied by heart failure), or tamponade (distended neck veins, tachycardia, pulsus paradoxus).
- Pseudohypotension may be seen if flow to either or both subclavian arteries is compromised. Look for unequal blood pressure in the arms and document the presence of peripheral pulses carefully. Absent or changing pulses suggests extension of the dissection.

- Auscultation may reveal aortic valve regurgitation and occasionally a pericardial friction rub. Descending aortic dissections may rupture or leak into the left pleural space and the effusion results in dullness in the left base.
- Neurologic deficits may be due to carotid artery dissection or compression (hemiplegia) or spinal artery occlusion (paraplegia with sensory loss).

Conditions associated with aortic dissection

• Hypertension	Smoking, dyslipidaemia, cocaine/crack
• Connective tissue disorders	Marfan's syndrome[1]
	Ehlers–Danlos syndrome
• Hereditary vascular disorders	Bicuspid aortic valve
	Coarctaion
• Vascular inflammation	Giant cell arteritis
	Takayasu arteritis
	Behçet's disease
	Syphillis
• Decceleration trauma	Car accident
	Falls
• Chest trauma	
• Pregnancy	
• Iatrogenic	Catheterization
	Cardiac surgery

1 Marfan's syndrome (arm span>height, pubis to sole>pubis to vertex, depressed sternum, scoliosis, high arched palate, upward lens dislocation, thoracic aortic dilation/aortic regurgitation, increased urinary hydroxyprolene (some).

Differential diagnosis

- The chest pain may be mistaken for acute MI and acute MI may complicate aortic dissection. Always look for other signs of dissection (see above), as thrombolysis will be fatal.
- Severe chest pain and collapse may also be due to pulmonary embolism, spontaneous pneumothorax, acute pancreatitis, and penetrating duodenal ulcer.
- Pulse deficits without backache should suggest other diagnoses: atherosclerotic peripheral vascular disease, arterial embolism, Takayasu's arteritis etc.
- Acute cardiac tamponade with chest pain is also seen in acute viral or idiopathic pericarditis and acute myocardial infarction with external rupture.

Aortic dissection: investigations

General

- **ECG** may be normal or non-specific (LVH, ST/T abnormalities). Look specifically for evidence of acute MI (inferior MI is seen if the dissection compromises the right coronary artery ostium).
- **Chest X-ray** may appear normal, but with hindsight is almost always abnormal. Look for widened upper mediastinum, haziness or enlargement of the aortic knuckle, irregular aortic contour, separation (>5 mm) of intimal calcium from outer aortic contour, displacement of trachea to the right, enlarged cardiac silhouette (pericardial effusion), pleural effusion (usually on left). Compare with previous films if available.
- **Bloods:** Base FBC, U&E, cardiac enzyme as well as cross match. A novel monoclonal antibody assay to smooth muscle myosin heavy chains can accurately differentiate an acute dissection from a MI.

Diagnostic

- **Echocardiography:** *transthoracic ECHO* may be useful in diagnosing aortic root dilatation, aortic regurgitation and pericardial effusion/tamponade. *Transoesophageal ECHO* (TOE) is the investigation of choice as it allows better evaluation of both ascending aorta and descending aorta, may identify origin of intimal tear, allows evaluation of the origins of the coronary arteries in relation to the dissection flap, and provides information on aortic insufficiency. It is not good at imaging the distal ascending aorta and proximal arch.
- **MRI angiography** is the gold standard for diagnosing aortic dissection. It has all the positive features of TOE and in particular also provides accurate information on all segments of ascending/arch/descending aorta, entry/exit sites and branch vessels. Images can be displayed in multiple views as well as reconstructed in three dimensions. However, there are a number of disadvantages including i) availability of service out-of-hours and cost; ii) presence of metallic valves, pacemakers may preclude patient from having an MRI; iii) monitoring of unstable patients in the scanner can be difficult and unsafe.
- **Spiral (helical) CT with contrast** allows three dimensional display of all segments of aorta and adjacent structures. True and false lumen are identified by differential contrast flow, enter and exit site of intimal flap can be seen as well as pleural and pericardial fluid. However it cannot demonstrate disruption of the aortic valve, which may be associated with ascending aortic dissection.
- **Angiography** using the femoral or axillary approach may demonstrate altered flow in the two lumens, aortic valve incompetence, and involvement of the branches and the site of the intimal tear. It is invasive and associated with a higher risk of complications in an already high-risk patient. It has largely been superseded by CT/MRI and TOE.

Selecting a diagnostic modality

- Confirm or refute a diagnosis of dissection.
- Is the dissection confined to the descending aorta or does it involve the ascending/arch?
- Identify extent, sites of enter and exit and presence and absence of thrombus.
- To see whether there is aortic regurgitation, coronary involvement or pericardial effusions.

Selecting a diagnostic modality

- Where available, TOE should be the first line investigation. It is safe and can provide all the information necessary to take the patient to the operating theatre.
- If TOE is not available or if it fails to provide the necessary information a spiral contrast CT should be performed.
- MRI should generally be reserved for follow-up images.
- Angiography is rarely used, but is of value if other modalities have failed to provide a diagnosis and/or extensive information is needed on branch vessels.

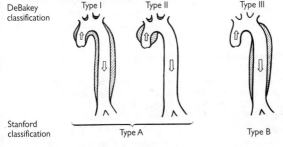

DeBakey classification

Type I   Type II   Type III

Stanford classification

Type A   Type B

Fig. 17.5 Clarification of aortic dissection.

Aortic dissection: management

Stabilize the patient

- If the diagnosis is suspected, transfer the patient to an area where full resuscitation facilities are readily available.
- Secure **venous access** with large bore cannulas (e.g. grey venflon).
- **Take blood** for FBC, U&Es, and cross match (10 units).
- When the diagnosis is confirmed or in cases with cardiovascular complications, **transfer to ITU**, insert an **arterial line** (radial unless the subclavian artery is compromised when a femoral line is preferred), **central venous line**, and **urinary catheter**.
- Immediate measures should be taken to correct blood pressure (see below).
- Adequate analgesia (diamorphine 2.5–10 mg IV and metoclopramide 10 mg IV).

Plan the definitive treatment

This depends on the type of dissection (see Fig. 17.5 p663) and its effects on the patient. General principles are:

- Patients with involvement of the ascending aorta should have **emergency surgical repair and BP control.**
- Patients with dissection limited to the descending aorta are managed initially medically with aggressive blood pressure control.

However, this may change in the near future with emerging encouraging data from deployment of endovascular stent-grafts.

Indications and principles for surgery

1 Involvement of the ascending aorta.
2 External rupture (haemopericardium, haemothorax, effusions).
3 Arterial compromise (limb ischaemia, renal failure, stroke).
4 Contraindications to medical therapy (AR, LVF).
5 Progression (continued pain, expansion of haematoma on further imaging, loss of pulses, pericardial rub or aortic insufficiency).

The aim of surgical therapy is to replace the ascending aorta, thereby preventing retrograde dissection and cardiac tamponade (main cause of death). The aortic valve may need reconstruction and resuspension unless it is structurally abnormal (bicuspid or Marfan's), where it is replaced.

Indications and principles for medical management

Medical therapy is the treatment of choice for:

- Uncomplicated type B dissection.
- Stable isolated arch dissection.
- Chronic (>2 weeks duration) stable Type B dissection.
  In all but those patients who are hypotensive, initial management is aimed at reducing systemic blood pressure and myocardial contractility. The goal is to stop spread of the intramural haematoma and to prevent rupture. The best guide is control of pain. Strict bed rest in a quiet room is essential.

Control blood pressure: (Reduce systolic BP to 100–120 mmHg).

- Start on IV β-blocker (if no contraindications) aiming to reduce the heart rate to 60–70/min (see table opposite).
- Once this is achieved, if blood pressure remains high, add a vasodilator such as sodium nitroprusside (see table opposite). Vasodilators in the absence of β-blockade may increase myocardial contractility and the rate of rise of pressure (dP/dt). Theoretically this may promote extension of the dissection.
- Further anti-hypertensive therapy may be necessary and other conventional agents such as calcium channel blockers, α-blockers and ACE inhibitors can be used.
- In patients with aortic regurgitation and congestive cardiac failure, myocardial depressants should not be given. Aim to control blood pressure with vasodilators only.

Hypotension may be due to haemorrhage or cardiac tamponade.

- Resuscitate with rapid intravenous volume (ideally colloid or blood, but crystalloid may be used also). A pulmonary artery wedge catheter (Swan–Ganz) should be used to monitor the wedge pressure and guide fluid replacement.
- If there are signs of aortic re.g.urgitation or tamponade, arrange for an urgent ECHO and discuss with the surgeons.

Emerging indications and principles for interventional therapy

There are increasing reports and short case series demonstrating favourable outcome (prognostic as well as symptomatic) data on using endovascular stent-grafts in management of primarily Type B and also to a lesser extent Type A aortic dissections.

On the basis of the current evidence endovascular stent-grafts should be considered to seal entry to false lumen and to enlarge compressed true lumen in the following situations:

- Unstable Type B dissection.
- Malperfusion syndrome (proximal aortic stent-graft and/or distal fenestration/stenting of branch arteries).
- Routine management of Type B dissection (under evaluation).

Cardiac tamponade: if the patient is relatively stable pericardiocentesis may precipitate haemodynamic collapse and should be avoided. The patient should be transferred to the operating theatre for direct repair as urgently as possible. In the context of tamponade and EMD or marked hypotension pericardiocentesis is warranted.

Long term treatment must involve strict blood pressure control.

Prognosis

- The mortality for untreated aortic dissection is roughly 20–30% at 24 hours and 65–75% at 2 weeks.
- For dissections confined to the descending aorta, short-term survival is better (up to 80%) but ~30–50% will have progression of dissection despite aggressive medical therapy and require surgery.

- Operative mortality is of the order of 10–25% and depends on the condition of the patient pre-operatively. Postoperative 5-year actuarial survival of up to 75% may be expected.

Medical therapy of aortic dissection	
β-blockade (aim for HR <60–70/min)	
Labetalol	20–80 mg slow IV injection over 10 min then 20–200 mg/hr IV, increasing every 15 min. 100–400 mg po q12h
Atenolol	5–10 mg slow iv injection then 50 mg PO after 15 min and at 12 hours, then 100 mg PO daily
Propranolol	0.5 mg iv (test dose), then 1 mg every 2–5 min. up to max 10 mg; repeat every 2–3 hrs. 10–40 mg po 3–4 times daily.
When HR 60–70 /min, (or if β-blocker contraindicated), add	
Nitroprusside	0.25–10 µg/kg/min iv infusion
Hydralazine	5–10 mg iv over 20 minutes 50–300 µg/min iv infusion 25–50 mg po q8h
GTN	1–10 mg/hr iv infusion
Amlodipine	5–10 mg po od.

Acute pericarditis: assessment

Presentation

- Typically presents as central chest pain—often pleuritic—relieved by sitting forward and can be associated with breathlessness.
- Other symptoms (e.g. fever, cough, arthralgia, rash, faintness/dizziness secondary to pain/↑HR) may reflect the underlying disease.
- A pericardial friction rub is pathognomonic. This may be positional and transient and may be confused with the murmur of TR or MR.
- Venous pressure rises if an effusion develops. Look for signs of cardiac tamponade (p672).

Investigations

ECG
- May be normal in up to 10%.
- *'Saddle-shaped' ST-segment elevation* (concave upwards), with variable T inversion (usually late stages) and *PR-segment depression* (opposite to p wave polarity). Minimal lead involvement to be considered typical includes I, II, aVL, aVF and V3–V6.
- ST-segement is always depressed in aVR, frequently depressed or isoelectric in V1 and sometimes in depressed in V2.
- May be difficult to distinguish from acute MI. Features suggesting pericarditis are:
  - Concave ST elevation (vs. convex).
  - All leads involved (vs. a territory e.g. inferior).
  - Failure of usual ST evolution and no Q waves.
  - No AV block, BBB, or QT prolongation.
- Early repolarization (a normal variant) may be mistaken for pericarditis. In the former, ST elevation occurs in pre-cordial and rarely in V6 or the limb leads, and is unlikely to show ST depression in V1 or PR segment depression.
- Usually not helpful in diagnosing pericarditis post-MI.
- The voltage drops as an effusion develops and in tamponade there is electrical alternans best seen in QRS complexes.

ECHO
- May demonstrate a pericardial collection.
- Useful to monitor LV function in case of deterioration due to associated myopericarditis.
- We recommend every patient has an ECHO prior to discharge to assess LV function.

Other investigations depend on the suspected aetiology.

All patients should have

- FBC and biochemical profile
- ESR and CRP (levels rise proportionate to intensity of disease)
- Serial cardiac enzymes (CK, CK-MB, troponin)—elevations indicate subpericardial myocarditis.
- CXR (heart size, pulmonary ooedema, infection)

Where appropriate

- Viral titres (acute + 2 weeks later)—and obtain virology opinion.
- Blood cultures.
- Autoantibody screen (RF, ANA, anti-DNA, complement levels).
- Thyroid function tests.
- Fungal precipitins (if immunosuppressed), ↑Mantoux test.
- Sputum culture and cytology.
- Diagnostic pericardial tap (culture, cytology).

Causes of acute pericarditis

- Idiopathic
- Infection (viral, bacterial, TB, and fungal)
- Acute myocardial infarction
- Dressler's syndrome, post-cardiotomy syndrome
- Malignancy (e.g. breast, bronchus, lymphoma)
- Uraemia
- Autoimmune disease (e.g. SLE, RA, Wegner's, scleroderma, PAN)
- Granulomatous diseases (e.g. sarcoid)
- Hypothyroidism
- Drugs (hydralazine, procainamide, isoniazid)
- Trauma (chest trauma, iatrogenic)
- Radiotherapy.

Acute pericarditis: management

General measures

- **Admit?** Depends on clinical picture. We recommend admission of most patients for observation for complications especially effusions, tamponade and myocarditis. Patients should be discharged when pain free.
- **Bed rest.**
- **Analgesia:** NSAIDS are the mainstay. Ibuprofen is well tolerated and increases coronary flow (200–800 mg qds). Aspirin is an alternative (600 mg qds po). Indomethacin should be avoided in adults as it reduces coronary flow and has marked side effects. Use PPI (lansoprazole 30 mg od) to minimise GI side effects. Opoid analgesia may be required. Colchicine used as monotherapy or in addition to NSAIDs may help settle pain acutely and prevent recurrence.
- **Steroids:** these may be used if the pain does not settle within 48 hours (e.g. prednisolone EC 40–60 mg po od for up to 2 weeks, tapering down when pain settles). Use in conjunction with NSAID and taper steroids first before stopping NSAID. It is also of value if pericarditis secondary to autoimmune disorders.
- **Colchicine:** anecdotal evidence suggests that either used as monotherpay or in conjunction with NSAIDs it may help to settle pain acutely and prevent relapses (1 mg/day divided doses). Stop if patient develops diarrhea, nausea. (1 mg stat, 500 mcg q6h for 48h).
- **Pericardiocentesis:** this should be considered for significant effusion or if there are signs of tamponade (p672).
- **Antibiotics:** these should be given only if bacterial infection is suspected.
- **Oral anticoagulants** should be discontinued (risk of haemo-pericardium). Patient should be given IV UFH, which is easier to reverse (IV protamine) if complications arise.

Cardiac tamponade: presentation

Cardiac tamponade occurs when a pericardial effusion causes haemodynamically significant cardiac compression. The presentation depends on the speed with which fluid accumulates within the pericardium. Acute tamponade may occur with 100–200 ml in a relatively restricted pericardial sac. Chronic pericardial collections may contain up to 1000 ml of fluid without clinical tamponade.

Causes

Acute tamponade

- Cardiac trauma
- Iatrogenic
  - Post-cardiac surgery
  - Post-cardiac catheterization•
  - Post-pacing/EP study
- Aortic dissection
- Spontaneous bleed
  - Anticoagulation
  - Uraemia
  - Thrombocytopenia
- Cardiac rupture post MI

'Sub-acute' tamponade

- Malignant disease
- Idiopathic pericarditis
- Uraemia
- Infections
- Bacterial
  - Tuberculosis
- Radiation
- Hypothyroidism
- Post pericardotomy
- SLE

Presentation

- Patients commonly present either with cardiac arrest (commonly electrical mechanical dissociation) or with hypotension, confusion, stupor, and shock.
- Patients who develop cardiac tamponade slowly are usually acutely unwell, but not in extremis. Their main symptoms include:
  - Breathlessness, leading to air hunger at rest.
  - There may be a preceding history of chest discomfort.
  - Symptoms resulting from compression of adjacent structures by a large effusion (i.e. dysphagia, cough, hoarseness, or hiccough).
  - There may be symptoms due to the underlying cause.
  - Insidious development may present with complications of tamponade including renal failure, liver and/or mesenteric ischaemia, and abdominal plethora.

Important physical signs

Most physical findings are non-specific. They include:
- Tachycardia (except in hypothyroidism and uraemia).
- Hypotension (± shock) with postural hypotension.
- Raised JVP (often >10 cm) with a prominent systolic x descent and absent diastolic y descent. If the JVP is visible and either remains static or rises with inspiration it indicates concomitant pericardial constriction (Kussmaul's sign).
- Auscultation may reveal diminished heart sounds. Pericardial rub may present and suggests a small pericardial collection.
  for pulsus paradoxus, (a decrease in the palpable pulse and
  c BP of >10 mmHg on inspiration). This may be so marked that

the pulse and Korotkoff sounds may be completely lost during inspiration. This can be measured using a BP cuff[1] or arterial catheter if in situ already. Other conditions that can cause a pulsus paradoxus include: acute hypotension, obstructive airways disease, and pulmonary embolus.

- Other physical signs include cool extremities (ears, nose) tachypnoea, hepatomegaly and signs of the underlying cause for the pericardial effusion.

Causes of hypotension with a raised JVP

- Cardiac tamponade
- Constrictive pericarditis
- Restrictive pericarditis
- Severe biventricular failure
- Right ventricular infarction
- Pulmonary embolism
- Tension pneumothorax
- Acute severe asthma
- Malignant SVC obstruction and sepsis (e.g. lymphoma).

---

1 Teaching point: To establish presence of pulsus paradoxus non-invasively inflate BP cuff to 15 mmHg above highest systolic pressure. Deflate cuff gradually until first beats are heard and hold pressure at that level concentrating on disappearance and reappearance of sounds with respiration (bump-bump, silence-silence, bump-bump, where noise reflects expiration). Continue to deflate slowly paying attention to same pattern until all beats are audible. The difference between the initial and final pressure should be greater than 10 mmHg.

Cardiac tamponade: management

Tamponade should be suspected in patients with hypotension, elevated venous pressure, falling BP, ↑HR and ↑RR (with clear chest), pulsus paradoxus especially if predisposing factors are present.

Investigations

- *Chest X-ray:* the heart size may be normal (e.g. in acute haemopericardium following cardiac trauma). With slower accumulation of pericardial fluid (>250 ml) the cardiac silhouette will enlarge with a globular appearance. The size of the effusion is unrelated to its haemodynamic significance. Look for signs of pulmonary oedema.
- *ECG:* usually shows a sinus tachycardia, with low voltage complexes and variable ST segment changes. With large effusions 'electrical alternans' may be present with beat-to-beat variation in the QRS morphology resulting form the movement of the heart within the pericardial effusion.
- *Echocardiography* confirms the presence of a pericardial effusion. The diagnosis of tamponade is a clinical one. ECHO signs highly suggestive of tamponade include: i) chamber collapse during diastole (RA, RV, RV outflow tract), ii) marked variation in transvalvular flow, iii) dilated IVC with little or no diameter change on respiration.
- If available, examine the central venous pressure trace for the characteristic exaggerated *x* descent and absent *y* descent.

Management

Following confirmation of the diagnosis:
- While preparing for drainage of the pericardial fluid, the patient's circulation may temporarily be supported by loading with IV colloid (500–1000 ml stat) and starting inotropes (i.e. Adrenaline).
- In patients with an adequate blood pressure, cautious systemic vasodilatation with hydralazine or nitroprusside in conjunction with volume loading, may increase forward cardiac output. This is not to be recommended routinely as it may cause acute deterioration.
- The effusion should be urgently drained (see p698 for pericardiocentesis) guided by echo or fluoroscopy. **In the event of circulatory collapse drainage must happen immediately without imaging.**
- Surgical drainage is indicated if the effusion is secondary to trauma.
- Avoid intubation and positive pressure ventilation as this reduces CO.
- In patients with cardiac arrest chest compression has little or no value, as there is no room for additional filling.
- Uraemic patients will also need dialysis.
- The cause of the effusion should be established (see p669). Pericardial fluid should be sent for cytology, microbiology including TB, and if appropriate Hb, glucose, and amylase.

Further management is of the underlying cause.

Special cases
1 **Recurrent pericardial effusion:** in some cases pericardial effusion recurs. This requires either a change in the treatment of the underlying cause or a formal surgical drainage procedure such as a surgical pericardial window or pericardiectomy.
2 **Low pressure tamponade:** seen in the setting of dehydration. The JVP is not raised, right atrial pressure is normal and tamponade occurs even with small volumes of pericardial fluid.
   - The patient may respond well to IV fluids.
   - If there is a significant pericardial collection this should be drained.

Practical procedures

Central line insertion

You will need the following
- Sterile dressing pack and gloves.
- 10 ml and 5 ml syringe with green (21G) and orange (25G) needles.
- Local anaesthetic (e.g. 2% lignocaine).
- Central line (e.g. 16G long Abbocath® or Seldinger catheter.
- Saline flush.
- Silk suture and needle.
- No 11 scalpel blade.
- Sterile occlusive dressing (e.g. Tegaderm®).

Risks
- Arterial puncture (remove and apply local pressure).
- Pneumothorax (insert chest drain or aspirate if required).
- Haemothorax.
- Chylothorax (mainly left subclavian lines).
- Infection (local, septicaemia, bacterial endocarditis).
- Brachial plexus or cervical root damage (over enthusiastic infiltration with local anaesthetic).
- Arrhythmias.

General procedure
- The basic technique is the same whatever vein is cannulated.
- Lie the patient supine (±head down tilt).
- Turn the patient's head away from the side you wish to cannulate.
- Clean the skin with iodine or chlorhexidine: from the angle of the jaw to the clavicle for internal jugular vein (IJV) cannulation and from the midline to axilla for the subclavian approach.
- Use the drapes to isolate the sterile field.
- Flush the lumen of the central line with saline.
- Identify your landmarks (see p679 and p681).
- Infiltrate skin and subcutaneous tissue with local anaesthetic.
- Have the introducer needle and Seldinger guide-wire within easy reach so that you can reach them with one hand without having to release your other hand. Your fingers may be distorting the anatomy slightly making access to the vein easier and if released it may prove difficult to relocate the vein.
- With the introducer needle in the vein, check that you can aspirate blood freely. Use the hand that was on the pulse to immobilize the needle relative to the skin and mandible or clavicle.
- Remove the syringe and pass the guide wire into the vein; it should pass freely. If there is resistance, remove the wire, check that the needle is still within the lumen and try again.
- Remove the needle leaving the wire within the vein and use a sterile swab to maintain gentle pressure over the site of venepuncture to prevent excessive bleeding.
- With a No.11 blade make a nick in the skin where the wire enters, to facilitate dilatation of the subcutaneous tissues. Pass the dilator over the wire and remove, leaving the wire *in situ*.

- Pass the central line over the wire into the vein. Remove the guide-wire, flush the lumen with fresh saline and close off to air.
- Suture the line in place and cover the skin penetration site with a sterile occlusive dressing.

Measuring the CVP—tips and pitfalls

- When asked to see a patient at night on the wards with an abnormal CVP reading, it is a good habit to always re-check the zero and the reading yourself.
- Always do measurements with the mid-axillary point as the zero reference. Sitting the patient up will drop the central filling pressure (pooling in the veins).
- Fill the manometer line being careful not to soak the cotton wall stopping. If this gets wet it limits the free-fall of saline or dextrose in the manometer line.
- Look at the rate and character of the venous pressure. It should fall to its value quickly and swing with respiration.
- If it fails to fall quickly consider whether the line is open (i.e. saline running in), blocked with blood clot, positional (up against vessel wall-ask patient to take some deep breaths), arterial blood (blood tracks back up the line). Raise the whole dripstand (if you are strong), and make sure that the level falls. If it falls when the whole stand is elevated it may be that the CVP is very high.
- It is easier, and safer, to cannulate a central vein with the patient supine or head down. There is an increased risk of air embolus if the patient is semi-recumbent.

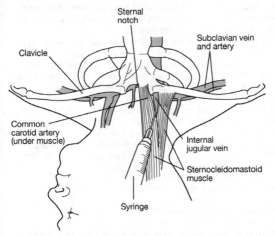

Fig. 18.1 Technique for catheterization at the internal jugular and subclavian sites. Reproduced with premission from McGee DC, Gould MK (2003). Preventing complications of central venous catheterization. *N Engl J Med* **348**: 1123–1133.

Internal jugular vein cannulation

The internal jugular vein (IJV) runs just postero-lateral to the carotid artery within the carotid sheath and lies medial to the SCM in the upper part of the neck, between the two heads of SCM in its medial portion and enters the subclavian vein near the medial border of the anterior scalene muscle (see Fig.18.2). There are three basic approaches to IJV cannulation: medial to sternocleidomastoid (SCM), between the two heads of SCM, or lateral to SCM. The approach used varies and depends on the experience of the operator and the institution.

- Locate the carotid artery between the sternal and clavicular heads of SCM at the level of the thyroid cartilage; the IJV lies just lateral and parallel to it.
- Keeping the fingers of one hand on the carotid pulsation, infiltrate the skin with L.A. thoroughly, aiming just lateral to this and ensuring that you are not in a vein.
- Ideally first locate the vein with a blue or green needle. Advance the needle at 45° to the skin, with gentle negative suction on the syringe, aiming for the ipsilateral nipple, lateral to the pulse.
- If you fail to find the vein, withdraw the needle slowly, maintaining negative suction on the syringe (you may have inadvertently have transfixed the vein). Aim slightly more medially and try again.
- Once you have identified the position of the vein, change to the syringe with the introducer needle, cannulate the vein and pass the guidewire into the vein (see p685).

Tips and pitfalls

- Venous blood is dark, and arterial blood is pulsatile and bright red!
- Once you locate the vein, change to the syringe with the introducer needle, taking care not to release your fingers from the pulse; they may be distorting the anatomy slightly making access to the vein easier and if released it may prove difficult to relocate the vein.
- The guide wire should pass freely down the needle and into the vein. With the left IJV approach, there are several acute bends that need to be negotiated. If the guide wire keeps passing down the wrong route, ask your assistant to hold the patient's arms out at 90° to the bed, or even above the patient's head, to coax the guide wire down the correct path.
- For patients who are intubated or requiring respiratory support it may be difficult to access the head of the bed. The anterior approach may be easier (see Fig.18.2) and may be done from the side of the bed (the left side of the bed for right-handed operators, using the left hand to locate the pulse and the right to cannulate the vein).
- The IJV may also be readily cannulated with a long Abbocath®. No guide wire is necessary, but as a result, misplacement is commoner than with the Seldinger technique.
- When using an Abbocath®, on cannulating the vein, remember to advance the sheath and needle a few mm to allow the tip of the plastic sheath (~1 mm behind the tip of the bevelled needle) to enter the vein. Holding the needle stationary, advance the sheath over it into the vein.
- Arrange for a CXR to confirm the position of the line.

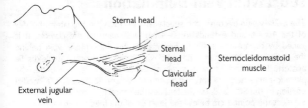

(a) Surface anatomy of external and internal jugular veins

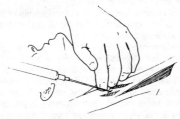

(b) Anterior approach: the chin is in the midline and the skin puncture is over the sternal head of SCM muscle

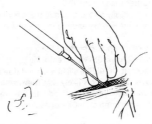

(c) Central approach: the chin is turned away and the skin puncture is between the two heads of SCM muscle

Fig. 18.2 Internal jugular vein cannulation.

Subclavian vein cannulation

The axillary vein becomes the subclavian vein (SCV) at the lateral border of the 1st rib and extends for 3–4 cm just deep to the clavicle. It is joined by the ipsilateral IJV to become the brachiocephalic vein behind the sternoclavicular joint. The subclavian artery and brachial plexus lie posteriorly separated from the vein by the scalenus anterior muscle. The phrenic nerve and the internal mammary artery lie behind the medial portion of the SCV and, on the left, lies the thoracic duct.

- Select the point 1 cm below the junction of the medial third and middle third of the clavicle. If possible place a bag of saline between the scapulae to extend the spine.
- Clean the skin with iodine or chlorhexidine.
- Infiltrate skin and subcutaneous tissue and periosteum of the inferior border of the clavicle with local anaesthetic up to the hilt of the green (21G) needle, ensuring that it is not in a vein.
- Insert the introducer needle with a 10 ml syringe, guiding gently under the clavicle. It is safest to initially hit the clavicle, and 'walk' the needle under it until the inferior border is just cleared. In this way you keep the needle as superficial to the dome of the pleura as possible. Once it has just skimmed underneath the clavicle, advance it slowly towards the contralateral sternoclavicular joint, aspirating as you advance. Using this technique the risk of pneumothorax is small, and success is high.
- Once the venous blood is obtained, rotate the bevel of the needle towards the heart. This encourages the guide-wire to pass down the brachiocephalic rather than up the IJV.
- The wire should pass easily into the vein. If there is difficulty, try advancing during the inspiratory and expiratory phases of the respiratory cycle.
- Once the guide wire is in place, remove the introducer needle, and pass the dilator over the wire. When removing the dilator, note the direction that it faces; it should be slightly curved downwards. If it is slightly curved upwards, then it is likely that the wire has passed up into the IJV. The wire may be manipulated into the brachiocephalic vein under fluoroscopic control but if not available it is safer to remove the wire and start again.
- After removing the dilator pass the central venous catheter over the guide wire, remove the guide wire, and secure as above.
- A chest X-ray is mandatory after subclavian line insertion to exclude a pneumothorax and to confirm satisfactory placement of the line, especially if fluoroscopy was not employed.

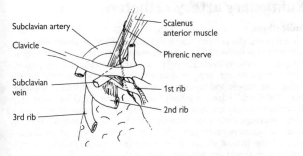

Subclavian artery

Clavicle

Subclavian vein

3rd rib

Scalenus anterior muscle

Phrenic nerve

1st rib

2nd rib

Fig. 18.3 The subclavian vein and surrounding structures.

Pulmonary artery catheterization

Indications

PA catheters (Swan–Ganz catheters) allow direct measurement of a number of haemodynamic parameters that aid clinical decision-making in critically ill patients (evaluate right and left ventricular function, guide treatment and provide prognostic information). The catheter itself has no therapeutic benefit and there have been a number of studies showing increased mortality (and morbidity) with their use. Consider inserting a PA catheter in any critically ill patient, after discussion with an experienced physician, if the measurements will influence decisions on therapy, (and not just to reassure yourself). Careful and frequent clinical assessment of the patient should always accompany measurements and PA catherisation should not delay treatment of the patient.

General indications (not a comprehensive list) include:
- Management of complicated myocardial infarction.
- Assessment and management of shock.
- Assessment and management of respiratory distress (cardiogenic vs. non-cardiogenic pulmonary oedema).
- Evaluating effects of treatment in unstable patients (e.g. inotropes, vasodilators, mechanical ventilation, etc).
- Delivering therapy (e.g. thrombolysis for pulmonary embolism, prostacyclin for pulmonary hypertension, etc).
- Assessment of fluid requirements in critically ill patients.

Equipment required
- Full resuscitation facilities should be available and the patient's ECG should be continuously monitored.
- Bag of heparinised saline for flushing the catheter and transducer set for pressure monitoring. (Check that your assistant is experienced in setting up the transducer system BEFORE you start).
- 8F introducer kit (pre-packaged kits contain the introducer sheath and all the equipment required for central venous cannulation).
- PA catheter: Commonly a triple lumen catheter, that allows simultaneous measurement of RA pressure (proximal port) and PA pressure (distal port) and incorporates a thermistor for measurement of cardiac output by thermodilution. Check your catheter before you start.
- Fluoroscopy is preferable, though not essential.

General technique
- Do not attempt this without supervision if you are inexperienced.
- Observe strict aseptic technique using sterile drapes, etc.
- Insert the introducer sheath (at least 8F in size) into either the internal jugular or subclavian vein in the standard way. Flush the sheath with saline and secure to the skin with sutures.
- Do not attach the plastic sterile expandable sheath to the introducer yet but keep it sterile for use later once the catheter is in position (the catheter is easier to manipulate without the plastic covering).

• Flush all the lumens of the PA catheter and attach the distal lumen to the pressure transducer. Check the transducer is zeroed (conventionally to the mid axillary point). Check the integrity of the balloon by inflating it with the syringe provided (1–2 ml air) and then deflate the balloon.

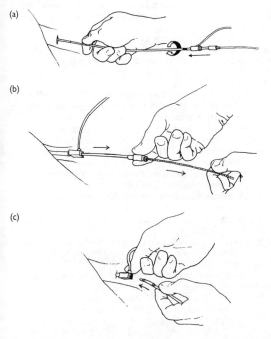

(a)

(b)

(c)

Fig. 18.4 Pulmonary artery catheterization. (a) The sheath and dilator are advanced into the vein over the guige-wire. A twisting motion makes insertion easier. (b) The guidewire and dilator are then removed. The sheath has a haemostatic valve at the end preventing leakage of blood. (c) The PA catheter is then inserted through the introducer sheath into the vein.

Insertion technique

- Flush all the lumens of the PA catheter and attach the distal lumen to the pressure transducer. Check the transducer is zeroed (conventionally to the mid axillary point). Check the integrity of the balloon by inflating it with the syringe provided and then deflate the balloon.

- Pass the tip of the PA catheter through the plastic sheath, keeping the sheath compressed. The catheter is easier to manipulate without the sheath over it; once in position, extend the sheath over the catheter to keep it sterile.

- With the balloon deflated, advance the tip of the catheter to approx 10–15 cm from the right IJV or SCV, 15–20 cm from the left (the markings on the side of the catheter are at 10 cm intervals: 2 lines = 20 cm). Check that the pressure tracing is typical of the right atrial pressure (Fig. 18.5).

- Inflate the balloon and advance the catheter gently. The flow of blood will carry the balloon (and catheter) across the tricuspid valve, through the right ventricle and into the pulmonary artery (see Fig. 18.5).

- Watch the ECG tracing closely whilst the catheter is advanced. The catheter commonly triggers runs of VT when crossing the tricuspid valve and through the RV. The VT is usually self limiting, but should not be ignored.

- If more than 15 cm of catheter is advanced into the RV without the tip entering the PA, this suggests the catheter is coiling in the RV. Deflate the balloon, withdraw the catheter into the RA, reinflate the balloon and try again using clockwise torque while advancing in the ventricle, or flushing the catheter with cold saline to stiffen the plastic. If this fails repeatedly, try under fluoroscopic guidance.

- As the tip passes into a distal branch of the PA, the balloon will impact and not pass further—the wedge position—and the pressure tracing will change (see Fig. 18.5).

- Deflate the balloon and check that a typical PA tracing is obtained. If not, try flushing the catheter lumen and if that fails, withdraw the catheter until the tip is within the PA and begin again.

- Reinflate the balloon slowly. If the PCW pressure is seen before the balloon is fully inflated, it suggests the tip has migrated further into the artery. Deflate the balloon, withdraw the catheter 1–2 cm and try again.

- If the pressure tracing flattens and then continues to rise, you have 'overwedged'. Deflate the balloon, pull back the catheter 1–2 cm and start again.

- When a stable position has been achieved, extend the plastic sheath over the catheter and secure it to the introducer sheath. Clean any blood from the skin insertion site with antiseptic and secure a coil of the PA catheter to the patient's chest to avoid inadvertent removal.

- Obtain a CXR to check the position of the catheter. The tip of the cathater should ideally be no more than 3–5 cm from the midline.

Normal values of right heart pressures and flows

Right atrial pressure	0–8 mmHg
Right ventricle	
systolic	15–30 mmHg
end diastolic	0–8 mmHg
Pulmonary artery	
systolic/diastolic	15–30/4–12 mmHg
mean	9–16 mmHg
Pulmonary capillary wedge pr.	2–10 mmHg
Cardiac index	2.8–4.2 L/min/m²

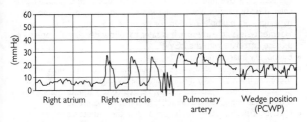

Fig. 18.5 Pressure tracings during pulmonary artery catheterization.

Tips and pitfalls

- Never withdraw the catheter with the balloon inflated.
- Never advance the catheter with the balloon deflated.
- Never inject liquid into the balloon.
- Never leave the catheter with the balloon inflated as pulmonary infarction may occur.
- The plastic of the catheter softens with time at body temperature and the tip of the catheter may migrate further into the PA branch. If the pressure tracing with the balloon deflated is 'partially wedged' (and flushing the catheter does not improve this), withdraw the catheter 1–2 cm and reposition.
- Sometimes it is impossible to obtain a wedged trace. In this situation one has to use the PA diastolic pressure as a guide. In health there is ~2–4 mmHg difference between PA diastolic pressure and PCWP. Any condition which causes pulmonary hypertension (e.g. severe lung disease, ARDS, long standing valvular disease) will alter this relationship.

- *Valvular lesions, VSDs, prosthetic valves, and pacemakers*: If these are present then seek advice from a cardiologist. The risk of SBE may be sufficiently great that the placement of a PA catheter may be more detrimental than beneficial.
- PEEP. Measurement and interpretation if PCWP in patients on PEEP depends on the position of the catheter. Ensure the catheter is below the level of the left atrium on a lateral CXR. Removing PEEP during measurement causes marked fluctuations in haemodynamics and oxygenation and the pressures do not reflect the state once back on the ventilator.

Complications

- *Arrhythmias*: watch the ECG tracing closely whilst the catheter is advanced. The catheter commonly triggers runs of VT when crossing the tricuspid valve and through the RV. If this happens, deflate the balloon, pull back and try again. The VT is usually self-limiting, but should not be ignored.
- *Pulmonary artery rupture*: (~0.2% in one series). Damage may occur if the balloon is overinflated in a small branch. Risk factors include mitral valve disease (large v wave confused with poor-wedging), pulmonary hypertension, multiple inflations or hyperinflations of balloon. Haemoptysis is an early sign. It is safer to follow PA diastolic pressures if these correlate with the PCWP.
- Pulmonary infarction.
- *Knots*: usually occur at the time of initial placement in patients where there has been difficulty in traversing the RV. Signs include loss of pressure tracing, persistent ectopy, resistance to catheter manipulation. If this is suspected, stop manipulation and seek expert help.
- *Infection*: risks increase with length of time the catheter is left *in situ*. Pressure transducer may occasionally be a source of infection. Remove the catheter and introducer in replace only if necessary.
- *Other complications*: complications associated with central line insertion, thrombosis and embolism, balloon rupture, intracardiac damage.

Indications for temporary pacing

1. Following acute myocardial infarction

- Asystole.
- Symptomatic complete heart block (CHB) (any territory).
- Symptomatic 2° heart block (any territory).
- Trifascicular block—alternating LBBB and RBBB.
  —1° heart block + RBBB + LAD.
  —new RBBB and left posterior hemiblock.
  —LBBB and long PR interval.
- After anterior MI —asymptomatic CHB.
  —asymptomatic 2° (Mobitz II) block.
- Symptomatic sinus bradycardia unresponsive to atropine.
- Recurrent VT for atrial or ventricular overdrive pacing.

2. Unrelated to myocardial infarction

- Symptomatic sinus or junctional bradycardia unresponsive to atropine (e.g. carotid sinus hypersensitivity).
- Symptomatic 2° heart block or sinus arrest.
- Symptomatic complete heart block.
- Torsades de pointes tachycardia.
- Recurrent VT for atrial or ventricular overdrive pacing.
- Bradycardia dependent tachycardia.
- Drug overdose (e.g. verapamil, β-blockers, digoxin).
- Permanent pacemaker box change in a pacing-dependent patient.

3. Before general anaesthesia

- The same principles as for acute MI (see above).
- Sinoatrial disease, 2° (Wenckebach) heart block only need prophylactic pacing if there are symptoms of syncope or pre-syncope.
- Complete heart block.

Transvenous temporary pacing

- The technique of temporary wire insertion is described on p692.
- The most commonly used pacing mode and the mode of choice for life-threatening bradyarrhythmias is ventricular demand pacing (VVI) with a single bipolar wire positioned in the right ventricle.
- In critically ill patients with impaired cardiac pump function and symptomatic bradycardia (especially with right ventricular infarction), cardiac output may be increased by up to 20% by maintaining atrio-ventricular synchrony. This requires two pacing leads, one atrial and one ventricular, and a dual pacing box.

Epicardial temporary pacing

- Following cardiac surgery, patients may have *epicardial wires* (attached to the pericardial surface of the heart) left in for up to 1 week in case of post-operative bradyarrhythmia. These are used in the same way as transvenous pacing wires, but the threshold may be higher.

Table 18.1 Indications for temporary transvenous cardiac pacing

Emergency/acute
- *Acute myocardial infarction:* (Class I: ACC/AHA)[3]
- Asystole
- Symptomatic bradycardia (sinus bradycardia with hypotension and type I 2nd degree AV block with hypotension not responsive to atropine)
- Bilateral bundle branch block (alternating BBB or RBBB with alternating LAHB/LPHB)
- New or indeterminate age bifascicular block with first degree AV block
- Mobitz type II second degree AV block

Bradycardia not associated with acute myocardial infarction
- Asystole
- 2nd or 3rd degree AV block with haemodynamic compromise or syncope at rest
- Ventricular tachyarrhythmias secondary to bradycardia

Elective
- Support for procedures that may promote bradycardia
- General anaesthesia with:
  2nd or 3rd degree AV block
  Intermittent AV block
  1st degree AV block with bifascicular block
  1st degree AV block and LBBB
- Cardiac surgery
  Aortic surgery
  Tricuspid surgery
  Ventricular septal defect closure
  Ostium primum repair
- Rarely considered for coronary angioplasty (usually to right coronary artery)

Overdrive suppression of tachyarrhythmias

Reproduced with permission from Gammage, MD (2000). Temporary cardiac pacing. *Heart* **83**: 715–720.

Temporary ventricular pacing

- *Cannulate a central vein*: the wire is easiest to manipulate via the RIJ approach but is more comfortable for the patient via the right subclavian (SC) vein. The LIJ approach is best avoided as there are many acute bends to negotiate and a stable position difficult to achieve. Avoid the left subclavicular area as this is the preferred area for permanent pacemaker insertion and should be kept 'virgin' if possible. The femoral vein may be used (incidence of DVT and infection is high).
- *Insert a sheath* (similar to that for PA catheterization) through which the pacing wire is to be fed. Pacing wires are commonly 5F or 6F and a sheath at least one size larger is necessary. Most commercially available pacing wires are pre-packed with an introducer needle and plastic cannula similar to an Abbocath® which may be used to position the pacing wire. However the cannula does not have a haemostatic seal. The plastic cannula may be removed from the vein, leaving the bare wire entering the skin, once a stable position has been achieved. This reduces the risk of wire displacement but also makes repositioning of the wire more difficult should this be necessary, and infection risk is higher.
- Pass the wire through the sterile plastic cover that accompanies the introducer sheath and advance into the upper right atrium (see Fig. 18.6) but do not unfurl the cover yet. The wire is much easier to manipulate with gloved hands without the hindrance of the plastic cover.
- Advance the wire with the tip pointing towards the right ventricle; it may cross the tricuspid valve easily. If it fails to cross, point the tip to the lateral wall of the atrium and form a loop. Rotate the wire and the loop should fall across the tricuspid valve into the ventricle.
- Advance and rotate the wire so that the tip points inferiorly as close to the tip of the right ventricle (laterally) as possible.
- If the wire does not rotate down to the apex easily, it may be because you are in the coronary sinus rather than in the right ventricle. (The tip of the wire points to the left shoulder). Withdraw the wire and re-cross the tricuspid valve.
- Leave some slack in the wire; the final appearance should be like the outline of a sock with the 'heel' in the right atrium, the 'arch' over the tricuspid and the 'big toe' at the tip of the right ventricle.
- Connect the wire to the pacing box and check the threshold. Ventricular pacing thresholds should be <1.0 V but threshold up to 1.5 V is acceptable if another stable position cannot be achieved.
- Check for positional stability. With the box pacing at a rate higher than the intrinsic heart rate, ask the patient to take some deep breaths, cough forcefully and sniff. Watch for failure of capture and if so reposition the wire.
- Set the output to 3 V and the box on 'demand'. If the patient is in sinus rhythm and has an adequate blood pressure set the box rate to just below the patient's rate. If there is complete heart block or bradycardia set the rate at 70–80/min.
- Cover the wire with the plastic sheath and suture sheath and wire securely to the skin. Loop the rest of the wire and fix to the patient's skin with adhesive dressing.

- When the patient returns to the ward, obtain a CXR to confirm satisfactory positioning of the wire and to exclude a pneumothorax.

Checklist for pacing wire insertion

- Check the screening equipment and defibrillator are working.
- Check the type of pacing wire: atrial wires have a pre-formed 'J' that allows easy placement in the atrium or appendage and is very difficult to manipulate into a satisfactory position in the ventricle. Ventricular pacing wires have a more open, gentle 'J'.
- Check the pacing box (single vs. dual or sequential pacing box) and leads to attach to the wire(s). Familiarize yourself with the controls on the box: you may need to connect up in a hurry if the patient's intrinsic rhythm slows further.
- Remember to don the lead apron before wearing the sterile gown, mask and gloves

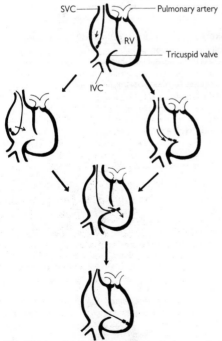

Fig. 18.6 Insertion of a ventricular pacing wire (see text for details) Reproduced with permission from Ramrakha P, Moore K (2004) *Oxford Handbook of Acute Medicine*. 2nd ed. Oxford: Oxford University Press.

Temporary atrial pacing

- The technique of inserting an atrial temporary wire is similar to that of ventricular pacing.
- Advance the atrial wire until the 'J' is reformed in the right atrium.
- Rotate the wire and withdraw slightly to position the tip in the right atrial appendage. Aim for a threshold of <1.5 V.
- If atrial wires are not available, a ventricular pacing wire may be manipulated into a similar position or passed into the coronary sinus for left atrial pacing.

A–V sequential pacing

In critically ill patients with impaired cardiac pump function and symptomatic bradycardia (especially with right ventricular infarction), cardiac output may be increased by up to 20% by maintaining atrioventricular synchrony. This requires two pacing leads, one atrial and one ventricular, and a dual pacing box.

Patients most likely to benefit from AV sequential pacing

- Acute MI (especially RV infarction).
- 'Stiff' left ventricle: aortic stenosis, HCM, hypertensive heart disease, amyloidosis.
- Low cardiac output states (cardiomyopathy).
- Recurrent atrial arrhythmias.

Temporary pacing: complications

1. Ventricular ectopics or VT

- Non-sustained VT is common as the wire crosses the tricuspid valve (especially in patients receiving an isoprenaline infusion) and does not require treatment.
- Try to avoid long runs of VT and if necessary withdraw the wire into the atrium and wait until the rhythm has settled.
- If ectopics persist after the wire is positioned, try adjusting the amount of slack in the wire in the region of the tricuspid valve (either more or less).
- Pacing the right ventricular outflow tract can provoke runs of VT.

2. Failure to pace and/or sense

- It is difficult to get low pacing thresholds (<1.0 V) in patients with extensive myocardial infarction (especially of the inferior wall), cardiomyopathy or who have received class I antiarrhythmic drugs. Accept a slightly higher value if the position is otherwise stable and satisfactory.
- If the position of the wire appears satisfactory and yet the pacing thresholds are high, the wire may be in a left hepatic vein. Pull the wire back into the atrium and try again, looking specifically for the ventricular ectopics as the wire crosses the tricuspid valve.
- The pacing threshold commonly doubles in the first few days due to endocardial oedema.
- If the pacemaker suddenly fails, the most common reason is usually wire displacement.
- Increase the pacing output of the box.
- Check all the connections of the wire and the battery of the box.
- Try moving the patient to the left lateral position until arrangements can be made to reposition the wire.

3. Perforation

- A pericardial rub may be present in the absence of perforation (especially post-MI).
- *Presentation*: pericardial chest pain, increasing breathlessness, falling blood pressure, enlarged cardiac silhouette on CXR, signs of cardiac tamponade, left diaphragmatic pacing at low output.
- *Management :*
  - If there are signs of cardiac tamponade arrange for urgent ECHO and reposition the wire.
  - Monitor the patient carefully over the next few days with repeat ECHOs to detect incipient cardiac tamponade.

4. Diaphragmatic pacing

- High output pacing (10 V), even with satisfactory position of the ventricular lead may cause pacing of the left hemidiaphragm. At low voltages this suggests perforation (see above).
- Right hemidiaphragm pacing may be seen with atrial pacing and stimulation of the right phrenic nerve.
- Reposition the wire if symptomatic (painful twitching, dyspnoea).

Complications of temporary pacing

- Complications associated with central line insertion
- Ventricular ectopics
- Non-sustained VT
- Perforation
- Pericarditis
- Diaphragmatic pacing
- Infection
- Pneumothorax.

Pericardial aspiration

Equipment

Establish peripheral venous access and check that full facilities for resuscitation are available. Pre-prepared pericardiocentesis sets may be available. You will need:

- Trolley as for central line insertion with iodine or chlorhexidine for skin, dressing pack, sterile drapes, local anaesthetic (lignocaine 2%), syringes (including a 50 ml), needles (25G and 22G), No 11 blade, and silk sutures
- Pericardiocentesis needle (15 cm, 18G) or similar Wallace cannula.
- J-guide wire (≥80 cm, 0.035 diameter)
- Dilators (up to 7 French)
- Pigtail catheter (≥60 cm with multiple sideholes, a large Seldinger-type CVP line can be used if no pigtail is available).
- Drainage bag and connectors.
- Facilities for fluoroscopy or echocardiographic screening.

Technique

- Position the patient at ~30°. This allows the effusion to pool inferiorly within the pericardium.
- Sedate the patient lightly with midazolam (2.5–7.5 mg iv) and fentanyl 50–200 µg iv) if necessary. Use with caution as this may drop the BP in patients already compromised by the effusion.
- Wearing a sterile gown and gloves, clean the skin from mid-chest to mid-abdomen and put the sterile drapes on the patient.
- Infiltrate the skin and subcutaneous tissues with local anaesthetic starting 1–1.5 cm below the xiphisternum and just to the left of midline, aiming for the left shoulder and staying as close to the inferior border of the rib cartilages as possible.
- The pericardiocentesis needle is introduced into the angle between the xiphisternum and the left costal margin angled at ~30°. Advance slowly aspirating gently and then injecting more lignocaine every few mm, aiming for the left shoulder.
- As the parietal pericardium is pierced, you may feel a 'give' and fluid will be aspirated. Remove the syringe and introduce the guide wire through the needle.
- Check the position of the guide wire by screening. It should loop within the cardiac silhouette only and not advance into the SVC or pulmonary artery.
- Remove the needle leaving the wire in place. Enlarge the skin incision slightly using the blade and dilate the track.
- Insert the pigtail over the wire into the pericardial space and remove the wire.
- Take specimens for microscopy, culture (and inoculate a sample into blood culture bottles), cytology and haematocrit if blood stained (a FBC tube; ask the haematologists to run on the coulter counter for rapid estimation of Hb).

- Aspirate to dryness watching the patient carefully. Symptoms and haemodynamics (tachycardia) often start to improve with removal of as little as 100 ml of pericardial fluid.
- If the fluid is heavily blood stained, withdraw fluid cautiously–if the pigtail is in the right ventricle, withdrawal of blood may cause cardiovascular collapse. Arrange for urgent Hb/haematocrit .
- Leave on free drainage and attached to the drainage bag.
- Suture the pigtail to the skin securely and cover with a sterile occlusive dressing.

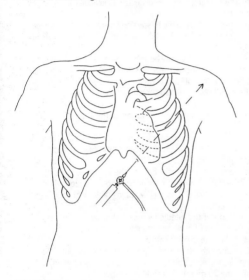

Fig. 18.7 Pericardial aspiration. Reproduced with permission from Ramrakha P, Moore K (2004). *Oxford Handbook of Acute Medicine.* 2nd ed. Oxford: Oxford University Press.

Aftercare

- Closely observe the patient for recurrent tamponade (obstruction of drain) and repeat ECHO.
- Discontinue anticoagulants.
- Remove the drain after 24 hours or when the drainage stops.
- Consider the need for surgery (drainage, biopsy or pericardial window) or specific therapy (chemotherapy if malignant effusion, antimicrobials if bacterial, dialysis if renal failure, etc).

Tips and pitfalls

1. *If the needle touches the heart's epicardial surface*, you may feel a 'ticking' sensation transmitted down the needle: withdraw the needle a few mm, angulate the needle more superficially and try cautiously again, aspirating as you advance.

2. *If you do not enter the effusion, and the heart not encountered:*
- Withdraw the needle slightly and advance again aiming slightly deeper, but still towards the left shoulder.
- If this fails, try again aiming more medially (mid clavicular point or even supra-sternal notch).
- Consider trying the apical approach (starting laterally at cardiac aped and aiming for right shoulder), if echo confirms sufficient fluid at the cardiac apex).

3. *If available, intrathoracic ECG* can be monitored by a lead attached to the needle as it is advanced. This is seldom clinically useful in our experience. Penetration of the myocardium results in ST elevation, suggesting the needle has been advanced to far.

4. *Difficulty in inserting the pigtail:*
- This may be because of insufficient dilatation of the tract (use a larger dilator).
- Holding the wire taught (by gentle traction) while pushing the catheter may help; take care not to pull the wire out of the pericardium.

5. *Haemorrhagic effusion vs blood:*
- Compare the Hb of the pericardial fluid to the venous blood Hb.
- Place some of the fluid in a clean container; blood will clot whereas haemorrhagic effusion will not as the 'whipping' action of the heart tends to defibrinate it.
- Confirm the position of the needle by first withdrawing some fluid and then injecting 10–20 ml of contrast; using fluoroscopy see if the contrast stays within the cardiac sillhouette.
- Alternatively if using echo guidance, inject 5–10 ml saline into the needle looking for 'microbubble contrast' in the cavity containing the needle tip. Injecting 20 ml saline rapidly into a peripheral vein will produce 'contrast' in the right atrium and ventricle and may allow them to be distinguised from the pericardial space.
- Connect a pressure line to the needle; a characteristic waveform will confirm penetration of the right ventricle.

Complications of pericardiocentesis

- Penetration of a cardiac chamber (usually right ventricle)
- Laceration of an epicardial vessel
- Arrhythmia (atrial arrhythmias as the wire is advanced, ventricular arrhythmias if the RV is penetrated)
- Pneumothorax
- Perforation of abdominal viscus (liver, stomach, colon)
- Ascending infection.

DC cardioversion

Relative contraindications

- Digoxin toxicity.
- Electrolyte disturbance ($\downarrow Na^+$, $\downarrow K^+$, $\downarrow Ca^{2+}$, $\downarrow Mg^{2+}$, acidosis).
- Inadequate anticoagulation and chronic AF.

Check list for DC cardioversion

- Defibrillator: **Check this is functioning with a fully equipped arrest trolley to hand in case of arrest.**
- Informed consent: unless life-threatening emergency).
- 12 lead ECG: AF, flutter, SVT, VT, signs of ischaemia or digoxin. If ventricular rate is slow have an external (transcutaneous) pacing system nearby in case of asystole.
- Nil by mouth: For at least 4 hours.
- Anticoagulation: Does the patient require anticoagulants ? Is the INR > 2.0 ? (Has it been so for >3 wks ?)
- Potassium: Check this is >3.5 mmol/L.
- Digoxin: Check there are no features of digoxin toxicity. If taking ≥250 µg/day check that renal function and recent digoxin level are normal. If there are frequent ventricular ectopics, give iv Mg^{2+} 8 mmol.
- Thyroid function: Treat thyrotoxicosis or myxoedema first.
- IV access: Peripheral venous cannula.
- Sedation: Short general anaesthesia (propofol) is preferable to sedation with benzodiazepine and fentanyl. Bag the patient with 100% oxygen.
- Select energy: (see table opposite).
- Synchronization: Check this is selected on the defibrillator for all shocks (unless the patient is in VF or haemodynamically unstable). Adjust the ECG gain so that the machine is only sensing QRS complexes and not P or T waves
- Paddle placement: Conductive gel pads should be placed between the paddles and the skin. Position one just to the right of the sternum and the other to the left of the left nipple (ant.-mid axillary line), Alternatively place one anteriorly just left of the sternum, and one posteriorly to the left of midline. There is no convincing evidence for superiority of one position over the other.
- Cardioversion: Check no one is in contact with the patient or with the metal bed. Ensure your own legs are clear of the bed! Apply firm pressure on the paddles.
- Unsuccessful: Double the energy level and repeat up to 360 J. Consider changing paddle position. If prolonged sinus pause or ventricular arrhythmia during an elective procedure, stop.
- Successful: Repeat ECG. Place in recovery position until awake. Monitor for 2–4 hrs and ensure effects of sedation have passed. Patients should be accompanied home by friend or relative if being discharged.

Complications of DC cardioversion

- Asystole/bradycardias
- Ventricular fibrillation
- Thromboembolism
- Transient hypotension
- Skin burns
- Aspiration pneumonitis.

Suggested initial energies for DC shock for elective cardioversion

Sustained VT	200 J.	Synchronized
Atrial fibrillation	50–100 J.	Synchronized
Atrial flutter	50 J.	Synchronized
Other SVTs	50 J.	Synchronized

- If the initial shock is unsuccessful, increase the energy (50, 100, 200, 360 J) and repeat.
- If still unsuccessful consider changing paddle position and try 360 J again. It is inappropriate to persist further with elective DC cardioversion.

1. Anticoagulation

The risk of thromboembolism in patients with chronic AF and dilated cardiomyopathy is 0–7% depending on the underlying risk factors.

Increased risk
- Prior embolic event
- Mechanical heart valve
- Mitral stenosis
- Dilated left atrium.

Low risk
- Age <60 years
- No underlying heart disease
- Recent onset AF (<3 days).

Anticoagulate patients at risk with warfarin for at least 3–4 weeks. For recent onset AF (1–3 days), anticoagulate with iv heparin for at least 12–24 hours and, if possible, exclude intra-cardiac thrombus with a trans-oesophageal ECHO prior to DC shock. If there is thrombus, anticoagulate with warfarin as above. For emergency cardioversion of AF (<24 hrs), heparinise prior to shock.

The risk of systemic embolism with cardioversion of atrial flutter and other tachyarrhythmias is very low, provided there is no ventricular thrombus, since the co-ordinated atrial activity prevents formation of clot. Routine anticoagulation with warfarin is not necessary but we would recommend heparin before DC shock as the atria are often rendered mechanically stationary for several hours after shock even though there is co-ordinate electrical depolarization.

After successful cardioversion, if the patient is on warfarin, continue anticoagulation for at least 3–4 weeks. Consider indefinite anticoagulation if there is intrinsic cardiac disease (e.g. mitral stenosis) or recurrent AF.

2. Special situations

Pregnancy DC shock during pregnancy appears to be safe. Auscultate the fetal heart before and after cardioversion and if possible, fetal ECG should be monitored.

Pacemakers There is a danger of damage to the pacemaker generator box or the junction at the tip of the pacing wire(s) and endocardium. Position the paddles in the anteroposterior position as this is theoretically safer. Facilities for back-up pacing (external or transvenous) should be available. Check the pacemaker post-cardioversion—both early and late problems have been reported.

Intra-aortic balloon counterpulsation

Indications
- Cardiogenic shock post MI.
- Acute severe mitral regurgitation.
- Acute ventricular septal defect.
- Preoperative (ostial left coronary stenosis).
- Weaning from cardiopulmonary bypass.
Rarely
- Treatment of ventricular arrhythmias post-MI.
- Unstable angina (as a bridge to CABG).

Contraindications
- Aortic regurgitation.
- Aortic dissection.
- Severe aorto-iliac atheroma.
- Bleeding diathesis.
- Dilated cardiomyopathy (if patient not a candidate for transplantation).

Complications
- Aortic dissection.
- Arterial perforation.
- Limb ischaemia.
- Trombocytopenia.
- Peripheral embolism.
- Balloon rupture.

Principle
The device consists of a catheter with a balloon (40 ml size) at its tip which is positioned in the descending thoracic aorta. The balloon inflation/deflation is synchronized to the ECG. The balloon should inflate just after the dicrotic notch (in diastole) thereby increasing pressure in the aortic root and increasing coronary perfusion. The balloon deflates just before ventricular systole, thereby decreasing afterload and improving left ventricular performance (see Fig.18.8).

Counterpulsation has a number of beneficial effects on the circulation:
- Increased in coronary perfusion in diastole.
- Reduced LV end diastolic pressure.
- Reduced myocardial oxygen consumption.
- Increased cerebral and peripheral blood flow.

The IAB cannot assist the patient in asystole or VF; it requires a minimum cardiac index of 1.2–1.4 L/min/m^2, often necessitating additional inotropes.

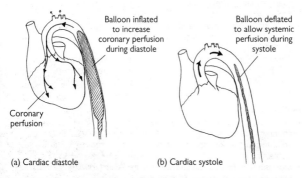

Balloon inflated to increase coronary perfusion during diastole

Balloon deflated to allow systemic perfusion during systole

Coronary perfusion

(a) Cardiac diastole   (b) Cardiac systole

Fig.18.8 Reproduced with permission from Ramrakha P, Moore K (2004) *Oxford Handbook of Acute Medicine* 2nd ed. Oxford: Oxford University Press.

Technique

Balloon insertion

Previous experience is essential. Formerly, a cut-down to the femoral artery was required, but newer balloons come equipped with a sheath which may be introduced percutaneously. Using fluoroscopy, the balloon is positioned in the descending thoracic aorta with the tip just below the origin of the left subclavian artery. Fully anticoagulate the patient with iv heparin. Some units routinely give iv antibiotics (flucloxacillin) to cover against *Staph.* infection.

Triggering and timing

The balloon pump may be triggered either from the patient's ECG (R-wave) or from the arterial pressure waveform. Slide switches on the pump allow precise timing of inflation and deflation during the cardiac cycle. Set the pump to 1:2 to allow you to see the effects of augmentation on alternate beats (see Fig. 18.9)

Trouble-shooting

- Seek help from an expert! There is usually an on-call cardiac perfusionist or technician, senior cardiac physician or surgeon.
- Counterpulsation is inefficient with heart rates over 130/min. Consider anti-arrhythmics or 1:2 augmentation instead.
- Triggering and timing: for ECG triggering, select a lead with most pronounced R wave; ensure that the pump is set to trigger from ECG not pressure; permanent pacemakers may interfere with triggering—select a lead with negative and smallest pacing artefact. Alternatively, set the pump to be triggered from the external pacing device. A good arterial waveform is required for pressure triggering; the timing will vary slightly depending on the location of the arterial line (slightly earlier for radial artery line cf. femoral artert line). Be guided by the

haemodynamic effects of balloon inflation and deflation rather than precise value of delay.
- Limb ischaemia: exacerbated by poor cardiac output, adrenaline, noradrenaline, and peripheral vascular disease. Wean off and remove the balloon.
- Thrombocytopenia: commonly seen; does not require transfusion unless there is overt bleeding and returns to normal once the balloon is removed. Consider prostacyclin infusion if platelet counts fall below 100×10^9/L.

IABP removal
- The patient may be progressively weaned by gradually reducing the counterpulsation ratio (1:2, 1:4, 1:8, etc) and/or reducing the balloon volume and checking that the patient remains haemodynamically stable.
- Stop the heparin infusion and wait for the ACT (activated clotting time) to fall <150 sec (APTT <1.5 normal).
- Using a 50 ml syringe, have an assistant apply negative pressure to the balloon.
- Pull the balloon down until it abuts the sheath; do not attempt to pull the balloon into the sheath.
- Withdraw both balloon and sheath and apply firm pressure on the femoral puncture site for at least 30 minutes or until the bleeding is controlled.

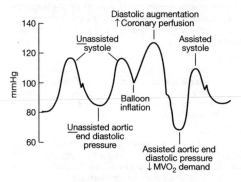

Fig.18.9 Arterial waveform variations during IABP therapy.

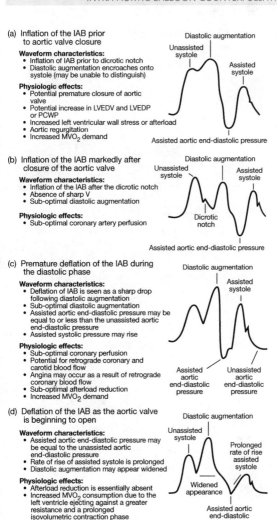

(a) Inflation of the IAB prior to aortic valve closure

Waveform characteristics:
- Inflation of IAB prior to dicrotic notch
- Diastolic augmentation encroaches onto systole (may be unable to distinguish)

Physiologic effects:
- Potential premature closure of aortic valve
- Potential increase in LVEDV and LVEDP or PCWP
- Increased left ventricular wall stress or afterload
- Aortic regurgitation
- Increased MVO$_2$ demand

Labels on waveform: Diastolic augmentation; Unassisted systole; Assisted systole; Assisted aortic end-diastolic pressure

(b) Inflation of the IAB markedly after closure of the aortic valve

Waveform characteristics:
- Inflation of the IAB after the dicrotic notch
- Absence of sharp V
- Sub-optimal diastolic augmentation

Physiologic effects:
- Sub-optimal coronary artery perfusion

Labels on waveform: Diastolic augmentation; Unassisted systole; Assisted systole; Dicrotic notch; Assisted aortic end-diastolic pressure

(c) Premature deflation of the IAB during the diastolic phase

Waveform characteristics:
- Deflation of IAB is seen as a sharp drop following diastolic augmentation
- Sub-optimal diastolic augmentation
- Assisted aortic end-diastolic pressure may be equal to or less than the unassisted aortic end-diastolic pressure
- Assisted systolic pressure may rise

Physiologic effects:
- Sub-optimal coronary perfusion
- Potential for retrograde coronary and carotid blood flow
- Angina may occur as a result of retrograde coronary blood flow
- Sub-optimal afterload reduction
- Increased MVO$_2$ demand

Labels on waveform: Diastolic augmentation; Assisted systole; Assisted aortic end-diastolic pressure; Unassisted aortic end-diastolic pressure

(d) Deflation of the IAB as the aortic valve is beginning to open

Waveform characteristics:
- Assisted aortic end-diastolic pressure may be equal to the unassisted aortic end-diastolic pressure
- Rate of rise of assisted systole is prolonged
- Diastolic augmentation may appear widened

Physiologic effects:
- Afterload reduction is absent
- Increased MVO$_2$ consumption due to the left ventricle ejecting against a greater resistance and a prolonged isovolumetric contraction phase
- IAB may impede left ventricular ejection and increase the afterload

Labels on waveform: Diastolic augmentation; Unassisted systole; Prolonged rate of rise assisted systole; Widened appearance; Assisted aortic end-diastolic pressure

Fig.18.10 Timing errors. (a) Early inflation; (b) late inflation; (c) early deflation; (d) late deflation.

Index